PROGRESS IN
CLINICAL NEUROSCIENCES

VOLUME 25

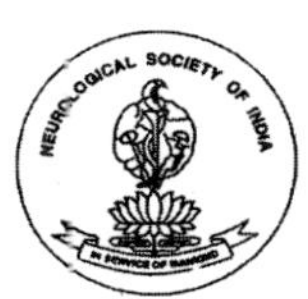

Neurological Society of India

PROGRESS
IN
CLINICAL
NEUROSCIENCES

VOLUME 25

Editors

DEEPU BANERJI

APOORVA PAURANIK

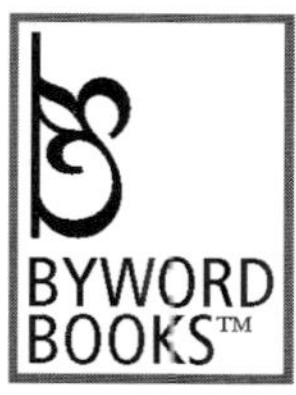

BYWORD BOOKS™

ISBN 978-81-8193-078-1

The typeface used on the cover is a Fell Type digitally reproduced by Igino Marini (www.iginomarini.com)

Cover design
NETRA SHYAM

Typeset by
JACOB THOMAS

Published by
BYWORD BOOKS PRIVATE LIMITED
Virat Bhavan, Mukherjee Nagar Commercial Complex, Delhi 110009
email: bywordbooks@gmail.com
website: www.bywordbooks.in

Printed at
Indraprastha Press (CBT), New Delhi 110002

Contents

SKULL BASE SURGERY

NEUROENDOSCOPY

SPINAL SURGERY

CLINICAL NEUROLOGY

Preface

It is a privilege to be the editors of *Progress in Clinical Neurosciences, Volume 25* for the second year. Volume 24, with the introduction of colour pictures, was highly appreciated.

We have tried to maintain the quality of this scientific publication of NSI. This year, we have a joint NSI–CNS conference and some high-quality, original and researched clinical and technical work has been contributed by international and national faculty.

We have continued with theme-based topics. This edition contains interesting topics covering neurovascular surgery, skull base surgery, recent developments in endoscopic neurosurgery and newer techniques in spinal surgery. Topics of general interest include fluid and electrolyte imbalance in the neuro-ICU and radiation biology. The section on clinical neurology has newer views and updates on neuroinfection, demyelination, stroke and headache. As in the past, we have tried to present new authors with wide experience in their fields.

We would like to thank all the authors for their contributions and prompt response to editorial queries. We would like to put on record our appreciation for our publisher Byword Books for a highly professional approach to bringing out this publication.

2 December 2010

DEEPU BANERJI
Convener, CME

APOORVA PAURANIK
Co-convener, CME

List of contributors

ATUL AGARWAL
Neurology Clinic, 55 Ravindrapalli, Faizabad Road, Lucknow;
formerly Department of Neurology, C.S.M. Medical University (KGMC), Lucknow, Uttar Pradesh;
dratul1@rediffmail.com

PUNIT AGRAWAL
The Ohio State University Department of Neurology, Ohio, USA; punit.agrawal@osumc.edu

LISSA BAIRD
Department of Neurosurgery, Louisiana State University Health Sciences Center, Shreveport, LA, USA

ANIRBAN DEEP BANERJEE
Department of Neurosurgery, Louisiana State University Health Sciences Center, Shreveport, LA, USA

DEEPU BANERJI
Department of Neurosurgery, Fortis Hospital, Mulund, Mumbai, Maharashtra;
deepu.banerji@gmail.com

R.N. BHATTACHARYA
Department of Neurosurgery, AMRI Hospital, Dhakuria, Kolkata, West Bengal;
rnb@amrihospitals.in

VLADIMIR DADASHEV
Department of Neurosurgery, Emory University School of Medicine, Atlanta, GA, USA

JOY DESAI
Department of Neurology, Jaslok Hospitals and Research Centre, Mumbai, Maharashtra;
desaijoy@gmail.com

SANJEEV DEVESHWAR
Moses Cone Health System, Neurointerventional Radiology, 1200 N. Elm Street, Greensboro, NC, USA;
tonydev00@msn.com

SANJAY S. DHALL
Department of Neurological Surgery, Emory University, Atlanta, GA, USA

SALVATORE DI MAIO
Clinical Fellow in Cerebrovascular and Skull Base Neurosurgery, Harborview Medical Center
University of Washington, Seattle, WA, USA; sdimaio@u.washington.edu

T.N. DUBEY
Department of Neurology, Hamidiya Hospital, Bhopal, Madhya Pradesh;
drtndubey@gmail.com

MANUEL FERRIERA
Department of Neurological Surgery, Harborview Medical Center, Box 359766 Seattle, WA, USA;
manuelf3@u.washington.edu

RABINDRANATH GARCIA-LOPEZ
Department of Neurological Surgery, Harborview Medical Center, Box 359766 Seattle, WA, USA

AJAY GARG
Department of Neuroradiology, Neurosciences Centre, All India Institute of Medical Sciences, New Delhi

ATUL GOEL
Department of Neurosurgery, K.E.M. Hospital and Seth G.S. Medical College, Mumbai;
atulgoel62@hotmail.com

COL S.P. GORTHI
Senior Advisor, Medicine and Neurology, Command Hospital (CC), Lucknow, Uttar Pradesh;
pgorthi2002@yahoo.com

ADRIANA IOACHIMESCU
Departments of Neurosurgery and Medicine, Emory University School of Medicine, Atlanta, GA, USA

V.K. JAIN
Department of Neurosurgery, Sir Ganga Ram Hospital, New Delhi; vkjneuro2004@yahoo.com

RAKESH JALALI
Department of Radiation Oncology, Neuro-Oncology Group, Tata Memorial Hospital, Mumbai,
Maharashtra; rjalali@tmc.gov.in

NARAYAN JAYASHANKAR
Dr Balabhai Nanavati Hospital, SV Road, Vile Parle (West), Mumbai, Maharashtra

VIJAYAKUMAR JAVALKAR
Department of Neurosurgery, Louisiana State University Health Sciences Center, Shreveport, LA, USA;
vjaval@lsuhsc.edu

MATHEW JOSEPH
Department of Neurological Sciences, Christian Medical College, Vellore, Tamil Nadu;
mjoseph@cmcvellore.ac.in

SANDEEP JULKA
Department of Endocrinology, CHL-Apollo Hospital, Indore, Madhya Pradesh;
sandeep_julka@yahoo.com

SHASHANK SHARAD KALE
Department of Neurosurgery, All India Institute of Medical Sciences, New Delhi;
skale67@gmail.com

SAMIR K. KALRA
Department of Neurosurgery, Sir Ganga Ram Hospital, New Delhi

ELINA KARI
Department of Otolaryngology, Emory University School of Medicine, Atlanta, GA, USA

MANU KOTHARI
Department of Anatomy, K.E.M. Hospital and Seth G.S. Medical College, Parel, Mumbai, Maharashtra

DANIEL C. LU
Department of Neurological Surgery, University of California, Los Angeles, CA, USA

SHASHWAT MISHRA
Department of Neurosurgery, Neurosciences Center, All India Institute of Medical Sciences, New Delhi;
gyrusrectus@gmail.com

S.K. MISHRA
Department of Neurosurgery, AMRI Hospital, Dhakuria, Kolkata, West Bengal

K.P. MORWANI
Dr Balabhai Nanavati Hospital, SV Road, Vile Parle (West), Mumbai, Maharashtra

GAURAV MUKERJI
Neurosurgery Unit, N.S.C.B. Medical College, Apex Hospital and Research Centre, Jabalpur,
Madhya Pradesh

PRAVEEN V. MUMMANENI
Department of Neurological Surgery, University of California, San Francisco, CA;
505 Parnassus Ave. Rm. M779 San Francisco, CA, USA; mummanenip@neurosurg.ucsf.edu

ANIL NANDA
Department of Neurosurgery, Louisiana State University Health Sciences Center in Shreveport,
1501 Kings Highway, PO Box 33932, Shreveport, LA, USA; ananda@lsuhsc.edu

ARVIND NANDA
Department of Interventional Neuroradiology, Indraprastha Apollo Hospitals, New Delhi

R. LAKSHMI NARASIMHAN
Madras Institute of Neurology, Madras Medical College, Chennai, Tamil Nadu;
lakshmineuro@gmail.com

NELSON OYESIKU
Departments of Neurosurgery and Medicine, Emory University School of Medicine, Atlanta, GA, USA
noyesik@emory.edu

DACHLING PANG
Kaiser Permanente Medical Center, Department of Paediatric Neurosurgery, 280 W. MacArthur Blvd., Oakland, CA, USA; PangTV@aol.com

VIJAY PARIHAR
Neurosurgery Unit, N.S.C.B. Medical College, Apex Hospital and Research Centre, Jabalpur, Madhya Pradesh

SUSHIL PATKAR
Department of Neurosurgery, Bhartiya Vidyapeeth Medical College and Poona Hospital, Pune, Maharashtra; patneuro@hotmail.com

M. PRASAD
Department of Neurosurgery, AMRI Hospital, Dhakuria, Kolkata, West Bengal

DINESH RAMANATHAN
Department of Neurological Surgery, Harborview Medical Center, Box 359766 Seattle, WA, USA

HARSH RASTOGI
Department of Interventional Neuroradiology, Indraprastha Apollo Hospitals, New Delhi; harshrastogi@rediffmail.com

MICHAEL HERBAS ROCHA
Department of Neurological Surgery, Harborview Medical Center, Box 359766 Seattle, WA, USA

SURESH SANKHLA
Dr Balabhai Nanavati Hospital, SV Road, Vile Parle (West), Mumbai, Maharashtra; A-503, Chaitanya Towers, Appasaheb Marathe Marg, Prabhadevi, Mumbai, Maharashtra; sankhlasuresh@gmail.com

MANVINDER SAPPAL
Department of Neurology, Dayanand Medical College, Ludhiana, Punjab

LALIGAM N. SEKHAR
Department of Neurological Surgery, University of Washington, Harborview Medical Center; President, World Federation of Skull Base Societies 2008-2012, 325 9th Avenue Box 359924, Seattle, WA, USA; lsekhar@u.washington.edu

PRAMOD SETHI
Moses Cone Health System and Partner, Guilford Neurological Associates; psethi@guilfordneurologic.com

GNANA SHANMUGAM
Madras Institute of Neurology, Madras Medical College, Chennai, Tamil Nadu

RAVIKIRAN SHENOY
Neurosurgery Unit, N.S.C.B. Medical College, Apex Hospital and Research Centre, Jabalpur, Madhya Pradesh

SNEHAL SHEREKAR
Neurosurgery Unit, N.S.C.B. Medical College, Apex Hospital and Research Centre, Jabalpur, Madhya Pradesh

GAGANDEEP SINGH
Department of Neurology, Dayanand Medical College, Ludhiana, Punjab;
gagandeep_si@yahoo.co.uk

ASHISH SURI
Department of Neurosurgery, Neurosciences Center, All India Institute of Medical Sciences, New Delhi;
surineuro@gmail.com

VIVEK TIWARI
Neuro-Oncology, Tata Memorial Hospital, Mumbai, Maharashtra

KEKI E. TUREL
Department of Neurosurgery, New Wing, Bombay Hospital, Marine Lines, Mumbai, Maharashtra;
kekiturel@rediffmail.com

SARAH WISE
Department of Otolaryngology, Emory University School of Medicine, Atlanta, GA, USA

YAD RAM YADAV
Neurosurgery Unit, NSCB Medical College, Apex Hospital and Research Centre, Jabalpur,
Madhya Pradesh; yadavyr@yahoo.co.in

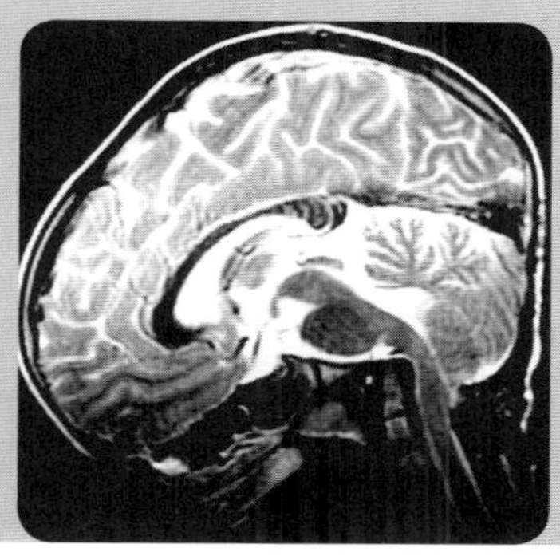

General neuroscience

1

Sodium–water disorders in a neuro ICU

MATHEW JOSEPH

Abnormalities in sodium and water balance are common in a general inpatient population and even more frequent in the setting of critical care neurology and neurosurgery, as this homoeostasis is controlled primarily by the central nervous system (CNS). Hyponatraemia has been found to have a significantly worse outcome in hospitalized patients,[1] though a partial explanation of this phenomenon could be that hyponatraemia was found in the sickest patients. No data are currently available on the incidence of these abnormalities in patients with primarily CNS disease.

This review describes the normal control of sodium and water, followed by the clinical features of sodium abnormalities. The pathophysiology, diagnosis and treatment of the major abnormalities are discussed, including algorithms for the diagnosis of hyponatraemia.

Normal sodium–water homoeostasis

Sodium metabolism is primarily controlled by the renin–angiotensin–aldosterone pathway, whereas water metabolism is controlled by arginine vasopressin (AVP), also called the antidiuretic hormone (ADH). AVP is a 9-amino acid peptide secreted by magnocellular neurons in the supraoptic and paraventricular nuclei of the hypothalamus and transported down the pituitary stalk to be released in the posterior pituitary gland. Normal levels are <4 pg/ml; it is metabolized by vasopressinases in both the liver and kidneys, and has a half life of ~35 minutes.[2]

The primary input into these nuclei is from hypothalamic osmoreceptors located in the subfornicial organ (outside the blood–brain barrier). Secondary input is from medullary cardiovascular centres responding to baroreceptors located in the cardiac atria, aorta and carotid arteries, as well as the carotid bodies and area postrema.[3,4] The osmoreceptors maintain serum osmolality in a tight range, between 280 and 295 mOsm/kg; an increase of as little as 2% causes a significant increase in urine osmolality because of water reabsorption, and a decrease of 2% causes maximal dilution of urine because of water excretion. An increase in osmolality also stimulates the thirst mechanism. The non-osmotic stimulus from the cardiovascular system requires a much larger change of 10%–20% in circulating volume or blood pressure to influence AVP secretion. AVP production is also stimulated to some degree by nausea, hypoxia, hypercapnia, stress, hypoglycaemia and intermittent positive pressure ventilation (IPPV), and can be diminished by opioids.[2]

AVP acts on the V2 receptors located on the cells of the renal collecting ducts, stimulating the movement of aquaporin-2 water channels from the intracellular vesicles to the apical plasma membrane to promote reabsorption of water. AVP also has a long-term effect on the expression of the aquaporin-2 gene to increase water channels.

Although the primary control of AVP secretion is in response to serum osmolality, the number of different factors that can affect secretion make dysregulation of water metabolism and the resulting hyponatraemia a common problem in the ICU.

Effects of abnormal sodium levels

The effects of hyponatraemia on all tissues in the body depend on the following two factors:

- Severity of the hyponatraemia
- The rate of decline of serum sodium levels: the effect of an acute drop in serum sodium levels has much more significant clinical consequences than a slower decline, and therefore patients with chronic hyponatraemia often remain asymptomatic at sodium levels that would otherwise cause devastating effects in an acute setting.

Although hyponatraemia affects all tissues of the body, its major consequences result from the effect on the brain. When serum osmolality drops, water enters the brain cells from the extracellular space along the osmotic gradient, causing neuronal dysfunction and brain oedema, with potentially lethal consequences. A decreased level of consciousness, seizures and raised pressure are common manifestations. If hyponatraemia develops slowly, the brain cells adapt by releasing various solutes from the brain, thus preventing the formation of the osmotic gradient that moves water into the cells.[5] The substances

that can be moved out of the cell include K+, Na+, Cl– and organic osmolytes, including amino acids, myoinositol and creatine.[6] The opposite process occurs during the correction of hyponatraemia, as serum tonicity normalizes. As the levels at which symptoms of hyponatraemia develop vary with the rate of decline, it is not possible to define a particular sodium concentration that results in clinical consequences.

Early symptoms of hyponatraemia are headache, irritability, nausea and confusion, which progress to hyporeflexia, drowsiness, seizures, coma and eventually brainstem compression caused by herniation and death. It must be emphasized again that the symptoms a patient has at a particular serum sodium concentration depend to a large extent on how acutely the level has decreased—in a study of 100 patients with severe hyponatraemia of <120 mEq/L, 29% of patients with an acute fall had seizures, against only 6% of those in whom the hyponatraemia had developed over >3 days.[7]

The correction of symptomatic hyponatraemia is a medical emergency and will be discussed later in this chapter. A disastrous consequence of rapid correction of chronic hyponatraemia is osmotic demyelination syndrome (previously known as central pontine myelinolysis), in which demyelination occurs in the pons, cerebellum and basal ganglia. This was first attributed to correction of hyponatraemia by Kleinschmidt–DeMasters and Norenberg in 1981.[8] Myelin shows marked destruction with relative preservation of axon cylinders. The pathogenesis of this phenomenon is not fully understood. One theory is that in chronic hyponatraemia a sudden rise in serum sodium leads to brain cell shrinkage, and in order to maintain volume the cell begins to take up the osmolytes it had earlier removed to adjust to the serum hypotonicity.[9] These organic osmolytes are thought to be protective for intracellular proteins and DNA and, because it takes time to accumulate these compounds, cell damage occurs when the serum hypotonicity corrects rapidly.[9] It is also possible that the process is related to blood–brain barrier damage in these areas with immune-mediated destruction of myelin, as the concentration of IgG is high in the areas of demyelination, and dexamethasone has been used successfully to prevent these lesions in rats.[10] Therefore, correction of hyponatraemia requires close calibration and monitoring. Osmotic demyelination is much more common in patients with chronic hyponatraemia, and is unlikely to occur during correction of acute hyponatraemia, especially if the serum sodium is >120 mEq/L.

Acute hypernatraemia can theoretically cause brain cell shrinkage, but the phenomenon has not been well studied experimentally or clinically. Symptoms are initially similar to those of hyponatraemia with thirst, irritability and lethargy proceeding to hyper-reflexia, seizures, coma and death. These clinical features are not well defined, as the sodium levels often increase only in patients in whom the thirst mechanism is not functional because of hypothalamic damage, and these patients are usually already unconscious.

Hyponatraemia

In order to accurately diagnose and treat hyponatraemia it is essential to have a rational diagnostic algorithm for the various causes. The easiest way of understanding hyponatraemia is to divide the patients on the basis of serum tonicity. It is not the purpose of this review to discuss all the causes of hyponatraemia, and therefore the focus will be on the commonest causes seen in neurological patients.

Classification of hyponatraemia on the basis of serum tonicity

Hypertonic hyponatraemia: This is caused by the presence of osmotically active compounds in the serum that in turn cause an osmotic movement of water from the intracellular to the extracellular fluid, diluting the sodium, although the serum remains hyperosmolar. Common particles responsible are glucose, mannitol and contrast agents.

Isotonic hyponatraemia: Also known as pseudo-hyponatraemia, it is primarily seen in marked hyperlipidaemia or hyperproteinaemia. Normally these compounds constitute ~7% of serum, with the remainder being aqueous. When this non-aqueous component of the serum increases, the amount of water (and therefore the quantity of sodium per unit volume of serum) decreases. The sodium concentration per unit of water is not low, and this is primarily a measurement artefact. The low sodium values in these patients have no clinical significance, but the clinician must be aware of this entity.

Hypotonic hyponatraemia: Sodium is the main osmotically active solute in normal serum, and therefore this is the syndrome most frequently seen in patients. Patients in this group are further divided on the basis of their volume status into hypervolaemic, euvolaemic and hypovolaemic. The common differential diagnoses are listed in Table 1.

Once the more obvious causes listed in Table 1 are ruled out, one is left with the diagnostic conundrum of figuring out if the patient has cerebral salt wasting (CSW) or syndrome of inappropriate antidiuretic hormone secretion

Table 1. Volume-based differential diagnosis of hypotonic hyponatraemia (modified from Bradshaw and Smith, 2008[11])

Hypovolaemic	Euvolaemic	Hypervolaemic
Cerebral salt wasting	SIADH	SIADH
Diuretics	Thiazide diuretics	Cardiac failure
Diarrhoea/vomiting	Hypocortisolism	Cirrhosis
Blood loss	Hypothyroidism	Acute renal failure
Mineralocorticoid deficiency	Iatrogenic	Iatrogenic

(SIADH). CSW (although not by that name) was the first syndrome to be described, but soon more and more cases of SIADH began to be reported to the point at which all patients with idiopathic hyponatraemia were considered to have SIADH. The pendulum began to swing the other way in the late 1980s when hyponatraemic patients were demonstrated to have a contracted extracellular volume which was not compatible with the water retention expected in SIADH, and most neurosurgical hyponatraemias were automatically said to be due to CSW. We have now reached a balanced state in most neurosurgical practices (although SIADH still dominates with most general medical physicians) in which the existence of both entities is acknowledged and a logical diagnostic process can be followed to differentiate between them.

CSW

Pathophysiology: The exact mechanism that causes natriuresis and hypovolaemia in these patients is not completely understood, but probably involves a combination of circulating natriuretic factors and disruption of neural input to the kidney.[12] Increased levels of atrial natriuretic peptide and brain natriuretic peptide can cause increased glomerular filtration and decreased sodium reabsorption, leading to natriuresis. The proximal tubule is the site where the bulk of sodium reabsorption occurs, and the sympathetic nervous system input has a considerable influence on its function. Any impairment of function would again lead to increased urinary sodium loss. The contraction of volume may actually stimulate the baroreceptors to increase the secretion of ADH, which would then prevent effective concentration of the urine.

Diagnosis: It must be demonstrated that the patient has hypotonic hyponatraemia, natriuresis and a contracted blood volume, and diagnostic criteria have been well defined as follows:[12–14]

- Serum sodium <135 mEq/L
- Serum osmolality <275 mOsm/kg
- Urine spot sodium >40 mEq/L
- Hypovolaemia.

Treatment: CSW is usually a transient phenomenon, and the goal of treatment is to replace lost sodium. A treatment protocol for neurosurgery patients with hyponatraemia and natriuresis developed at the author's institution is to administer normal saline to correct the volume deficit, and to transfuse blood if the haematocrit is <27% (again to assist in building up volume).[13,14] The serum sodium in most patients is corrected within 72 hours on this regimen. Hypertonic saline may be added in cases of severely symptomatic hyponatraemia. In occasional patients, it may be necessary to administer fludrocortisone to correct and maintain serum sodium.

SIADH

Pathophysiology: Increased secretion of ADH, even in the presence of a hypotonic serum, causes continuing reabsorption of water. Patients with SIADH often reach a steady state of urinary sodium excretion in which the administration of even normal saline results in the excretion of sodium and worsening of the hyponatraemia.

Diagnosis: The secretion of ADH in the absence of an osmotic stimulus has a large number of possible causes, as detailed in Table 2.[4,15] If none of these causes is found, then the patient may be said to have primary SIADH. The criteria for diagnosis of SIADH laid down in 1967 by Bartter and Schwartz are still valid today.[16] In summary, these diagnostic criteria are as follows:

- Hypotonic (osmolality <280 mOsm/L) hyponatraemia (Na+ <135 mEq/L)
- Urine sodium >18 mEq/L (most authors now use >40 mEq/L)[13,14]
- Normal thyroid, renal and adrenal function
- Clinical euvolaemia.

Treatment: If identified, the underlying cause of the SIADH (as listed in Table 2) should be treated. The hyponatraemia is managed with the following modalities of treatment:

- Fluid restriction to 1000 ml a day is all that is needed in asymptomatic or mildly symptomatic patients for a gradual correction of serum sodium. However, this is often not possible due to patient discomfort or because the underlying medical condition does not permit a decrease in administered fluid (hypotension, subarachnoid haemorrhage, risk of stroke, or renal impairment).

- Hypertonic saline may be used to correct sodium in more severely symptomatic patients and in those for whom fluid restriction is not possible.

- AVP receptor antagonists promise to be an effective means of treatment for SIADH. They block action at the V2 receptor, promoting excretion of free water. The compounds under trial, collectively known as the vaptans, include tolvaptan, lixivaptan and conivaptan (the last drug has been approved by the FDA for use in hospital patients). Conivaptan has been shown to markedly increase serum sodium in patients with euvolaemic or hypervolaemic hyponatraemia.[17,18]

Table 2. Common causes of SIADH

Malignancies

Bronchogenic carcinoma, mesothelioma

Carcinomas of the gut or urinary system

Thymoma

Hodgkin's disease, acute leukaemia, lymphosarcoma

Uterine carcinoma

Nasopharyngeal carcinoma

CNS

Meningitis, encephalitis

Trauma, subarachnoid haemorrhage

Stroke, hypoxia, sinus thrombosis

Vasculitis, multiple sclerosis

Tumour, abscess

Chest disorders

Tuberculosis, mycoplasma, acute pneumonia, fungal infections

Respiratory failure, COPD, IPPV

Asthma, cystic fibrosis

Drug induced

ACE inhibitors

Cyclphosphamide, vincristine

Phenothiazines, tricyclics

Carbamazepine

Morphine, barbiturates

Serotonin reuptake inhibitors

Omeprazole

Ecstasy

Others

Prolonged severe exercise

Old age

Idiopathic

Diagnostic algorithm for the cause of hyponatraemia in a neuro ICU

As disorders of sodium and water are often caused by hypothalamic dysfunction, it is emphasized again that other endocrine functions must be checked and corrected if necessary. The author has seen patients with hyponatraemia who became normal or even later manifested a diabetes insipidus on correction of thyroid and adrenal status.

- Once underlying causes have been ruled out, the algorithm shown in Fig. 1 should be followed to establish a diagnosis. Supplementary investigations have been described to demonstrate the volume-contracted state in CSW (increase in albumin, haematocrit or bicarbonate) or SIADH (decreased uric acid, urea) but have limited utility. Occasionally, it may prove impossible to definitely identify the cause of the hyponatraemia using these criteria. In these cases, one might have to perform a diagnostic therapeutic trial, with close clinical and laboratory monitoring to avoid harm to the patient. This therapeutic trial for diagnosis is based on the fact that in a

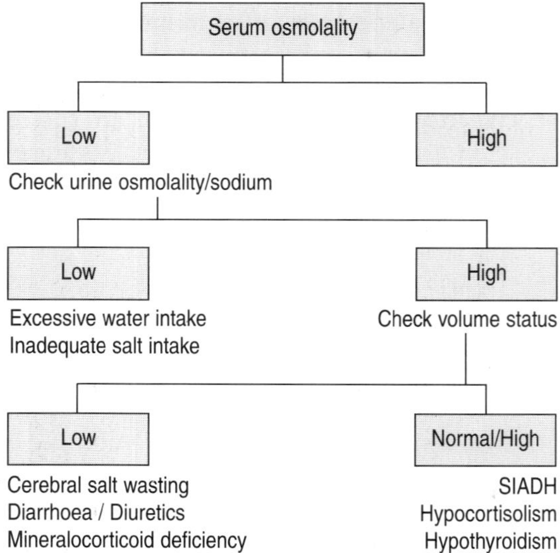

Fig. 1. Diagnostic algorithm for hypotonic hyponatremia (modified from multiple sources[12–14])

patient with SIADH administration of normal volumes of isotonic saline results in worsening of hyponatraemia due to a steady state of sodium as described earlier. The author's practice is to do the following:

—First raise the serum sodium using hypertonic saline to at least 125 mEq/L or whatever higher level is necessary for the patient to be awake and able to guard his or her airway.

—After this, administer normal fluid volumes (safer than fluid restriction in most patients) and watch the trend of the sodium. If it

- Increases – CSW
- Remains almost the same or drops by only 1 or 2 mEq/L add fludrocortisone – if sodium increases – CSW
- Decreases – SIADH.

Rate of correction of hyponatraemia

When treating a patient the risks of hyponatraemia have to be balanced against the risks of correction. Both the severity of symptoms and the acuity of the hyponatraemia influence the rate at which the sodium can be corrected. Serum sodium must be measured frequently (every 2–4 hours) during the acute phase of correction.

A medical emergency constitutes a situation in which a patient develops severe hyponatraemia in <48 hours (the generally accepted definition of acute hyponatraemia) and is comatose, or having seizures. In these patients treatment with 3% saline can even be started at such a rate as to achieve an initial correction of 3–5 mEq/L per hour to avoid irreversible brain damage. In less severe acute hyponatraemia, the initial rate of increase should be no ≤1–2 Eq/L per hour. The correction rate can be slowed down once a level of 125 mEq/L has been reached.

In mildly symptomatic patients and those with chronic hyponatraemia an hourly increase of 0.5 mEq/L is recommended to minimize the risks of complications. Special care must be taken in young women who are particularly vulnerable to complications of rapid correction.[5]

Hypernatraemia

The main osmotically active substance in the body is sodium, so hypernatraemic states are always associated with hyperosmolar serum. For the purposes of diagnosis it is useful to consider three different scenarios that can result in hypernatraemia:

- Hypervolaemic hypernatraemia: This is an uncommon state usually caused by administration of hypertonic fluids or enteral feeds with insufficient free water. An increased intake of oral salt can sometimes be causative.
- *Inadequate fluid intake:* This is usually seen in unconscious patients or those who are unable to ingest water in response to thirst. A rare cause of inadequate fluid intake is damage to the thirst centres in the hypothalamus, usually seen after surgery in the region.
- *Increased water loss:* This is the commonest cause of hypernatraemia—the loss of free

water from the system. High blood sugar with glycosuria, gastrointestinal losses, hypokalaemia and hypercalcaemia can all cause loss of free water. In the absence of any of these conditions, water loss could result from insufficient AVP secretion or renal causes. Diabetes insipidus is a familiar cause of hypernatraemia.

Diabetes insipidus (DI)

Pathophysiology: DI can be divided into central (insufficient secretion of AVP) and nephrogenic (an abnormal response of the kidneys to available AVP) causes.

- Central DI can be congenital or result from any lesions that affect the hypothalamo–pituitary axis. Common causes are trauma, subarachnoid haemorrhage, tumours and surgery in the region, granulomatous disease, and some autoimmune conditions. DI does not manifest until at least 90% of the magnocellular neurons that produce AVP are destroyed. It is also seen as a preterminal event in brain death.
- Nephrogenic DI is caused by end-organ resistance of the kidney and can be congenital, arising from mutations of either the V2 receptor or aquaporin water channels. It may also be seen in severe hypercalcaemia and hypokalaemia.

Diagnosis: Once other causes of polyuria, such as high blood sugar levels, have been ruled out, DI can be diagnosed if the following factors occur:

- Serum sodium >145 mEq/L
- Polyuria with output of >3 ml/kg/hour (some authorities use >4 ml/kg/hour)
- Dilute urine with a specific gravity <1.005
- Polydipsia and polyuria in awake patients with intact thirst mechanisms or hypovolaemia in patients unable to drink water.

Treatment: Once central DI has been confirmed, the treatment consists of replacement of both the water deficit and the AVP deficiency.

- In awake patients with access to water, severe hypernatraemia rarely develops, as the thirst mechanism will ensure that the patient drinks enough water. In patients unable to drink adequately, either because of nausea or altered sensorium, hypotonic fluids may be administered either intravenously or through a nasogastric tube to correct the water deficit. Care must be taken during this process to not cause fluid overload.
- Definitive treatment consists of administration of desmopressin (1-deamino-8-D-arginine vasopressin, DDAVP) either intranasally or orally. In some patients, especially in the immediate postoperative period, the response to DDAVP is inconsistent. In these patients parenteral pitressin may be used, and in severe DI it may be administered as an infusion. As in the correction of hyponatraemia, rapid reduction of serum sodium can result in cerebral oedema. However, the risk is less in these patients since DI is usually diagnosed early and correction of acute hypernatraemia is unlikely to have complications.

DI after surgery in the suprasellar region

Postoperative DI can be transient, permanent or triphasic. Transient DI is thought to be caused by damage to the pituitary stalk, and resolves in a few days as full function of the AVP-producing neurons is resumed. DI might be permanent if the damage extends to the magnocellular neurons. A major determinant of the duration of DI is the level of section of the pituitary stalk—if it is near the median eminence then almost 100% of patients develop permanent DI. The classic triphasic response begins with transient DI. This is followed 5–7 days later by a period of SIADH, as AVP in the disintegrating cells is released, lasting up to 2 weeks.[19] After these stores are consumed, the third phase of permanent DI begins if enough of the magnocellular neurons have been destroyed.

Conclusion

Alterations of sodium and water metabolism are a common finding in the neurology ICU. A logical approach enables an accurate diagnosis in most cases. Rigorous monitoring of fluid status and electrolytes is an indispensable part of management, and knowledge of the complications associated with the abnormality and correction of tonicity improves patient outcome.

References

1. Anderson RJ, Chung HM, Kluge R, *et al.* Hyponatremia: A prospective analysis of its epidemiology and the pathogenetic role of vasopressin. *Ann Intern Med* 1985;**102**:164–8.
2. Sharman A, Low J. Vasopressin and its role in critical care. *Cont Education in Anaesth, Crit Care and Pain* 2008;**4**:134–7.
3. Robinson AG, Verbalis JG. The posterior pituitary. In: Larsen PR, Kronenberg HM, Melmed S, *et al.* (eds). *Williams Textbook of Endocrinology.* 10th ed. Philadelphia: WB Saunders; 2003:281–329.
4. Multz AS. Vasopressin dysregulation and hyponatremia in hospitalized patients. *Intensive Care Med* 2007;**22**:216–23.
5. Lien YH, Shapiro JI. Hyponatremia: Clinical diagnosis and management. *Am J Med* 2007;**120**: 653–8.
6. Lien YH, Shapiro JI, Chan L. Study of brain electrolytes and organic osmolytes during correction of chronic hyponatremia: Implications for the pathogenesis of central pontine myelinolysis. *J Clin Invest* 1991;**88**:303–9.
7. Arieff AI, Llach F, Massry SG. Neurological manifestations and morbidity of hyponatremia: Correlation with brain water and electrolytes. *Medicine* 1976;**55**:121–9.
8. Kleinschmidt-DeMasters BK, Norenberg MD. Rapid correction of hyponatremia causes demyelination: Relation to central pontine myelinolysis. *Science* 1981;**211**:1068–70.
9. Yancey PH, Clark ME, Hand SC, *et al.* Living with water stress: Evolution of osmolyte systems. *Science* 1982;**217**:1214–22.
10. Sugimura Y, Murase T, Takefuji S, *et al.* Protective effect of dexamethasone on osmotic-induced demyelination in rats. *Exp Neurol* 205;**192**:178–83.
11. Bradshaw K, Smith M. Disorders of sodium balance after head injury. *Cont Education in Anaesth, Crit Care and Pain* 2008;**8**:129–33.
12. Palmer BF. Hyponatremia in patients with central nervous system disease: SIADH versus CSW. *Trends Endocrinol Metab* 2003;**14**:182–87.
13. Sivakumar V, Rajshekhar V, Chandy MJ. Management of neurosurgical patients with hyponatremia and natriuresis. *Neurosurgery* 1994;**34**:269–74.
14. Damaraju SC, Rajshekhar V, Chandy MJ. Validation study of a central venous pressure based protocol for the management of neurosurgical patients with hyponatremia and natriuresis. *Neurosurgery* 1997;**40**: 312–16.
15. Adler SM, Verbalis JG. Disorders of body water homeostasis in critical illness. *Endocrinol Metab Clin N Am* 2006;**35**:873–94.
16. Bartter FC, Schwartz WB. The syndrome of inappropriate secretion of antidiuretic hormone. *Am J Med* 1967;**42**:790–806.
17. Ghali JK, Koren MJ, Taylor JR, *et al.* Efficacy and safety of oral conivaptan: A V1A/V2 receptor antagonist, assessed in a randomized placebo-controlled trial in patients with euvolemic or hypervolemic hyponatremia. *J Clin Endocrinol Metabol* 2006;**91**:2145–52.
18. Li-Ng M, Verbalis JG. Conivaptan: Evidence supporting its use in hyponatremia. *Core Evid* 2010;**15**:83–92.
19. Hollinshead WH. The interphase of diabetes insipidus. *Mayo Clin Proc* 1964;**39**:92–100.

2

Neurobiology of radiation and radiation-induced neurological complications

RAKESH JALALI, VIVEK TIWARI

Introduction

Radiotherapy (RT) is an integral component of the multimodal management of primary brain tumours. It has a potential impact on local control, symptom improvement, and progression-free survival of those with low-grade and benign neoplasms, and on overall survival in those with malignant brain tumours. Following maximal safe resection, adjuvant RT is indicated postoperatively for all high-grade primary brain tumours. For completely excised benign tumours, such as pituitary adenomas and benign meningiomas, upfront adjuvant RT has currently no role to play. For low-grade gliomas, with no residual tumour on neuroimaging, surveillance alone is a reasonable option. However, RT is recommended in such tumours either if a macroscopic residual tumour is evident on postoperative imaging or if tumour progression is documented on serial imaging. For tumours in the eloquent cortex where only a partial excision or biopsy is possible, radical RT is needed to improve the outcome.

The types of radiation used in clinical practice are mainly ionizing in nature and comprise:

- X-rays
- Gamma rays
- Beta radiations
- Protons and neutrons.

Out of these, the most widely used are X-rays in the form of linear accelerators and the latest modalities of high-precision treatment delivery, including 3-dimensional conformal RT (3D-CRT), stereotactic radiosurgery and radiotherapy (SRS and SRT), and intensity-modulated radiotherapy (IMRT). However, in many places in India, the major bulk of cancer patients requiring radiation receive conventional RT such as Co-60 gamma rays.

The basis of the radiation effect is DNA damage due to hydrolysis of the water molecules present in the body tissues. This takes place by complex mechanisms working in a direct as well as indirect manner.

Complications of RT in the CNS

RT-induced complications to the central nervous system (CNS) may occur after treatment for

- Primary brain tumours
- Metastatic brain tumours
- Prophylactic cranial RT (acute lymphoblastic leukaemia [ALL], lymphoma, small cell lung cancer)

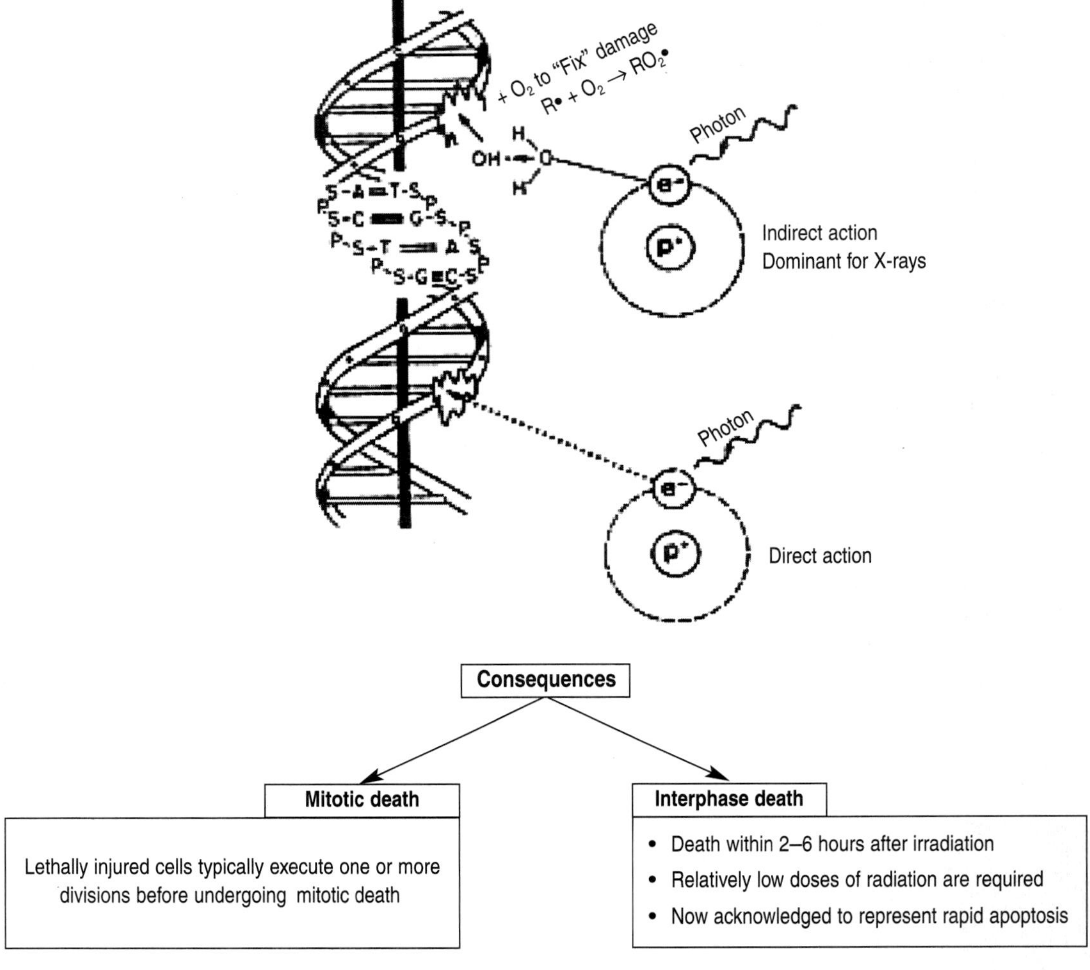

However, CNS complications may be encountered after treatment of head and neck cancers (temporal lobe necrosis, radiation myelitis).

Complications encountered in practice

Major
- Neuropsychological
- Neurological function
- Neurocognition
- Neuroendocrine impairment
- Radiation-induced second malignancy.

Relatively less common
- Cerebrovascular accidents (CVA)
- Radiation-induced necrosis
  —Radiation-induced optic neuropathy (RION)
  —Radiation myelitis
  —Skin toxicities (e.g. permanent hair loss).

Complications are mainly described according to the radiation portal (focal conformal RT, cranio-spinal irradiation [CSI] and whole brain radiation therapy [WBRT] or grade of the tumour (high and low grade). The grade and site of disease, age at presentation, radiation energy used (cobalt/linear accelerator) and intensity of treatment regimen (fraction schedule, total RT dose) are important factors in the development of acute and late complications.

Acute toxicities: Complications occur within 2 months of completion of treatment.

Late toxicities: Complications usually occur after 2–3 years; however, they may be observed even many years after completion of treatment.

Manifestations of neuronal injuries

- *Time frame*: 3 months to several years.
- *Histology:* pallor of white matter combined with cerebral oedema/demyelination, coagulation necrosis, vascular thickening, perivascular fibrosis, calcium deposition, fibrin deposition, fibrin exudation, chronic inflammatory exudates (Figs 1 and 2)
- *Target:* fine vasculature, oligodendrocytes
- End-point—necrosis, best seen in benign tumours.
- Threshold for changes 45 Gy/25# seen either as low-density areas on CT scan or localized masses with contrast enhancement
- MRI shows periventricular changes at doses of 24 Gy.

Neuropsychological function

- Neurological function is traditionally assessed by clinical examination such as assessment of Karnofsky performance status (KPS) and neurological performance status (NPS). These are simple tests, require minimum expertise and are used to detect any sensory or motor impairment.
- Numerous batteries of tests are used in clinical practice in India to evaluate neurocognitive and psychological function, such as the Weschsler intelligent scoring chart (WISC) Bhatia scoring system and Vithoba Paknikar (VP) in blind patients. Intelligence quotient (IQ) is described as global IQ (GQ) or full-scale IQ (FSIQ), performance IQ (PQ), memory IQ (MQ) and verbal IQ (VQ). These IQ scores are assessed by different verbal questionnaires and performance domains. In children below the age of 16 years, neuropsychological function is assessed by performing FSIQ, PQ and VQ, whereas in adults, MQ is also assessed. The total score depends on the tasks performed and total time taken.

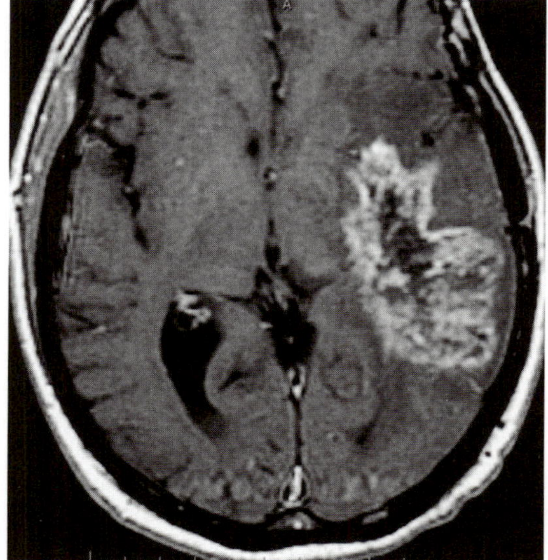

Fig. 1. Typical radiological (MRI) appearance of necrosis

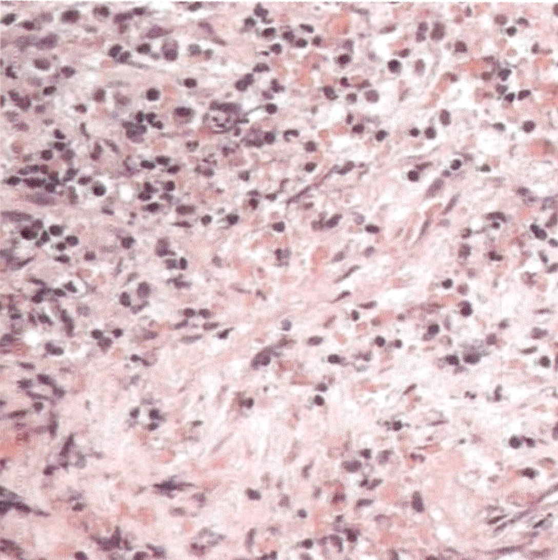

Fig. 2. Histopathological appearance of necrosis

There has, however, been a discrepancy in our understanding of the relationship of neuropsychological and neurocognitive functions with radiation *per se*, owing to a few basic but important facts.

- The majority of neurocognitive function assessment data have been obtained after either WBRT or CSI and showed deterioration of function after RT. However, these data were obtained from studies which mostly used a telecobalt machine and suboptimal radiation techniques. Thus, neuropsychological function should be evaluated in the light of modern RT techniques and newer assessment tools.
- IQ assessment is the benchmark for measuring changes in cognitive function. A decline in IQ is mostly the result of failure to learn at a rate that is appropriate for the age of the child, rather than from a loss of previously acquired knowledge.
- A considerable number of children and young adults may exhibit low IQ levels even before starting RT, suggesting that other factors such as tumour, surgery, etc. could also be responsible.[1]
- In several patients, a decline in IQ is associated with treatment-related risk factors such as young age at the time of treatment, long time since treatment, hydrocephalus, RT schedule, and dose and volume of the irradiated normal brain.
- Loss of cerebral white matter and failure to develop white matter at a rate appropriate for the developmental stage may be responsible for changes in IQ score.
- Decline in IQ function after CSI is estimated to be 4 points per year and is cumulative. Young age and radiation dose were the most significant factors influencing a fall in IQ score.[2]
- The decline in PQ is greater than that in VQ. However, the decline in IQ scores may be of a lesser magnitude after focal conformal RT (3D-CRT) as demonstrated in recent studies.[3] There is a paucity of prospective data on neuropsychological status in patients with brain tumours, especially among those who have undergone focal partial brain RT.[3]
- Studies with a relatively short follow up have shown the superiority of 3D-CRT with or without stereotactic guidance (SCRT) in maintaining long-term cognitive scores when compared to conventional RT.[4]
- After RT, reading appears to be affected more than other academic skills and may decline over time despite stable intellectual functioning. Mathematics and spelling performance remain stable. Supratentorial tumour location and multiple surgeries are predictive of a poorer reading performance.[1]
- A randomized controlled trial on CSI dose (36 Gy versus 23.6 Gy) showed that there was significantly less reduction in both neuropsychological and neuroendocrine function with a lower dose of CSI (23.6 Gy) compared with higher-dose CSI (36 Gy).[2] The study found that young age (<7 years) and higher radiation dose (>23.6 Gy) have a deleterious effect on cognitive function. However, patients with recurrent disease also had a significantly worse quality of life and poorer cognitive function.
- Prophylactic cranial radiation (PCI) in acute leukaemia (ALL) was shown to reduce neurocognitive function and was assessed by a randomized trial with long-term follow-up data.[3] Poorer performance after PCI was independent of the sex of the patient, time since treatment and age at diagnosis. The findings suggest that addition of 2400 cGy PCI in ALL increases the risk for mild global loss in intellectual and neuropsychological ability.[5]

Randomized trials have shown that young ALL patients treated with a lower dose of PCI (18 Gy) had significantly less reduction in full-scale, VQ and PQ as measured with the WISC scale, compared with those who received 24 Gy PCI.[5]

- Thus, reducing the dose of PCI from 2400 cGy to 1800 cGy reduces neurotoxicity to acceptable levels.

Our data

There is a relative paucity of data on cognitive function and its correlation with RT doses to different volumes of brain. It is especially imperative to study the possible correlation of RT doses with cognitive sequelae, so that modern techniques of 3D-CRT (e.g. stereotactic irradiation and intensity-modulated RT) can be used to their optimal potential. In an attempt to characterize the patterns of IQ scores with time after highly conformal cranial RT and how these scores are affected by age at the time of RT, and parenchymal dose–volume analysis, no difference has been found in neurocognitive outcomes on the basis of dose–volumes in the whole brain, frontal lobes or the right temporal lobe. In contrast, high doses of RT to the left temporal lobe seem to have a clear impact.[6]

The importance of the left temporal lobe and hippocampus in VQ and memory functions has been previously reported.[6] Left temporal lobe lesions have also been reported to produce a different pattern of results in the Weschler scores for IQ in adults.[7] The relevance of high dose–volumes ($\geq$43.2 Gy) seems greater than low dose–volumes with respect to the maintenance of cognition and could have relevance in planning conformal RT for benign and low-grade tumours. A smaller target volume and the reduction in margins may have the potential to reduce normal temporal lobe volumes receiving higher doses, thus reducing the risk of cognitive damage.[7]

Neurocognitive function is assessed by the Lowenstein Occupational Therapy Cognitive Assessment (LOTCA) battery of tests. The LOTCA is a direct observational and verbal communication method of assessment. The LOTCA was designed to measure the basic cognitive abilities and visual perception of clients with neurological dysfunction. It provides a profile of the client's cognitive status and establishes a baseline for the purpose of planning intervention goals and monitoring changes during treatment.[8]

Assessment of neurological function by activities of daily living (ADL)

Functional activity is assessed more objectively by measuring activities of daily living (ADL). ADL is a battery of tests done to assess the 'functional activity' of a person, essentially in terms of the degree of performance activity regarding movement, eating, cooking, self-care, bathing, dressing, etc. ADL is a validated method to assess the functional status of a patient. People with low scores are more dependent on others to help with the tasks of daily living than with those with higher scores. Depending on the performance activity, this evaluation also helps to identify patients who may require support for daily living, and assesses the efficacy of supportive care in improving their functional activity. ADL is most commonly assessed by the modified Barthel index (BI). However, the functional independence measurement and functional activity measurement (FIM FAM) scoring system is now being used to assess ADL as it is a comprehensive tool that encompasses cognitive parameters as well.

BI has been used to evaluate the efficacy of supportive care or any sort of intervention (RT or surgery), primarily in elderly patients with high-grade gliomas (HGG). BI has been shown to improve after RT in HGG and brain metastasis.

Data are sparse on BI score in paediatric patients with low-grade brain tumour treated with RT. However, in our prospective series, there was no deterioration in BI domain scores at 3-year follow up.[7]

Endocrine function

Assessment of neuroendocrine function is done by estimating the serum hormone levels of different hormones of the pituitary–hypothalamic axis (PHA). These include thyroid hormone (T3, T4, thyroid-stimulating hormone [TSH]), growth hormone (unstimulated and stimulated GH), sex hormone (luteinizing hormone [LH], follicle-stimulating hormone [FSH], testosterone), cortisol and prolactin hormone axis (prolactin).

RT to the brain has been implicated as one of the most important factors associated with neuroendocrine dysfunction on long-term follow up.[10] The radiation dose and volume of brain irradiated are significantly correlated. The majority of the findings are from either CSI or WBRT.[10]

- Both during WBRT and CSI, the PHA receives a high dose and thus functional impairment is expected even years after RT. GH seems to be the most sensitive hormone as its serum level is the first to decline after RT. A decline in the level of GH is followed by a decline in thyroid hormone-releasing hormone (THRH) and cortisol levels. Impairment of the circadian hormonal surge is considered an early sign of hormone axis deficit.[9] After conventional WBRT with a dose of more than 18 Gy, impairment of normal GH secretion is the first and most commonly recognized deficit.[9,10]
- In medulloblastoma, after a CSI dose of 36 Gy, 75% had hormone axis impairment with the majority (70%) having GH axis deficit, while the cortisol and thyroid axis were usually preserved.[11]
- It seems that HP axis deficiency is dose dependent and a lower radiation dose is associated with significantly less hormone axis deficiency.[9,12]

Prospective evaluation of endocrine function after focal RT has not been well studied. There is evidence of a 'dose–effect' relationship between RT dose and HP axis deficit.[9,12]

- As the HP axis is expected to be spared with focal RT, it is assumed that there will be a higher probability of preservation of endocrine function.

Among the literature on focal RT, paediatric patients suffering from germinoma treated with low-dose focal radiation (25 Gy) were shown to have preserved endocrine function.[13]

- SCRT is dosimetrically superior to other focal RT techniques as it requires a lesser planning target volume (PTV) margin.[14] Thus, it will be interesting to assess the status of endocrine function after treatment with SCRT.
- Long-term follow up of paediatric patients with brain tumour treated with proton beam therapy is needed to evaluate the extent of preservation of neuroendocrine function.

Second malignant neoplasms

Second malignancy data are obtained either from retrospective series, large randomized trials as secondary end-points, or recently from population-based surveillance epidemiology and end results (SEER) data.

- In the SEER data, the cumulative incidence of second cancer among all cancer patients was 5.0%, 8.4%, 10.8% and 13.7% at 5, 10, 15, and 25 years, respectively.
- Second malignancies after treatment of brain tumour with radiation are meningioma, sarcoma and glioma.

The relative risk of developing a second brain tumour after radiation compared with the incidence in the normal population was 9.38 (3.05–21.89).[15]

- The cumulative incidence of brain tumours at 20 years after cranial RT in ALL was 1.39% (95% CI, 0.63%–2.15%). Thus, second malignancy is relatively uncommon after RT for primary brain tumour.

Cerebrovascular accidents (CVA)

An increased incidence of cerebrovascular accidents (CVA) and related mortality has been reported in patients with pituitary adenoma treated with RT.[16] The possible risk factors include hypopituitarism, irradiation and extensive surgery, but none are proven causes at present.

Brada *et al.*[16] reported a 4.1-fold increased mortality from CVA in a series of 334 patients irradiated for pituitary tumour. However, the increased incidence of CVA may be related to endocrine dysfunction rather than the RT itself.

Radiation-induced necrosis

RT-induced necrosis is usually observed in 1%–2% after high-dose RT. However, RT-induced necrosis ('pseudoprogression') is increased by up to 14% after treatment of HGG with concurrent RT and temozolomide.[17]

This increased contrast enhancement after RT is called pseudoprogression. Pseudoprogression needs to be differentiated from true progression. Functional imaging may improve the non-invasive diagnosis of pseudoprogression, but randomized prospective studies are needed to evaluate the real impact of pseudoprogression and validate neuroradiological techniques that are able to make a reliable distinction between tumour recurrence and pseudoprogression.[18]

- *[18F]-3'-fluoro-3'-deoxy-L-thymidine:* 18F-3'-fluoro-3'-deoxy-L-thymidine (18F-FLT), the latest entity in the field of oncology, is a radiolabelled analogue of thymidine, and can be trapped within the cytosol after being monophosphorylated by thymidine kinase-1 (TK-1), a principal enzyme in the salvage pathway of DNA synthesis. It has been demonstrated in cell culture, animal models and clinical studies that the accumulation of 18F-FLT is closely associated with cellular proliferation.

18F-FLT PET may be more accurate than 18F-FDG PET in differentiating benign from malignant pulmonary lesions.

A detailed analysis of the heterogeneous tumour compartments on 18F-FLT permits differentiation of high-proliferating from low-proliferating tumour areas. Thus, 18F-FLT analysis allows for detection of the part of the tumour that is proliferating the most. Because the most proliferating part of the tumour is mainly responsible for tumour progression, 18F-FLT analysis enables a more precise estimation of the malignancy and may also serve as an accurate measure of antiproliferative treatment strategies.

Radiation myelitis

Radiation myelitis, though rare, is seen in patients with brain or posterior fossa tumours treated with CSI. There is a higher probability of myelitis with a higher RT dose (>50 Gy).[19]

In most cases, acute radiation myelitis is self-limiting. Late-onset myelitis is permanent and associated with significant neurological deficits.

Radiation-induced optic neuropathy (RION)

The optic chiasm is radiosensitive and blindness from damage is well documented. The risk of damage following RT is 1%–2% with a latency period of 2 months–4 years. Gadolinium MR has shown that the cause is injury to the vasa nervosum. The degree of risk is related to the dose and dose per fraction.

Radiation-induced optic neuropathy (RION) is a devastating late complication of radiotherapy to the anterior visual pathway resulting in acute, profound, irreversible visual loss. It is thought to be a result of radiation necrosis of the anterior visual pathway. Visual loss may be unilateral or bilateral; simultaneous or sequential. Cumulative doses of radiation that exceed 50 Gy or single doses to the anterior visual pathway of more than 10 Gy are usually required for RION to develop.[20]

- The risk increases (by 3%–7%) at doses of 55–60 Gy and becomes more substantial (>7%–20%) for doses >60 Gy when fractionations of 1.8–2.0 Gy are used.[20]

For single-fraction SRS, RION is rare for a Dmax <8 Gy, increases in the range of 8–12 Gy, and becomes >10% in the range of 12–15 Gy.

- *Radiation tolerance of structures to single-fraction treatment:* Radiation-related optic neuropathy was picked up earliest by a delay or reduction in the amplitude of visual evoked potentials <10 Gy: No RION; 10–15 Gy: 26.7%; >15 Gy: 77.8%.[20]

Conclusion

In this era of evidence-based and highly precise radiation techniques, it is imperative to have an understanding of the basis of the radiation *per se*, and apply it to improve treatment strategy and related policies. In case of CNS tumours, it becomes all the more challenging to counter complications and achieve the ideal outcome with respect to the neuropsychological, cognitive and neuroendocrine parameters, as these contribute immensely towards the patient's overall well-being and quality of life. Therefore, it is of the utmost importance to formulate evidence-based guidelines and also maintain an individualized approach to the aim of treatment, modalities used and delivery of radiation.

References

1. Carpentieri SC, Waber DP, Pomeroy SL, *et al.* Neuropsychological functioning after surgery in children treated for brain tumor. *Neurosurgery* 2003; **52**:1348–57.
2. Mulhern RK, Kepner JL, Thomas PR, *et al.* Neuropsychologic functioning of survivors of childhood medulloblastoma randomized to receive conventional or reduced-dose craniospinal irradiation: A pediatric oncology group study. *J Clin Oncol* 1998;**16**:1723–8.
3. Conklin HM, Li C, Xiong X, *et al.* Predicting change in academic abilities after conformal radiation therapy for localized ependymoma. *J Clin Oncol* 2008;**26**:3965–70.
4. Jalali R, Goswami S, Sarin R, *et al.* Neuropsychological status in children and young adults with benign and low-grade brain tumors treated prospectively with focal stereotactic conformal radiotherapy. *Int J Radiat Oncol Biol Phys* 2006;**66**: S14–S19.
5. Jankovic M, Masera G, Brouwers P, *et al.* Association of 1800 cGy cranial irradiation with intellectual function in children with acute lymphoblastic leukaemia. *The Lancet* 1994;**344**:224–7.
6. Dobbins C, Russell EW. Left temporal lobe brain damage pattern on the Wechsler Adult Intelligence Scale. *J Clin Psychol* 1990;**46**:863–8.
7. Jalali R, Mallick I, Dutta D, *et al.* Factors influencing neurocognitive outcomes in young patients with benign and low-grade brain tumors treated with stereotactic conformal radiotherapy. *Int J Radiat Oncol Biol Phys* 2010;**77**:974–9.
8. Katz N, Itzkovich M, Avrtbuch S, *et al.* The Loewenstein occupational therapy cognitive assessment (LOTCA) battery for brain injured patients: Reliability and validity. *Am J Occup Ther* 1989;**43**:184–92.
9. Dutta D, Shah N, Gupta T, Munshi A, *et al.* Prospective analysis of endocrine function in children with residual/recurrent low grade brain tumours treated with high precision stereotactic conformal radiotherapy. *J Clin Oncol* 2008;**26** (Suppl):[abstr 2049].
10. Heikens J, Michiels EM, Behrendt H, *et al.* Long-term neuro-endocrine sequelae after treatment for childhood medulloblastoma. *Eur J Cancer* 1998;**34**: 1592–7.
11. Abstracts from the Third Quadrennial Meeting of the World Federation of Neuro-Oncology (WFNO) and the Sixth Meeting of the Asian Society for Neuro-Oncology (ASNO). *Neuro Oncol* 2009;**11**: 871–970.
12. Agha A, Sherlock M, Brennan S, *et al.* Hypothalamic-pituitary dysfunction after irradiation of non-pituitary brain tumors in adults. *J Clin Endocrinol Metab* 2005;**90**:6355–60.
13. Daphne A, Brian T, William MM, *et al.* Radiation therapy for intracranial germ cell tumors. *Int J Radiat Oncol Biol Phys* 2003;**56**:511–18.
14. Murthy V, Jalali R, Sarin R, *et al.* Stereotactic conformal radiotherapy for posterior fossa tumours: A modelling study for potential improvement in therapeutic ratio. *Radiotherapy and Oncology* 2003; **67**:191–8.
15. Minniti G, Traish D, Ashley S, *et al.* Risk of second brain tumor after conservative surgery and radiotherapy for pituitary adenoma: Update after an additional 10 years. *J Clin Endocrinol Metab* 2005; **90**:800–4.
16. Brada M, Ashley S, Ford D, *et al.* Cerebrovascular mortality in patients with pituitary adenoma. *Clin*

Endocrinol (Oxf) 2002;**57**:713–7.

17. Clarke JL, Abrey LE, Karimi S, *et al.* Pseudo-progression (PsPr) after concurrent radiotherapy (RT) and temozolomide (TMZ) for newly diagnosed glioblastoma multiforme (GBM). *J Clin Oncol* 2008;**26**:(Suppl);[abstr 2025].

18. Chaskis C, Neyns B, Michotte A, *et al.* Pseudo-progression after radiotherapy with concurrent temozolomide for high-grade glioma: Clinical observations and working recommendations. *Surg Neurol* 2009;**72**:423–8.

19. Schultheiss TE. Spinal cord radiation tolerance: doctrine vs data. *Int J Radiat Oncol Biol Phys* 1994;**30**:735–6.

20. Danesh-Meyer HV. Radiation induced optic neuropathy. *J Clin Neurosci* 2008;**15**:95–100.

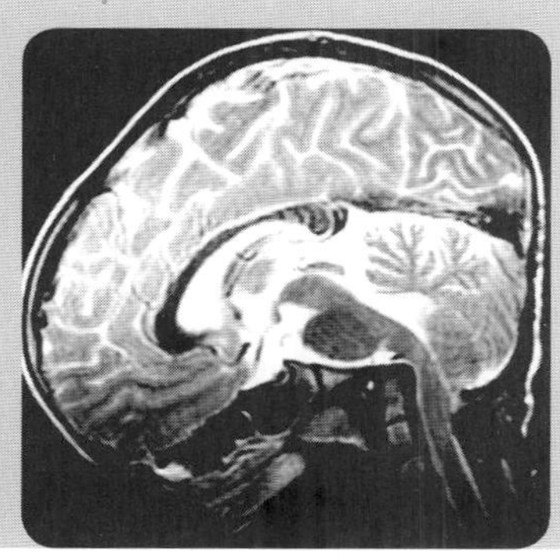

Embryology

3

Conceptual essentials of neuraxial embryogenesis

MANU KOTHARI, ATUL GOEL

Robert Persig, in *Zen and the Art of Motorcycle Maintenance*, applauds the quality of 'unstuckness'. The science of embryogenesis has yielded, after over 3 centuries of ceaseless work, the realization that in essence, animal embryogenesis is not only unknown but unknowable, being but a discipline of retrospection and mumbo jumbo of Greek and Latin terms. Hence, the title of this foray into what a neurosurgeon should know about the development of the central nervous system (CNS), or better, the neuraxis. As clinicians and neurosurgeons, we need to get unstuck from standard, or even advanced, descriptions of embryogenesis, to evolve concepts that reveal the what, why and wherefrom of a 100 trillion-celled human that starts from a single, featureless cell called the zygote.

Parsimonious Nature fashions a 1 mm flea and a 30,000 mm long whale through the prototypic homeobox, making both invertebrate and vertebrate embryogenesis essentially identical. The game plan is to make the zygote create, by cell multiplication and differentiation, first an embryonic plate that, folding on itself, creates the embryonic tube, which is good enough to create a limbless python on the one hand and a limbed

dinosaur on the other. The thalidomide tragedy taught us that the limbs are the offshoots of a basic embryonic cylinder. Each animal form is homeobox-wise simply and, biblically speaking, made 'fearfully and wonderfully'. The homeobox simplicity has further extended the Burnetian fact that 'all DNA is depressingly alike', as also that a typical animal cell, from eel to elephant, and bacteria to Buddha, has refused to give up its self-sameness during its stay on the earth for the past 5.3 billion years. The biblical fearful wondrousness lies in the invariable variability of every single animal form and of its varied components. No two cerebral hemispheres have ever been or will be alike, a fact only achievable by each developing cerebrum conversing with all the cerebra of the past, present and future— beyond all limits of time and space. Each dermatoglyphic fingerprint is cosmically designed. Burnet has generalized that each developing neurone knows which way to grow and to which neurones to connect.[1] The unfathomability of developmental mechanisms has been summed up well by Slack in his scholarly history of the scope and limitations of embryological research and texts.[2] He proposes the following:

- Molecular biology has yet to make a major contribution to our understanding of early development.
- Embryonic development is terribly complicated. It is a historical sequence of hierarchical decisions by which one state of systems leads to another.
- The models put forward for this process are of more use to us as an aid for clear thinking than as a possible explanation of reality.
- While the naïve reductionist molecular biologist is never going to explain how an egg becomes an animal, the sophisticated system analysts are left to wonder whether the phenomenon is real.

The homeobox mechanism decrees that all mammalian embryos are completely formed identically when 25 mm long. In this mini universe there is enough clear room for the chordi tendinae of the cardiac valves, on the one hand, and the lacrimal puncta on the other. Organogenesis is complete by 8 weeks of intrauterine life. The ensuing foetal stage is one of growth and not so much of development.

The following points are an attempt to summarize neuraxial development. The brevity below presupposes that the reader knows the initial and elementary embryological sequences leading to the formation of the embryonic tube that fashions the whole organism from head to foot.

- For the sake of descriptive convenience the neuraxis, from lamina terminalis (cephalic end) to filum terminale (caudal end), is a single, monolithic entity, divided into the so-called fore-, mid- and hindbrains, and the spinal cord.
- The foregoing must apply to the neuraxial cavity comprising the cerebral canal and the ventricles.
- One-tenth of the neuraxis is neurones; nine-tenth is varied neuroglia. Each neurone must be fully clothed by 10 neuroglial cells serving as a highly intelligent and dynamic blood–neurone bridge.

- Cross-sectionally, the neuraxial tube is similar all along its length, comprising the neuraqual cavity floored by the so-called ependymal cells, next to which is the mantle zone, surrounded by the marginal zone. The apparent externalization of grey matter on the cerebral/cerebellar surfaces is Nature's device to seek a wider neuronal spread, by making the mantle zone migrate to the surface. The neural tube does not turn inside-out at any stage.
- In a similar fashion, the cerebellar foliation and cerebral gyration (thus sulcation) is a neuraxial way of conveying a 'cap area' into an extensive 'turban area'. The gyration is a tridimensional cosmic event, for no two gyral patterns have ever been alike, as is the case with fingerprints.
- The crossing of most neuraxial fibres to offer contralateral cerebral control is Nature's way of a non-space demanding vertical commissure. The fibres to and from the tip of the left little finger will cross to the right side to instantly touch and communicate with the fibres to and from the tip of the right little finger. Nature is amazingly economical and efficient.
- The ontogeny of the neuraxis rigidly follows and repeats the neuraxial phylogeny, whereby from fish to man, every step is discernible and connected, be it paleo-, archi- or neoneuraxis.
- The neuraxis closely imitates the embryo in 'asking' the surface neural crest cells to fashion the leptomeninges to cover the neuraxis and the contained neuraqua, thereby rendering the neuraxis protected and essentially weightless, akin to the amniotic-fluid-held foetus. The neuraxis begets, as it were, the meninges, which then acquire maternal status to be so named—pia mater and arachnoid mater. Pia-arachnoid are neuraxial versions of amnion-chorion.
- The dorsal neural tube is a remarkable imitation of the ventral gut-tube. The embryonic plate's inner layer folds on itself to create the endodermal tube. The plate's dorsal ectoderm sinks to betube itself and get detached from the mother ectoderm to place

itself dorsal to the gut. The two romantically meet when the descending hypophyseal diverticulum meets the ascending palatal diverticulum to fashion the postero-anterior pituitary. The gut diverticula create the glands of the gastrointestinal tract. The neuraxial diverticula at its cervical end create the hemispheres, the pineal, the pituitary, and the optical systems.

- The (presumably protective) bony systems, namely, the skull and vertebral column, do not contain the neuraxis, but like a sleeve or cap, cover it, being sequential to the formation of the neuraxis. Every impression on the cranial inner surface has been caused by the brain surface, as the skull developed around it. The anatomy texts—*Gray's Anatomy* and beyond—are full of foramina of the skull through which blood vessels and nerves allegedly pass to and fro. In non-controvertible reality, the mandibular nerve does not pass through the foramen ovale, which has cast itself around the preformed mandibular nerve. The vertebrae form around the cord and the nerves that are in proximity with the cord, to create an illusion of the intervertebral foramen. Neither the nerves nor the cord segments are intervertebral. Each vertebra is intersegmental, the nerves between the two vertebrae representing correctly the somatic as well as spinal cord segments.

- Strange as it may seem, cleft palate and cleft-neuraxis are mirror images. Cleft palate, occurring in 1 in 1000 births, is a part of the normal distribution of the degree of fusion of the two palatal processes. Likewise, when the neuroectodermal folds fuse, some 'fail' to do so to give rise to spina bifida, meningocele, meningomyelocele, and even anencephaly. In a similar manner, abdominal dehiscence, called exomphalos minor/major, is a mimicry of split neuraxis, and vice versa. Nature exercises no terror of error but only exerts the forces of herdity, which dictates herd distribution of the so-called anomaly (e.g. 'My child has spina bifida because yours does not'). Even the phenomenon of cancer is herdistically governed;

one in five humans have it. The occurrence of cancer in one human spares four others from it. More specifically, say, acute lymphoblastic leukaemia (ALL) in one person spares 49,999 others of its occurrence—generation after generation, country after country, its incidence being steady at 1 in 50,000.

- It is a tradition in embryology to call the dorsal mantle zone as alar lamina and the ventral mantle zone as basal lamina. The former is 'sensory' in that its axons stay in/terminate in the neuraxis. The basal laminar cells are 'motor', as their axons leave the neuraxis. Nearly 96% of the neuraxis is alar laminar in cellular origin. The cerebellum and the cerebra lacking any neurons whose axons leave the CNS are described as purely alar.

- The CNS is not so much central as intermediate. Its affective/cognitive arm is all the sensory receptors and its effective/conative/motor arm is the muscle cells. The sensory receptors (S), the neurons (N) and the muscle cells (M) comprise the SNM complex made up in Leblond's pioneering classification of cell populations as postmitotic/non-divisible/perennial cells.[3] Their inherent normal indivisibility precludes their susceptibility to abnormal divisibility, otherwise known as 'cancer'.

The other overlooked aspect of the SNM complex is that during thymic maturation in intrauterine life, when dividing cells of the body present their 'selfhood' credentials to the thymus to make it destroy 'forbidden lymphocytic clones', the SNM cells fail to get the forbidden clones rejected and hence remain highly susceptible to autoimmune onslaught. Hence, the problem of uveitis and sympathetic ophthalmitis after eye injury or of autoimmune encephalomyelitis when some neuronal protein from within or 'vaccinationally' from without manages to enter the circulation and invite the thymic wrath.

The SNM complex, unlike its dividing cellular brethren, has to be connected precisely point-to-point, like in the electronic printed circuits. This fact, added to the indivisibility of the components of the complex, makes them poor repairers of injuries. They are unlikely to allow stem cell implants to offer neoneurons after neuraxial loss, lest the neoneurons precipitate encephalomyelitis. It is possible that the first thing that the injured neuraxis does is to clog the injured neural fibres from growing and entering the circulation. Stem cells, as therapy for neuraxial injury, do not seem to have a viable future. Modern medicine and cytology do not 'know' what a cell is. Blessed with this incurable ignorance, it is surprising that the as-yet undefinable stem cell is being mooted as a panacea for a wide range of problems. Modern medicine has proved to be a doer without being a knower. Stem-cell therapy has arrived to camouflage its intellectual bankruptcy and pump up its earnings on the one hand, and its flagging credibility on the other.

References

1. Burnet FM. *Cellular immunology.* London: Cambridge University Press; 1969:39.
2. Slack JMW. *From egg to emryo—determinative events in early development.* London: Cambridge University Press; 1983.
3. Leblond CP. *Classification of cell populations on the basis of their proliferative behaviour.* National Cancer Institute Monograph; 1964:14.

4

Embryology of the cranio-vertebral junction and congenital malformations in the region

DACHLING PANG

The bony cranio-vertebral junction (CVJ) can be conceptually divided into two component parts with respect to the governance of intersegmental movements and functional space for the nervous system. The first is the central pivot comprising the dens and C_2 vertebral body. The second comprises two ringed structures surrounding the central pivot, albeit eccentrically. The ringed structures are the foramen magnum, which consists of the basiocciput (clivus) and exocciput (including the occipital condyles), and the atlantal ring, with its anterior and posterior arches and lateral masses. These two superimposing rings transmit the lower brainstem and upper cervical spinal cord, while permitting limited rotatory and flexion–extension motions upon each other and around the dental pivot. Straddling these two rings and anchoring upon them are the stabilizing ligaments, viz. the alar and apical dental ligaments at the up-side of the pivot, the transverse atlantal ligament (TAL) across the main dental shaft, and the arching mantle of the tectorial membrane and cruciate ligament, strapping the clivus to the whole of the dens–axis assembly.

In keeping with the functional anatomy of the CVJ, the two main themes of clinical interest are instability and neural compression. Clinically significant developmental anomalies affecting, respectively, the 'pivot' and 'rings' also happen to follow this thematic division. Anomalies of the central pivot usually lead to instability, although basilar impression and a retroflexed dens can cause neural impingement. Anomalies of the surrounding rings result in deformity and crowding, but hypoplasia and aplasia of component parts can result in a weakened frame and loss of ligamentous anchorage. This chapter deals first with the normal development and genetic control of this region, followed by the embryogenesis, clinical relevance, and treatment of congenital malformations of the CVJ.

Embryology of the CVJ: The pre-somitic stage

At gastrulation, epiblastic cells from the embryonic plate caudal to the head process invaginate through the primitive streak to form mesoderm on each side of the neural plate, while cells from both sides of the dorsal lip of Hensen's node migrate through the primitive pit to integrate into the midline notochord. The

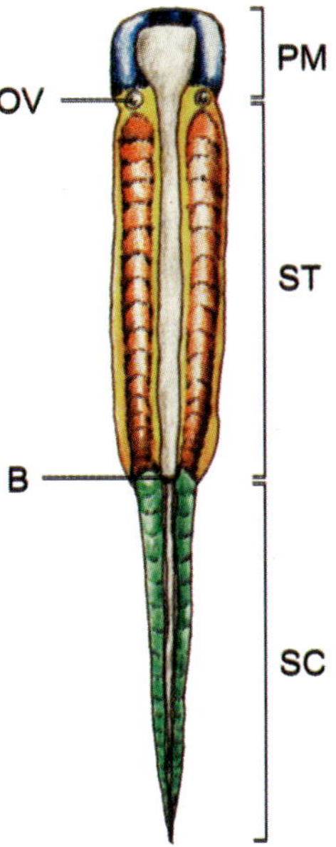

Fig. 1. Vertebrate embryonic plate around gastrulation showing the three main regions of the body plan: The prechordal mesoderm (PM) is anterior to the otic vesicle (OV). Posterior to the OV to the blastopore (B) is the somitic region of the trunk (ST), caudal to which is the caudal (tail) somitic region (SC).

embryonic plate thus elongates by new additions to its rear (caudal) aspect.[1]

The anterior–posterior (rostro-caudal) polarity of the embryo is determined very early during gastrulation. The prechordal mesoderm rostral to the otic vesicle (and notochord) forms most of the bones and muscles of the head and face without ever developing somites. Caudal to this tissue is the somitic region, which extends along the body axis down to the tip of the tail (Fig. 1). The anterior somitic region from the otic vesicle to the blastopore (future anus) corresponds to the future body axis from the occiput to the anus. Here, the epiblastic cells condense to form the parachordal mesoderm on each side of the notochord following systematic ingression movements through the primitive streak. This initially homogeneous column of cells, also called presomitic mesoderm (PSM) or segmental plate, subsequently segregates into segmental clusters called somites, which will eventually give

rise to the smooth muscle of the dermis, the axial musculature, the vertebral column, and support structures of the peripheral nervous system. After blastopore closure and complete regression of the primitive streak, the gastrulating region for the tail is restricted to a small region called the tail bud, located at the caudal tip of the primitive streak. The tail bud functions as a blastema of undifferentiated cells.[2,3] The pre-somitic mesoderm and later somites of the caudal and tail regions are therefore not formed by epiblastic ingression but by progenitor condensation *in situ*.

Primary segmentation: Somitogenesis

Before the appearance of somites, the PSM remains a column of loose mesenchyme without specific cellular polarity or stratification pattern alongside the lengthening notochord and neural plate.[4] During somitogenesis, the loose mesenchymal cells of the PSM undergo transformation into tightly apposed epithelial cells with definite polarity and orientation. A newly formed somite is a compact epithelial sphere ('somitomere') composed of a single layer of radially arranged cells with apices pointing towards a central lumen (somitocoele), which contains a few mesenchymal cells (Fig. 2).[5] The epithelial cells have polarized Golgi zones, basally

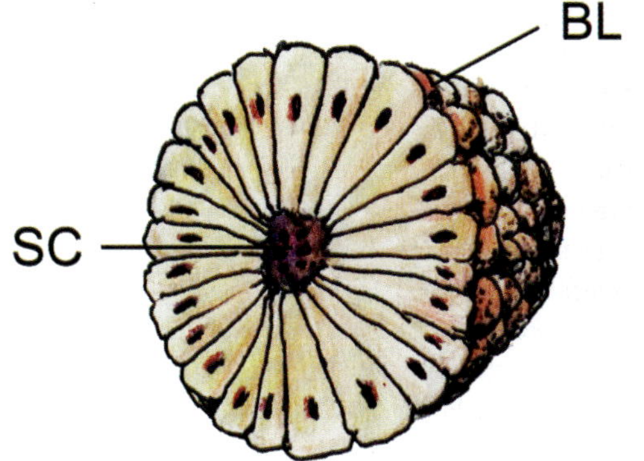

Fig. 2. Somite with radially arranged and polarized epithelial cells surrounding a central cavity, the somitocoele (SC), and enveloped by a basal lamina (BL).

aligned nuclei, and actin molecules near the luminal border, the entire sphere being enveloped by a collagen containing basal lamina.[6] This epithelial conversion of the PSM is aided by an increase in cell–cell adhesion mediated by a sharp but transient rise in the levels of the calcium-dependent adhesion molecule N-cadherin, of fibronectin and possibly cytotactin.[7]

Somitogenesis begins soon after internalization of the prochordal (head) mesoderm and continues through subsequent production of the body axis. The first somite forms immediately caudal to the otic vesicle, followed by sequential transformation such that a new pair of somites is regularly added in a rostro-caudal direction until a fixed species-specific number of somites is reached.[8] Thus, depending on the stage of gastrulation, the growing column of body mesoderm consists of a rostral section of mature somites already undergoing differentiation into sclerotomes and dermomyotomes, a middle section of new pre-differentiated epithelial somites, and a caudal section of pre-somitic mesoderm just rostral to the remaining primitive streak, the whole enterprise necessarily evolving in parallel with the neurulating neural plates (Fig. 3).

Current thinking regarding the mechanism of metameric transformation of the PSM follows what is called the 'clock and wavefront' model, first proposed by Cooke and Zeeman in 1976. In this model, PSM cells oscillate between a permissive and a non-permissive state for somite formation. These oscillations are phase-linked and controlled cell-autonomously by a 'segmentation clock'. Somitic formation is triggered when cells of the rostral PSM, while in the permissive phase of the 'clock', are hit by a wavefront of maturation (or determination) that slowly moves caudally along the embryonic axis. Thus, the clock generates a temporal periodicity that is translated spatially into the periodic boundaries of the somites.[4]

At the molecular level, the phasic oscillation of the segmentation clock is reflected by rhythmic expressions of a class of genes called cycling genes.[9] These genes include the *c-hairy* 1 family in fish, chick, frog and mouse, which encode transcription factors such as the split (HES) family and the glycosyl-transferase 'lunatic fringe', all tightly involved in the notch signalling pathway and its ligands, suggesting that periodic notch activation plays a critical role in the oscillator.[10,11] Also, these genes oscillate largely in synchrony in the PSM, suggesting they are downstream of a common cycling activator.

In chick and mouse embryos, the maturation or determination wave is generated by the

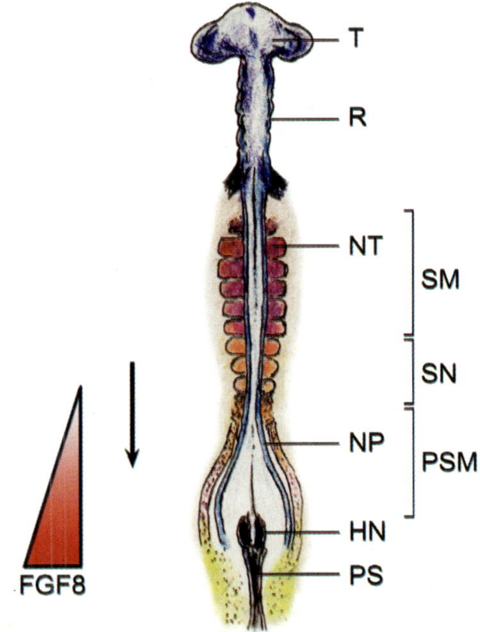

Fig. 3. Chick embryo during sequential somite formation at gastrulation. The rostral most mesoderm consists of matured somites (SM) already having undergone dorsoventral differentiation into dermomyotome and sclerotome, flanking the formed neural tubes (NT), followed by the newer pre-differentiated epithelial somites (SN), and the presomitic mesoderm (PSM) on each side of the unneurulated neural plate (NP).

HN=Hensen s node, PS=primitive streak, T=telencephalon, R=rhombencephalon. The red triangle shows the decreasing gradient of FGF8 (The Determination wavefront of somitogenesis) towards the somitogenic zone. Arrow indicates direction of sequential somites formation.

expression of genes, which include the fibroblast growth factor gene *fgf8*.[12] It is known that the caudal domain of the PSM is very high in the factor FGF8, which seems to actively maintain the mesenchymal identity of caudal PSM cells. The FGF8 gradient decreases towards the rostral axis, so that at the rostral domain of the PSM where somitogenesis is taking place, FGF8 level is very low (Fig. 3). Also, inhibition of somitogenesis is caused by over expression of *fgf8* in this region. Thus, the activation of epithelization of PSM cells is negatively regulated by FGF8, whose absence allows the PSM cells to become competent to respond to the clock signal and initiate somitic boundary formation.[13] The limit between the two domains of high (in the caudal PSM) and low (in the rostral PSM) *fgf8* expression therefore marks the determination wavefront of somitogenesis.[4]

Due to the constant caudal elongation of the body axis during gastrulation and the addition of new PSM cells with strong *fgf8* expression to the rear, the FGF8 gradient is continuously displaced caudally. Accordingly, the determination wave-front also moves slowly in a caudal direction along the body axis. This ensures that the old and new metameric boundaries, at both ends of a new somite, are separated by a distance corresponding to the caudal displacement of the determination wavefront during one period of oscillation of the segmentation clock.[9] The speed of new somite production is thus linked to the clock period, which is species-specific: 30 minutes for Zebrafish, 90 minutes for chick, and 120 minutes for mouse (Fig. 3).[14]

Differentiation of the somitic mesenchyme

Within hours after its formation, each somite starts differentiating along its dorso-ventral axis. Cells from its ventro-medial part lose their epithelial arrangement and migrate towards the notochord to form, with the luminal cells, the mesenchymal sclerotomes.[5,15] Together with the notochord, the sclerotomes provides exclusive material for the vertebral column. Cells from the dorsolateral part of the somite retain their epithelial arrangement to produce the dermomyotomes (Figs 4a and 4b). The dermomyotomes later subdivide into the dorsal dermatome immediately beneath the ectoderm to give rise to

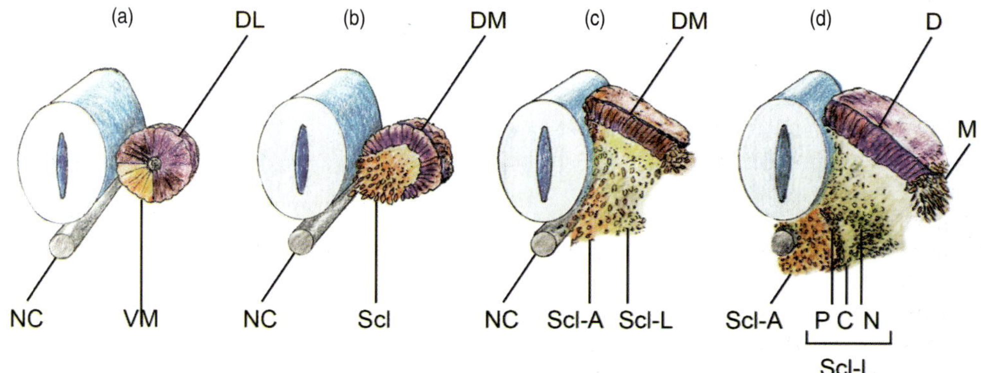

Fig. 4. Dorsoventral differentiation of somite. (a) Epithelial somite shows ventromedial cells (VM) destined to form the sclerotome and dorsolateral cells (DL) destined to become the dermomyotome. (b) Ventromedial sclerotome cells (Scl) de-epithelize from the somite and migrate towards the ventral notochord (NC). (c) Sclerotomal cells further subdivide into an axial cluster (Scl-A) surrounding the notochord, and lateral paired clusters (Scl-L) flanking the perichordal axial sclerotome. Dorsolateral somite retains its epithelial pattern to become the dermomyotome (DM). (d) The lateral sclerotome (Scl-L) forms a triangle next to the axial sclerotome. The three sides of the triangle become anlagen for the pedicle (P), neural arch (N), and the costal process (C), respectively. The dermomyotome also subdivides into the dermatome (D) and the lateral migrating myotome (M).

the dermis and its smooth muscles, whereas the disaggregated cells between the dermatome and the sclerotomes remain closely packed as the myotome, forming ultimately the axial skeletal muscles (Figs 4c and 4d).[1,15,16]

Whereas specification of the anterior–posterior pattern of the somite appears to be determined very early,[17–19] the dorsoventral values are not intrinsic to the somites. Thus, if the somite were to be surgically rotated dorsoventrally by 180°, sclerotomes still develop in the ventromedial position whereas the dermomyotomes remain dorsolateral. Moreover, a dorsally implanted notochord represses dermatomal but encourages sclerotomal formation, whilst notochord ablation completely prevents sclerotomal appearance.[1] These findings suggest that the dorsoventral differentiations of the somite depend on appositional instructions from the notochord, most likely through sonic hedgehog (*Shh*) expression.[20]

'Resegmentation' of the sclerotome

The term 'resegmentation' was originated by Remak in 1855 ('neugliederung') and remains a subject of controversies.[1,21,22] It refers to the fact that the early metameric boundaries between the somites are once again changed and 'reshuffled' during the development of the sclerotome, so that the later boundaries between the vertebral bodies do not match up with the original intersomitic clefts.[15]

During somitic differentiation, the ventromedial cells destined to become sclerotome subdivide into paired lateral clusters flanking the ventral aspects of the neural tube, and an unpaired median (axial) cluster surrounding the midline notochord (Fig. 5). The formation of the vertebral column takes place first in the lateral sclerotome, where a conspicuous subdivision into a densely packed caudal half and a more loosely cellular cranial half soon appear, separated by a fissure (of von Ebner).[23] The loose cranial half attracts, promotes and supports the

growth and expansion of peripheral nervous tissue from the neural tube and neural crests, but itself never chondrifies into vertebral parts (Fig. 6, middle). In contrast, the caudal densely packed mesenchyme of the lateral scleroderme soon takes on a triangular shape. The side of the triangle facing the axial perichordal sclerotome, which will become the future vertebral body, gives rise to the pedicle. The side facing dorsolaterally away from the axial sclerotome forms rudiments of the neural arch; and the side of the triangle facing ventrolaterally becomes the costal process (Fig. 4d).

Shortly after the specifications of the lateral sclerotome into its arcual, costal and pedicular components, the initially loosely meshed mesenchyme within the perichordal axial sclerotome also begins to show compartmentalization. A cell-dense zone develops at the same level as the dense caudal half of each lateral sclerotome, partly due to medial expansion of the lateral band of condensed tissues from the lateral sclerotome. The axial sclerotome in between these median dense zones remains loosely cellular. Later, the cranial-most layer of the axial dense zone, in line with von Ebner's fissure in the lateral sclerotome, becomes even more tightly packed and forms the

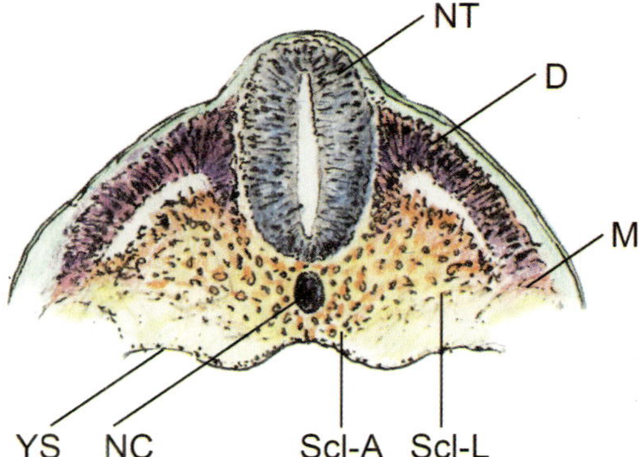

Fig. 5. Coronal section of chick embryo showing differentiating somite into axial or perichordal sclerotome (Scl-A) surrounding the notochord (NC), and lateral sclerotome (Scl-L) on both sides of the neural tube (NT).

D=dermatome, M=myotome, YS=yolk sac membrane

intervertebral boundary zone (IBZ) (Fig. 6, middle). This intervertebral boundary mesenchyme (IBM) ultimately forms the ring-like annulus fibrosus of the intervertebral disc, permanently enclosing a looser central core of nucleus pulposus made partly of notochordal remnants. The vertebral body itself is mainly made from chondrogenesis in the loose-cell zone of the perichordal sclerotome, now called the prevertebra,[1,15,24,25] although contributions from the condensed tissue adjacent to the IBZ have been observed.[21,26] As a final step, the pedicular anlagen from the lateral sclerotomes fuse with the chondrifying prevertebra of the axial sclerotome, while the neural arches surround the neural tube to complete the vertebral ring (Fig. 6, right). The costal component becomes the future transverse process but only in the thoracic region is it predestined to form ribs.

Thus, the neural arch of the vertebra is derived from the caudal–lateral part of a single somite.[21] However, labelling and transplantation experiments of half-somites have repeatedly demonstrated that each vertebral body is made up of

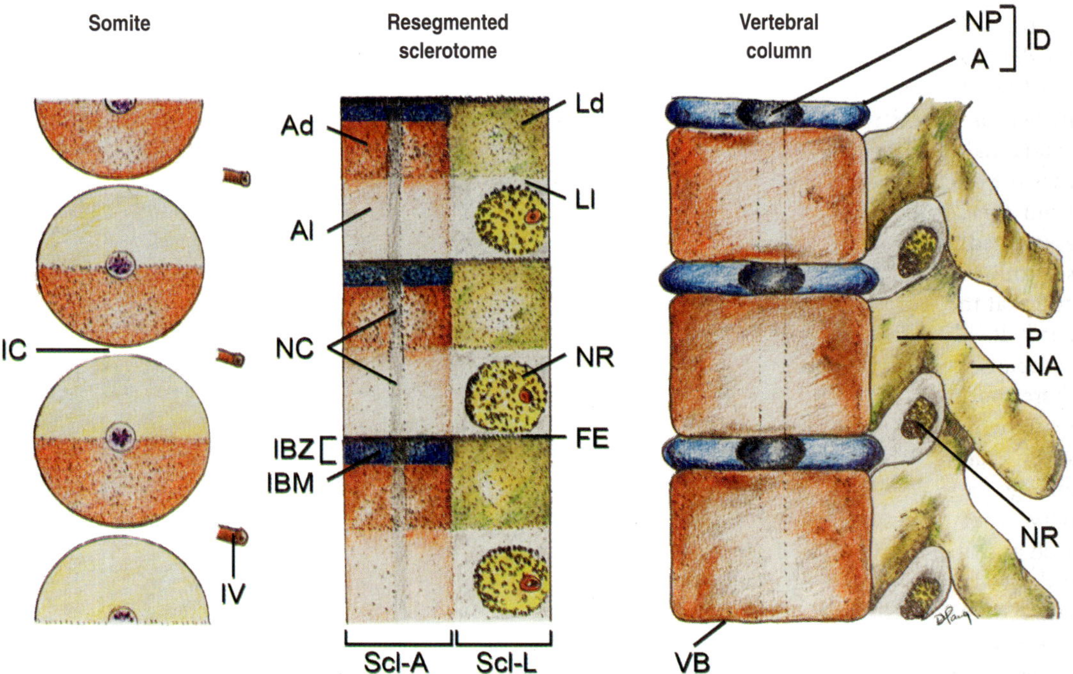

Fig. 6. Resegmentation of somites to form sclerotomes and changes of sclerotomal primordia to mature vertebral parts. The somitic and primordial origins and phenotypic parts are colour-matched, and the locations of the somites, resegmented sclerotomes, and vertebrae along the embryonic axis are approximately counter-registered. During re-segmentation, the sclerotome is formed from the caudal and rostral halves of two adjacent somites, such that the middle of the resegmented sclerotome lines up with the intersomitic cleft (IC). Both the axial sclerotome (Scl-A) and lateral sclerotome (Scl-L) develop dense and loose zones. The dense zone of the lateral sclerotome (Ld) becomes the neural arch (NA) and pedicle (P), which is attached to the rostral part of the vertebral body (VB) formed from chondrification of the loose (Al) and part of the dense zones (Ad) of the axial sclerotome. The rostral layer of the dense zone of the axial sclerotome soon forms the intervertebral boundary zone (IBZ) containing intervertebral boundary mesenchyme (IBM), which ultimately forms the annulus (A) and, together with notochord remnants (NC), the nucleus pulposus (NP) of the intervertebral disc (ID). The loose zone of the lateral sclerotome (Ll) does not form bone but promotes emergence of the nerve roots (NR). Thus, the neural arch is derived from a single somite but the vertebral body receives contributions for two adjacent somites. IV=intersomitic vessel

cells from the axial zones of two adjacent somites.[27,28] Although the exact boundary of individual somite participation is not known,[15] the juxtapositioning of axial and lateral sclerotomal components suggests that each vertebra probably comes from the caudal half of one somite and the rostral half of the somite below.[25] This will explain the slightly off-step registration between the levels of the somite and the re-segmented sclerotome[15,25,29] on the embryonic axis such that the middle of the resegmented sclerotome lines up with the original intersomitic cleft (Fig. 6, left and middle). Also, as the dense portion of the lateral sclerotome is in-line with the dense zone of the axial sclerotome adjacent to the IBZ, it makes perfect sense that the mature pedicle is joined to the cranial and not to the caudal half of the vertebral body.[15] It also follows that the spinal nerve, ganglion, and blood vessel from the corresponding somitic segment, being associated with the loose cranial half of the lateral sclerotome, must cross above its own neural arch, and that the corresponding segment of the spinal cord is always slightly more rostral to its companion vertebral body (Fig. 6, right). Given there are eight cervical somites but only seven resegmented axial sclerotomes and consequently seven cervical vertebrae, the C_1 nerve root emerges above the C_1 neural arch and the C_8 nerve root comes through below the C_7 neural arch and above the T1 neural arch, which in fact is derived from the C_8 somite. Finally, resegmentation of the sclerotome explains why the original 'pre-resegmented' intersomitic vessel ultimately enters the mid-point of the vertebral body as the segmental nutrient artery.

Special developmental features of the CVJ

The CVJ is the product of the occipital somites and the first three cervical somites. The proper number of occipital somites in vertebrates is debatable. Wilting *et al.*[30–32] thought there were five occipital somites in chick and mouse but conceded that the first somite either disappeared early or was an insignificant clan of cells that lacked sclerotomal lineage. Müller and O'Rahilly[25] studied staged human embryos and concluded that, in humans, there are only four occipital somites that participate in forming the skull base. The transitional zone between the skull and the cervical spine is thus taken to be between the fourth and fifth somites. During the fourth week of gestation, there are consequently 4 occipital, 8 cervical, 12 thoracic, 5 lumbar, 5 sacral, and 8-10 coccygeal somites—42 pairs all told.

Occipital somites (somites 1–4) and the proatlas

Following the general schema, the first three occipital somites give rise to an axial perichordal sclerotome and a lateral sclerotome, but no resegmentation takes place here. The axial sclerotomes never subdivide into dense and loose zones and therefore no IBM exists. They all eventually fuse into a unit that later chondrifies to become the rostral basioccipital.[25] The first three lateral occipital sclerotomes, like the vertebral sclerotomes, form dense and loose zones, and the loose zones of the second and third lateral occipital sclerotomes foster expansion of the upper and lower hypoglossal nerve roots and artery, whereas the corresponding dense zones form the bony hypoglossal canal.

Unlike the first three occipital somites, the fourth occipital (O_4) somite does show resegmentation. Its caudal dense zone combines with the cranial loose half of the first cervical somite to produce the transitional sclerotome called the proatlas (Fig. 7, left and middle).[25,29,33–36] The cranial region of the axial sclerotome of the proatlas soon fuses with the other three axial occipital sclerotomes to become the basion of the basioccipital,[36] but its most caudal portion, probably derived from the first cervical somite (somite 5), forms the anlage for the apical segment of the dens. Late in resegmentation, a boundary zone appears between this apical dental centrum and the loosely cellular prevertebra of the basioccipital, and the former soon detaches from the basioccipital and eventually becomes joined to the basal segment of the dens to complete the dental pivot (*see* below) (Fig. 7).[25,32] Herein lies the most unique feature of the transitional zone of the CVJ between somites 4 and 5, i.e. unlike other IBZs that form intervertebral discs, downstream activity of the proatlas' IBZ includes a physical severance of cells from the immediately adjacent loose perichordal zone of the basioccipital. This action, no doubt mediated by special cleavage genes, not only

allows the skull to become independent from the vertebral column, but also the final installation of the axis–dens assembly.

The lateral dense region of the proatlas becomes the two exoccipitals, which later form the two occipital condyles and the remainder of the anterolateral rim of the foramen magnum (Fig. 7). The lateral loose region promotes emergence of the C_1 nerve root. In humans, an additional arcuate cluster of dense proatlas cells ventral to the notochord, aptly called the hypochordal bow, gives rise to the bony anterior clival tubercle on the ventral surface of the basioccipital (Fig. 7).[25,36]

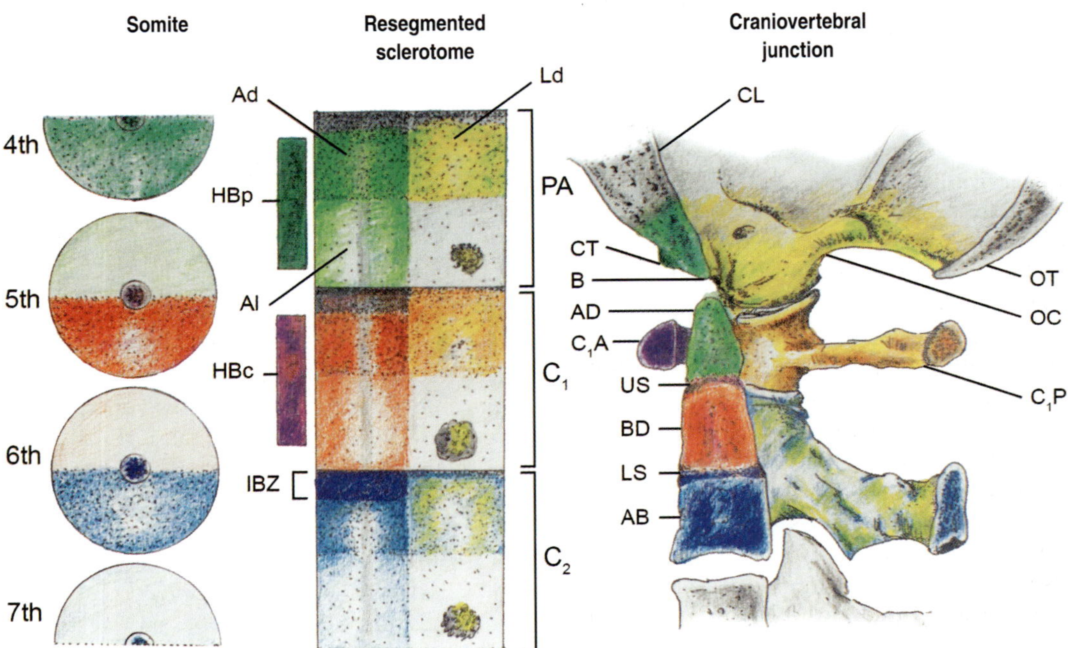

Fig. 7. Formation of the human cranio-vertebral junction. Sclerotomal primordia and their vertebral phenotypes are colour-matched. During resegmentation, the caudal half of the 4th somite (4th occipital somite) and rostral half of the 5th somite combine to form the proatlas sclerotome (PA). Derived from the proatlas are: the axial zones (Ad and Al) which become the basion (B) of the basioccipital or clivus (CL) and the apical segment of the dens (AD); the lateral dense zone (Ld) becomes the exoccipital comprising the occipital condyle (OC), and lateral rim and opisthion (OT) of the foramen magnum; the proatlas hypochordal bow (HBp) forms the ventral clival tubercle (CT). The C_1 resegmented sclerotome (C_1) comes from adjacent halves of the 5th and 6th somites. Derived from the C_1 sclerotome are: the axial zones form the basal segment of the dens (BD); the lateral zone forms the posterior atlantal arch (C_1P); the hypochordal bow (HBc) forms the anterior atlantal arch (C_1A). The C_2 resegmented sclerotome (C_2) comes from the 6th and 7th somites. From the C_2 sclerotome: the axial zone forms the C_2 vertebral body (AB); the lateral zone forms the neural arch of C_2 vertebra. The intervertebral boundary zone (IBZ) between the proatlas and C_1 sclerotome forms the upper dental synchondrosis (US) and the IBZ between the C_1 and C_2 sclerotomes forms the lower dental synchondrosis (LS).

First three cervical somites (somites 5–7)

Axial sclerotomes

During resegmentation, the caudal half of somite 5 and the cranial half of somite 6 combine to produce the first cervical sclerotome; likewise, the second cervical sclerotome is made up of corresponding parts of somites 6 and 7. In the axial region of these sclerotomes destined to form vertebral centra, dense and loose zones appear in regular succession as in the lower cervical sclerotomes. The loose prevertebral zone of the first cervical sclerotome gives rise to the basal segment of the dens, and that of the second cervical sclerotome becomes the body of the axis (Fig. 7). Unlike in the more caudal sclerotomes, however, where the dense IBZ ultimately becomes the annulus and nucleus pulposus of an intervertebral disc, the dense zones in the first two cervical sclerotomes do not form true intervertebral discs and soon disappear.[25] Their IBM gradually turns into the upper and lower dental synchondroses that ultimately cement the apical to the basal dens and the basal dens to the body of C_2, respectively (Fig. 7).

Thus after resegmentation, the human membranous axis consists of three median constituents that have been designated the apical dental segment from the caudal proatlas, the basal dental segment from the first cervical sclerotome, and the body of the axis from the second cervical sclerotome.[31,37–40] These three constituents chondrify simultaneously around 6 weeks' gestation but remain segregated by the more cellular upper and lower dental synchondroses. Ossification of the cartilaginous axis occurs in three chronological waves (Fig. 8). The first wave appears as a single ossification centre within the axial body at around 4 months' gestation. The second wave begins at 6 months' gestation as two separate ossification centres on each side of the basal dental segment.[41–44] At birth, these two centres integrate and fuse, and the main component of the dens should at least have begun to show bony fusion with the axis body, even

though a clear rarification may still be discernible at the lower synchondrosis until the fifth or sixth postnatal year (Figs 8 and 9). Occasionally, the basal dens remains bifid (dens bicornis) when the third wave of ossification arrives within the apical dens from 3 to 5 years of age (Figs 8–10).[37,42,45] Ossification of the dental tip and bony fusion of the upper synchondrosis are not completed until adolescence.[46–49]

Lastly, the apical ligament is almost certainly derived from the axial proatlas, and the alar and TALs from the axial component of the first cervical sclerotome in association with the basal dental segment.[25]

Lateral sclerotomes

The lateral dense zone of the first cervical sclerotome develops into the posterior arch of the atlas, whereas the lateral dense zone of the second cervical sclerotome forms the arch of the axis. Their respective loose zones promote outgrowths of the second and third cervical nerves and segmental arteries. The hypochordal bow of the first cervical sclerotome ventral to the notochord subsequently forms the anterior arch of the atlas (Fig. 7, middle and right).[25,36,40,50] No definite hypochordal bows are seen caudal to this level and equivalent cells in the lower segments appear to play no role in the formation of the vertebral column.

Genetic control of CVJ development

Hox genes: The control of rostrocaudal specification

After primary segmentation, the determination of the positional identity of the prevertebral segments along the embryonic axis, which in turn ordains the regional developmental specifications of the vertebral phenotypes, is controlled by Hox genes. The mammalian Hox genes encode transcription factors used in regulating the

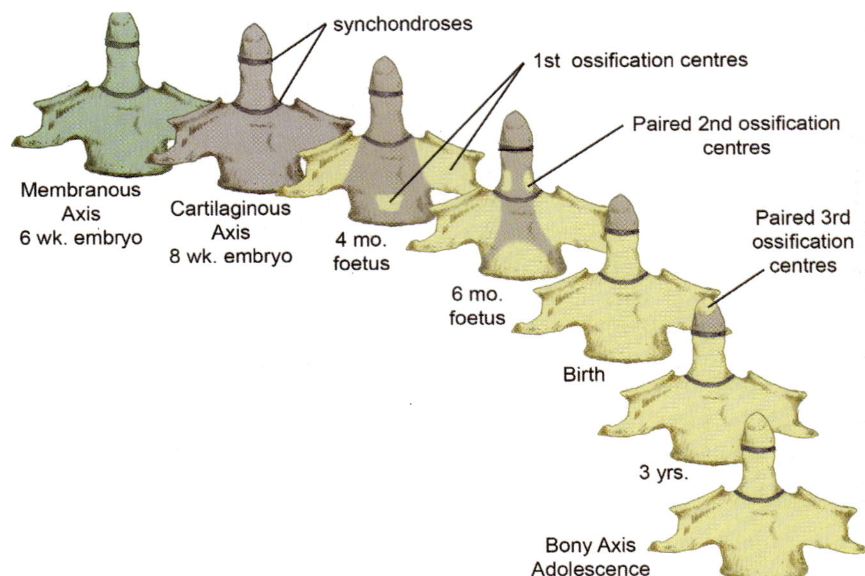

Fig. 8. The three developmental phases of the axis (C₂) and the 3 waves of ossification. The primordia for the dens components are assembled during the membranous phase. Upper and lower dental synchondroses are shown as dense lines. First wave of ossification at 4th foetal month consists of bilateral centres for the neural arches and a single centre for the centrum. Second wave at 6th foetal month consists of bilateral ossification centres for the basal dental segment. At birth, the basal dental centres should have integrated in the midline and begun to be fused to the centrum. Third wave of C₂ ossification occurs from 3–5 years postnatal life at the apical dental segment, which does not become fused to the basal dens till the sixth to ninth year, and fully formed during adolescence.

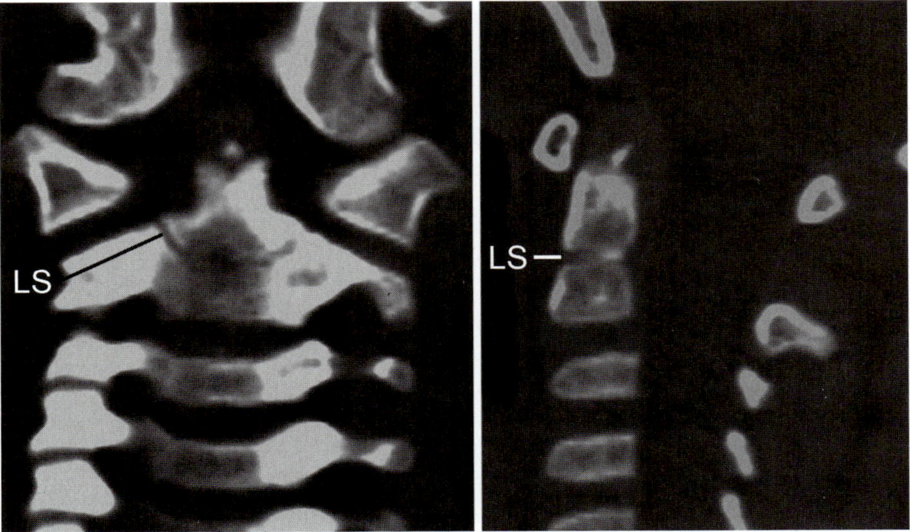

Fig. 9. State of ossification of the dens of a 4-year-old child. The tip of the basal dental segment is bicornuate from bilateral secondary ossification centres. Small density above this represents early third wave of ossification within the apical dental segment. Note lower dental synchondrosis (LS) in the coronal and sagittal views.

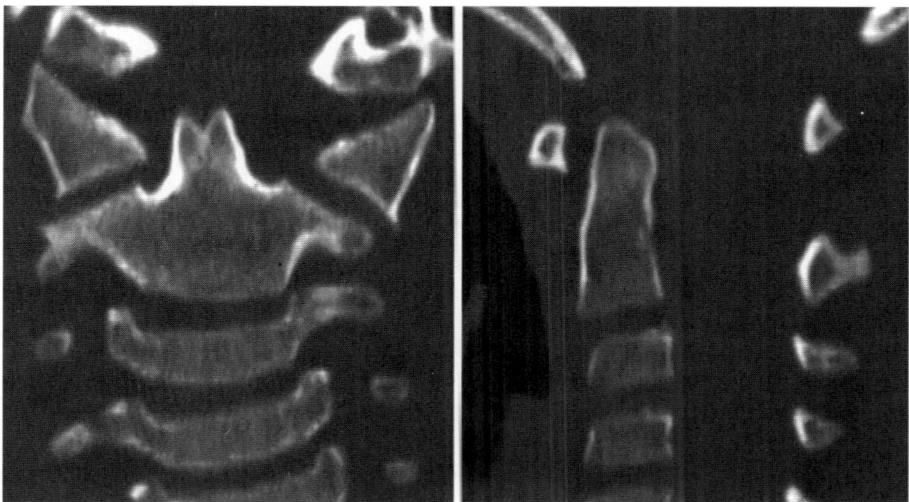

Fig. 10. Dens bicornis in a 7-year-old child. Lower synchondrosis has closed. Dens pivot is of normal height, suggesting the bifid tip is of the apical segment.

establishment of the body plan. They contain the phylogenetically highly conserved homeobox domain.[1,51,52] Mice and humans have 39 Hox genes distributed in four linkage clusters—Hox A, B, C and D—on four different chromosomes (chromosomes 6, 11, 15 and 2). The members of each cluster, designated by Arabic numerals, are also grouped vertically along the clusters because analogous members of each group are linked by common origin from a single ancestral gene, so that *Hox a4, b4, c4,* and *d4* are connected to the same phylogenetic origin and are called paralogues. The lower numbered paralogues are located on the anterior 3' axis of the chromosome and the higher numbered ones are on its posterior 5' locations (Fig. 11).

Hox genes are expressed in mesodermal and ectodermal cells along the body axis. Each gene has a characteristic and distinct anterior boundary of expression. A temporal and structural co-linearity exists between the position of a gene in a cluster and its expression pattern. Thus, genes from the more anterior 3' locations in the Hox clusters are expressed earlier and always occupy more anterior (cranial) expression domains than genes closer to the posterior 5'

location in the clusters (Fig. 11). For example, *Hox a3* has a more anterior expression domain than *Hox a-9* and similarly between *Hox d-4* and *Hox d-10.*

Functionally, only the anterior boundary of the Hox expression is important. As multiple genes have the same anterior expression boundary along the prevertebral axis, each metameric segment can be identified by its own characteristic combination of Hox gene expression domains, i.e. its own Hox code (Fig. 12). A specific Hox code acts as a master switch in determining the exact positional identity of a mesodermal segment along the body axis, and via regional idiosyncrasies in development, the Hox code thus becomes translated into a specific vertebral anatomy.[1,52,53]

The importance of the Hox code is illustrated by the severe abnormality in numbers and structures of vertebral segments when the code is altered by Hox gene mutations and teratogenic disturbance of Hox gene expressions. One example at the CVJ is the inactivation in mice of *Hox d-3,* an important component of the Hox code for the first cervical prevertebra. This results in a more caudal anterior boundary of *Hox d-3*

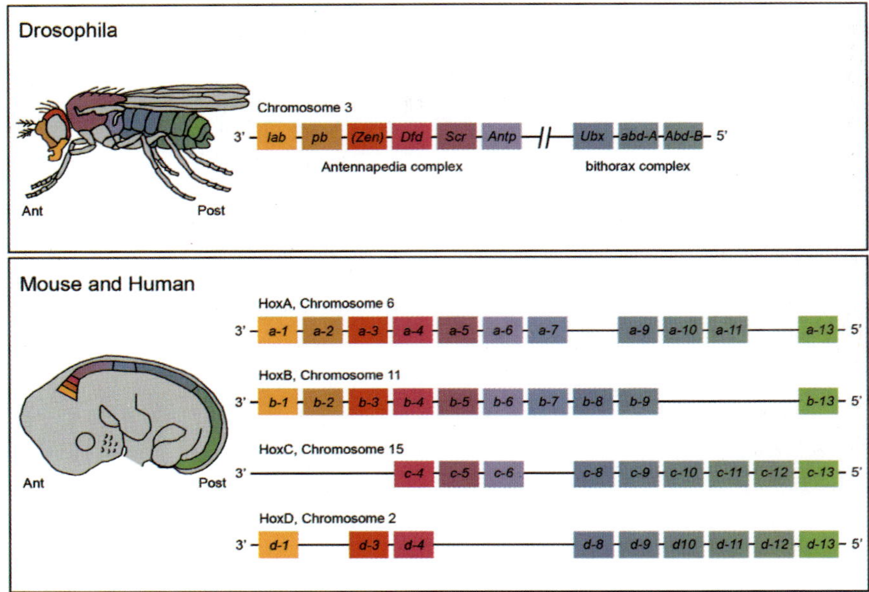

Fig. 11. Hox genes in mouse and human with their phylogenetic counterparts in drosophila. 39 Hox genes are involved in the mouse and human vertebral column, found in 4 clusters of Hox A, B, C and D on 4 chromosomes (6, 11, 15, and 2), designated by Arabic numbers within each cluster and arranged as paralogues, so that the lower numbered Hox paralogues such as *Hox a-1* and *Hox d-1* are located on the anterior 3' position of the chromosomes and the higher numbered paralogues are on the 5' posterior position of the chromosomes. There is also temporal and structural colinearity with the embryonic axis so that the lower numbered paralogues are expressed earlier and more anterior on the embryonic axis than the higher numbered paralogues. (*see* colour match between genes and their expression domains on the embryonic axis)

expression, shifting the transitional sclerotomal properties from C_1 to C_2 prevertebra and transforming the C_1 prevertebra to a more anterior (i.e. occipital) identity, producing mutant mice with atlas assimilation to the basioccipital.[54] This is called anterior homeotic transformation. Conversely, extension of an expression domain rostrally can transform prevertebral segments into a more caudal (posterior) identity, a phenomenon known as posterior homeotic transformation. This is exemplified in 'gain-of-function' transgenic mutation of the murine *Hox d-4* gene, also a component of the Hox code for the C_1 prevertebra, such that its expression domain is forced to extend towards the occipital somites. The exoccipital region of the transgenic mutant shows no occipital condyles but instead ectopic neural arches resembling cervical neural arches, and the basioccipital is fused to the apical dens, 'imitating' the behaviour of the atlas centrum.[33] Thus, an altered interpretation of axial position cues in the developing occipital somites leads to an imposition of cervical vertebral phenotype upon the occipital bones. These observations suggest that Hox gene abnormality may underlie many malformations in the CVJ.[29]

Pax 1: The resegmentation gene

The Pax family of regulatory genes is implicated in sclerotomal resegmentation. Pax genes in vertebrates all contain the highly conserved DNA sequence called 'paired-box'. Nine *Pax* genes have been identified; all except *Pax-1* and *Pax-9* are involved in development of the central neuraxis.[55] These two exceptions, especially *Pax-*

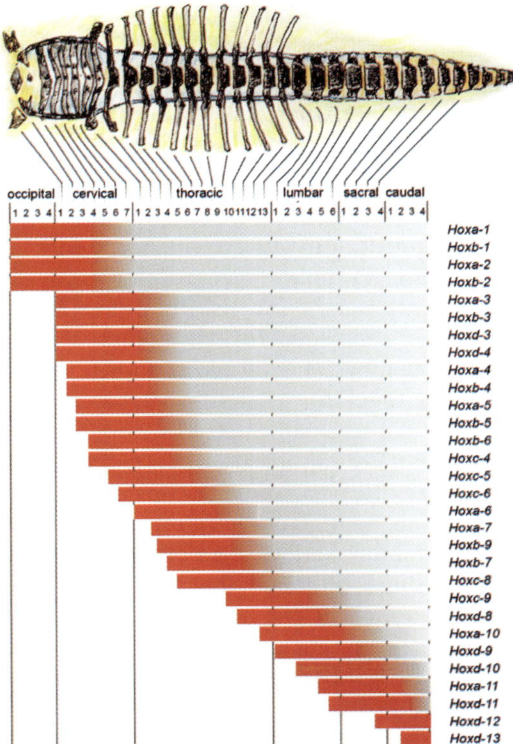

Fig. 12. Expression domains of *Hox* genes lined up with the mouse embryonic vertebral column. Only the anterior expression boundary (in red) is important, and since multiple genes have the same anterior expression boundary along the prevertebral axis, each prevertebral segment has its own combination of *Hox* gene expression domains (Hox code). For example, the Hox code for C_1 is Hox *a-1*, *b-1*, *a-2*, *b-2*, *a-3*, *b-3*, *d-3*, and *d-4*.

1 (*PAX-1* in the human homologue),[56] control boundary formation between tissues by keeping two cell populations separate, presumably because the transcription factor encoded by *Pax-1* differentially regulates cell surface molecules expressed by these two cell populations, and thereby divergently influences their respective fates. This scenario of cellular partitioning is a necessary condition for resegmentation, and *Pax-1* action at the future IBZ thus helps to demarcate the site and extent of sclerotomal segregation.

The downstream target gene for *Pax-1* is unknown, but may involve cell adhesion molecules, such as NCAM or cytotactin, or molecules that promote cell–cell communication, such as connexins.[56–59]

Pax-1 expression is detected very early in the pre-differentiated somites. Signals from the notochord and ventral floor plate of the neural tube, mediated by the SHH protein, induce the somite to divide into dermomyotome and the ventromedial sclerotome. This coincides with intense expression of *Pax-1* ventrally within the sclerotomal field, suggesting that *Pax-1* also plays a mediating role in the dorsoventral specification of somites.[20,32]

After somitic differentiation, *Pax-1* expression is noted within both the lateral and axial sclerotomes where its timing and fluctuating levels coincide with crucial events of resegmentation. For example, during condensation of the axial sclerotome into the loose and dense halves, *Pax-1* expression is weak within the loosely cellular prevertebrae but intense within the dense IBZ.[32,56] Later, with chondrification of the prevertebra to form the homogeneous vertebral body, *Pax-1* is further actively repressed in this location, but persists in high levels at the IBZ where partition of centra takes place, until formation of the intervertebral disc is well under way.[32] *Pax-1* level is also enhanced during condensation of the lateral sclerotome to form the neural arch.[26,60,61]

Conversely, normal fusion of certain adjacent sclerotomes takes place only when *Pax-1* expression is turned off. At the CVJ of chick embryos, *Pax-1* repression is timed exactly when the occipital sclerotomes fuse to form the basioccipital. The fusion of the two dens primordia with the axis body also coincides with the downregulation of the *Pax-1* gene.[32] Ectopic *Pax-1* expression disrupts normal assemblage of the dens–axis and basioccipital.[61] *Pax-1* is also highly expressed within the transitional zone between the proatlas and the first cervical sclerotome; it may thus also play a role in the separation of the head from the trunk.

Murine *Pax-1* mutants *undulated* show

multiple fusion of vertebral bodies and fusion of the dens with the anterior atlantal arch,[61] reminiscent of the human Klippel–Feil syndrome.[62] It is therefore conceivable that hyper- and hypo-segmentation defects in humans may be explained by over- and under-expression of *PAX-1* during vertebral development.

Basic types of developmental failure at the CVJ

Congenital osseous anomalies of the CVJ fall into the following four basic mechanisms of dysgenesis:

- Hyperplasia of primordium
- Aplasia/hypoplasia of primordium
- Disturbance of resegmentation
- Failure of midline integration of primordium.

Anomalies of the central pivot: Odontoid dysgeneses

The making of any part of the vertebral column requires the successful completion of three developmental phases: (i) The mesodermal primordium has to be properly formed and, in some cases, assembled during the membranous phase; (ii) the mesodermal primordium undergoes chondrification in the cartilaginous phase; and (iii) in the osseous phase, ossification takes place within the cartilaginous mould to complete the end-product. In the case of the dens–axis, there is a 4th phase, which involves bony fusion of the upper and lower dental synchondroses (Fig. 8). Developmental anomalies of the central pivot comprise various forms of odontoid dysplasia classifiable according to their probable pathogeneses, which, in turn are traceable to failure of one or more of the four developmental phases. Most clinical types are associated with instability, although basilar impression with or without a retroflexed odontoid can cause compression of the cervicomedullary junction.

Aplasia/hypoplasia of the axial sclerotome of proatlas and first cervical sclerotome

The odontoid process, or dens, develops from the axial sclerotome of the proatlas and first cervical sclerotome. Primordia of the apical and basal dental segments fuse with each other and with the C_2 centrum. Complete agenesis of both dental components is rare and usually occurs in the context of collagenopathy syndromes, such as spondyloepiphyseal and spondylometaphyseal dysplasias (Fig. 13). Agenesis or hypogenesis of just the basal segment results in a stumpy dental pivot with a floating apical ossicle (Fig. 14). Both types are associated with instability. By comparison, agenesis of the apical segment is the most common variety. Radiographically, the dens is short, although the TAL usually has adequate pivot height, and there is thus no

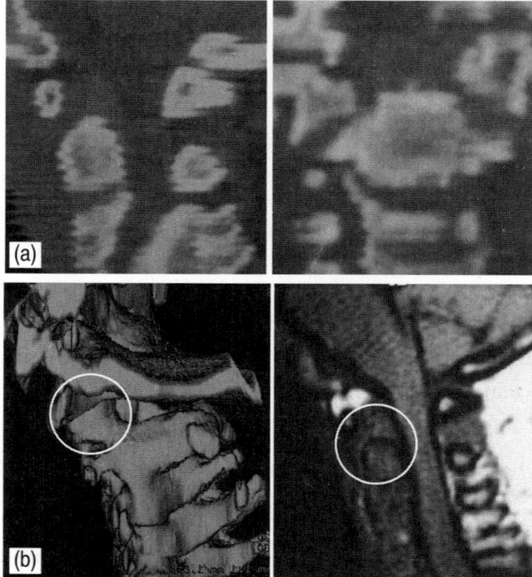

Fig. 13. Complete agenesis of the dens in a 10-year-old child with spondyloepiphyseal dysplasia. (a) CT sagittal and coronal views show no dental pivot although the centrum with a flat top does rise up above the expected level of the lower dental synchondrosis. (b) 3-D reconstruction and MR show the flat top of the centrum and potential for instability.

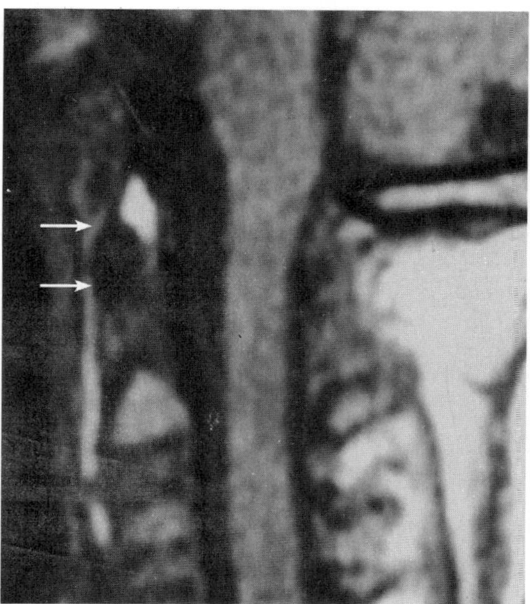

Fig. 14. Agenesis of basal dental segment with a stumpy C_2 centrum and a high-riding floating apical ossiculum (between arrows).

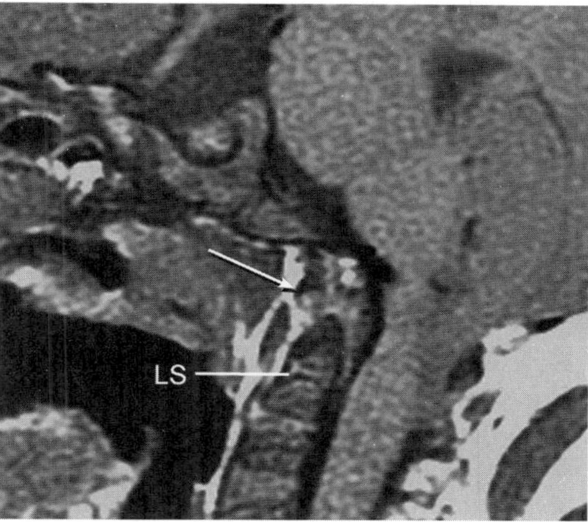

Fig. 15. Agenesis of apical dental segment, with a slightly short dental pivot but a definite basal segment (pointed) and a lower dental synchondrosis (LS). Arrow points to anterior arch of C_1. Note platybasia and Chiari I malformation.

instability (Fig. 15).

Complete odontoid agenesis in patients with collagenopathy or mucopolysaccharidosis, such as morquio's disease, may not be due to primordial failure as a completed cartilaginous mould of the dens has been seen *in situ*, where ossification was found to be defective because of the abnormal connective tissue production. Non-syndromic cases of odontoid agenesis may well be due to aplasia or hypoplasia of centrum primordia. Treatment of symptomatic cases is usually C_1–C_2 fusion.

Disturbance of the IBM of proatlas and first two cervical sclerotomes: os odontoideum and ossiculum terminale persistens

Aetiology

The abrogation of the IBZ during early resegmen-

tation, such as in the transgenic *undulated* mutant mice, causes abnormal fusion between sclerotomal units rather than lack of fusion.[32,56] The disaggregation of the distinct dental components seen in os odontoideum and ossiculum terminale persistens presumes that the respective IBZ between the proatlas and the first two cervical sclerotomes were initially demarcated but subsequent development of the upper and lower dental synchondroses was un-consummated.

os odontoideum

The question about whether os odontoideum represents a developmental anomaly or an un-united odontoid fracture has been debated endlessly in the literature. Proponents for the traumatic theory argue that the bases of most os odontoideum are above the 'expected base' of the normal dens, which is supposed to be below the level of the C_2 lateral masses,[29,39,48,63–67] and that there is often a 'cupola' bulging cranially from the axis stump that represents the bottom half of a fracture dens.[48] In countering, the developmentalists point out that transgenic mutant experiments repeatedly show vertebral primordia that suffer from aberrant development seldom evolve into the orthodox configuration of the normal phenotype, but instead become oddly shaped due to over-, under-, or even erratic growth, depending on the activities of local inducers.[25,32,56] The often expanded roundness of the os odontoideum, with its corrugated horn-like corners (Fig. 16a), can hardly be the expected visage of an unhealed odontoid fracture, with its compromised blood supply. In addition, os odontoideum has been found in identical twins[68] and families,[69] as well as among children with collagenopathies, and it frequently co-exists with other developmental bony anomalies of the skull base, all reinforcing the congenital theory. We believe that both aetiologies might be valid. It is possible the mesenchyme at the IBZ has failed to chondrify and therefore cannot ultimately undergo ossification and fusion. As the two dental components ossify on opposite sides of the IBZ and gain mechanical leverage, the persisting mesenchymal tissue could no longer withstand the stress caused by foetal movements, and the upper part separates as the loose os odontoideum. The evidence for either theory is selectively circumstantial, although the clinical implications are the same.

Ossiculum terminale persistens

The developmental origin of ossiculum terminale persistens is little disputed. The ossiculum represents an un-fused and detached apical dental segment, which comes from the proatlas centrum (Fig. 17).[39,48,70,71] The detachment is probably due to upper dental synchondrosis failure although late disturbance of the third wave of odontoid ossification may be responsible. The ossiculum is usually non-syndromic, although cases are seen with Morquio disease.

Clinical significance

Because the TAL straps around the basal segment of the dens, os odontoideum is at least potentially

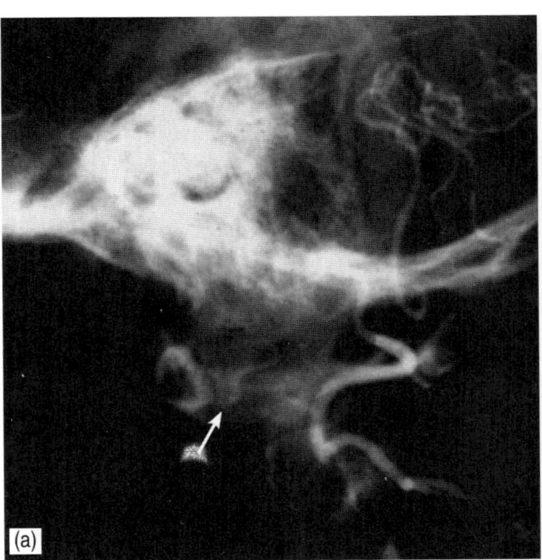
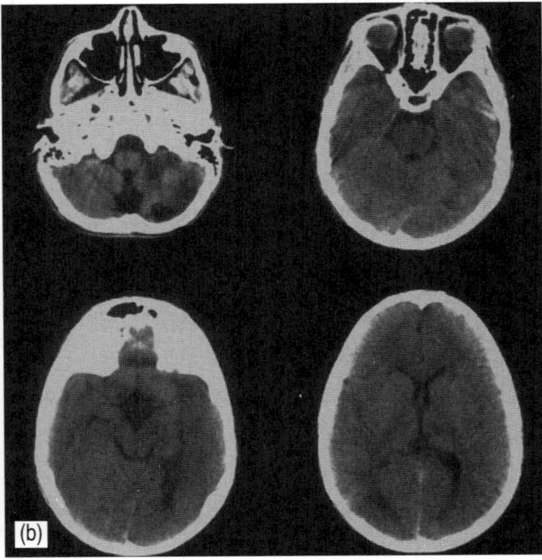

Fig. 16. os odontoideum in an 8-year-old child presented with multiple cerebellar and thalamic strokes. (a) Cerebral angiogram shows os odontoideum with a corrugated horn-like inferior edge (arrow) with anterior C_1–C_2 subluxation and stretch injury to the vertebral artery. (b) CT scans show multiple small infarcts of left cerebellar hemisphere and thalamus secondary to multiple vertebrobasilar emboli.

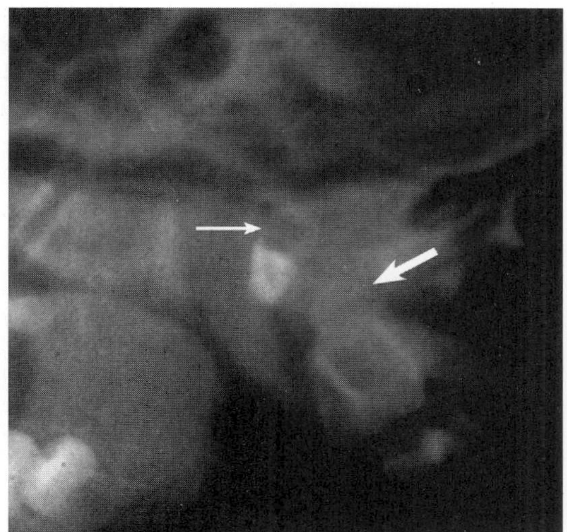

Fig. 17. Ossiculum terminale persistens (thin arrow), detached from the slightly shortened dental pivot formed by the basal dental segment (thick arrow).

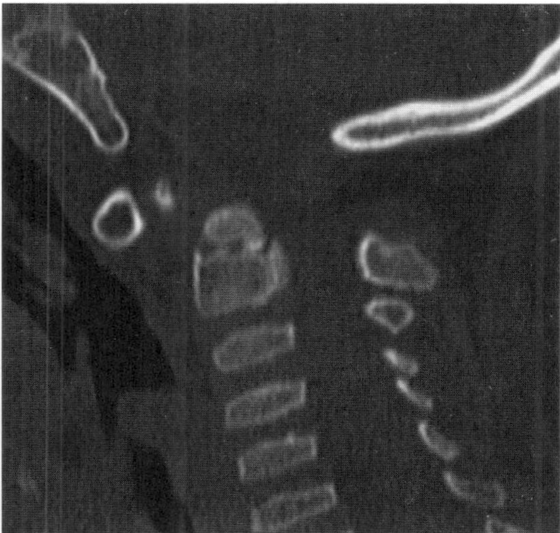

Fig. 19. Unstable ossiculum terminale with anterior C_1 subluxation. Note the short basal dental segment and an easily recognizable lower dental synchondrosis.

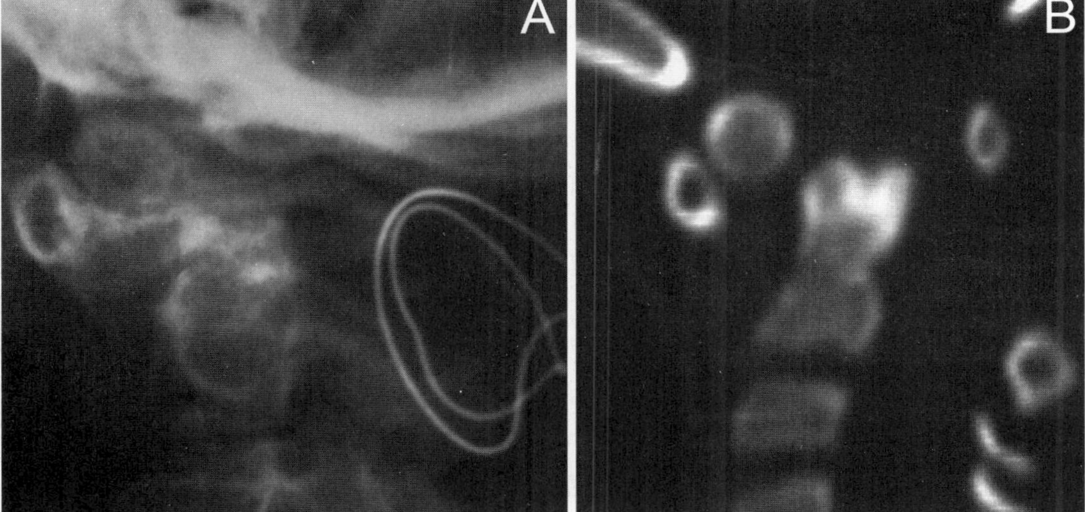

Fig. 18. Unstable os odontoideum with C_1–C_2 subluxation. (A) Shows widened ADI (13 mm) and a failed posterior bone fusion. (B) Shows another os with tall but jagged remaining dental pivot suggesting a traumatic aetiology.

unstable (Fig. 18) but not necessarily symptomatic. Symptoms vary from persistent neck pain, torticollis, transient quadriparesis, lower cranial neuropathies, to recurrent brain stem strokes caused by stretching of the vertebral arteries and basilar artery embolism (Fig. 16b).

Although most ossiculum terminales are stable anomalies[29,48] because the TAL's anchorage is not affected, our group has encountered cases in which the basal dental segment is hypoplastic and the dental pivot is short. Some of these are conducive to atlantoaxial subluxation and high cord compression (Fig. 19). In most cases, posterior C_1–C_2 fusion is adequate treatment.

Non-resegmentation of proatlas centrum: os avis

In this rare anomaly, the apical dental segment is attached to the basioccipital and is not fused to the main dental stem. The pivot is thus shortened but firmly fixed to the axis centrum, where a semi-lucent line representing the lower synchondrosis marks the successful integration of the two lower dens–axis components. This anomaly has been called 'dystopic os odontoideum' by von Torklus and Prescher[42,48,72] to distinguish it from the 'orthotopic os odontoideum' used by these authors to designate the common variety of os odontoideum. Their use of the term os odontoideum differs from ours in that they have included both the un-fused basal and un-fused apical dental segments.

Embryogenesis

In human malformations, it is not uncommon to find errant ontogeny reverting to a morphological pattern reminiscent of an organ's phylogenetic past. As case in point, a separate bone between the dens and the basioccipital resembling the attached ossiculum in the human anomaly is found in some fish and reptiles and many birds;[42,44,72–76] hence, our terminology of os avis. In higher vertebrates, this bone, the primordium of the apical dens, normally becomes detached from the basioccipital rim, which shares with it a common origin in the proatlas centrum. Failure of resegmentation of the proatlas centrum, in essence negating the necessary cleavage, prevents descent and subsequent joining of the apical segment with the centrum of the first cervical sclerotome to complete the dental pivot. The reason for this failure is unknown, but as proatlas resegmentation normally occurs at the transitional zone between somites 4 and 5, a caudal shift of this transitional zone along the body axis may affect the resegmentation process. In transgenic mouse mutant in which *Hox a-7* is expressed earlier and more rostrally in its anterior domain, the last occipital somite (O_4) is transformed (posteriorly) to become the atlas, bearing a 'proatlas' centrum that remains attached to the basioccipital. C_1 then becomes C_2 and acquires a complete centrum whereas C_2 is deleted of its normal dens.[1] This extra 'proatlas' bone in the murine mutant very much resembles the os avis in the human malformation and suggests that a Hox gene mutation causing posterior displacement of segmental identity may indeed underlie the genesis of the os avis.

Clinical significance

An os avis tends to be associated with neurological deterioration. The two patients with os avis described by Wollin[44] among 7 others with ossiculum terminale and os odontoideum are the only ones with symptoms, and both had a hypoplastic dental pivot. Both cases of os avis described by Menezes and Fenoy are symptomatic because of posterior dislocations of C_1 on C_2.[35] Of the two cases in our series, one had a hypoplastic dens and the atlantoaxial complex is extremely unstable on extension; the TAL is strapped against the os and therefore moves with the skull (Fig. 20). Our other case is associated with other CVJ anomalies, such as multiple hyposegmentation of vertebral bodies, short clivus, basilar impression, and a stenotic foramen magnum, even though the dens pivot is tall and sustaining for the TAL. The patient develops compressive symptoms (Fig. 21). In Wollin's cases, associated anomalies include a large median (third) occipital condyle (*see* below) and a hyperplastic anterior C_1 arch.[44]

Treatment of os avis depends on the other anomalies. Pure instability can be remedied with C_1–C_2 posterior fusion. An absent posterior C_1 arch or an occipitalized atlas would mandate

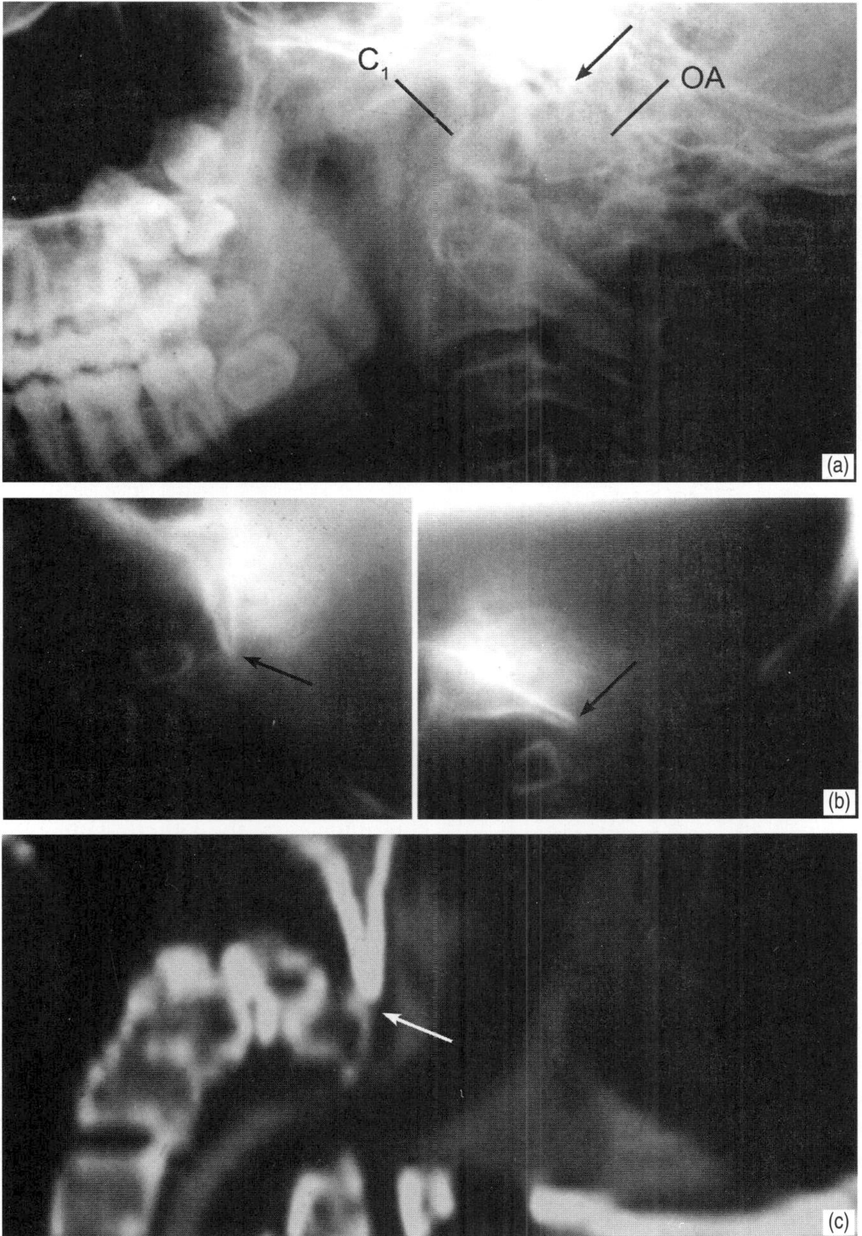

Fig. 20. os avis with severe posterior subluxation of skull and C_1 on C_2 producing quadriparesis. (a) The bone directly above the dental pivot is in fact a posteriorly shifted C_1 anterior arch (C_1). The os avis (OA) is just behind the C_1 arch, and is attached to the clivus marked by the arrow. Note posteriorly shifted posterior arch of C_1. (b) Flexion–extension polytomography shows relationship between C_1 arch, clivus, and os avis. Note attachment of the os with the clivus tip (arrow) and the unchanging (fixed) relationship with the clivus during flexion and extension. (c) CT myelogram shows spinal cord compression by the os avis during extension. Arrow marks attachment of os avis to clival tip.

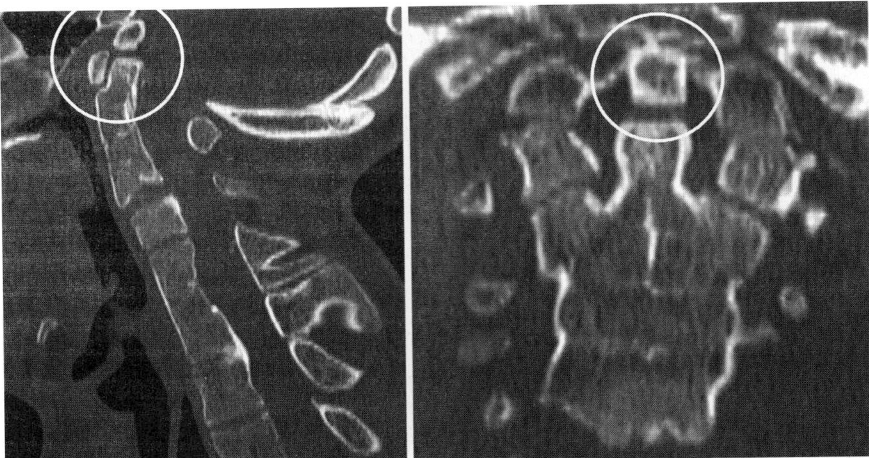

Fig. 21. Undescended apical dens still fused to the clivus (os avis). The dental pivot has a flat top but tall enough for the TAL and has no instability. Other anomalies such as multiple vertebral centra fusion, basilar invagination of the opisthion and stenosis by C_1 posterior arch cause compressive myelopathy.

inclusion of the occiput into the fusion. Concomitant neural compression caused by basilar impression or invagination of the opisthion may require simultaneous decompression.

Failure of midline integration of basal dental segment: The bifid dens

Aetiology

A completely bifid dens is an extremely rare entity. It is different from the 'dens bicornis' described by von Torklus and Gehle in which only the tip of the dens is bicornuate and the function of the otherwise well formed dental pivot is unaffected.[48] Dens bicornis results from aberrant distal ossification late in development. In true dental bifidity, the partition in the basal dental segment goes full length of the process to the lower synchondrosis. In one example, the bifid dens is accompanied by a dislocated ossiculum terminale (Fig. 22). In two others, one half of the split dental base is unattached to the centrum of C_2 and is floating free, whereas the body of C_2 is fused with that of C_3, which is itself bifid. The anterior C_1 arch is also un-fused in the midline (Fig. 23a). These examples suggest that the lack of midline integration occurs very early in development, probably in the mesenchymal prevertebral stage or during chondrification. The lack of midline integration in the primordium of the basal dental segment appears to interfere with fusion of the adjacent synchondrosis leading to a detached 'hemi-os' in two cases and an ossiculum terminale in the other. Also, faulty midline integration in the second example given here is not confined to the basal dens but also extends to the primordium of the C_3 centrum and the hypochordal bow of the first cervical sclerotome, which forms the anterior C_1 arch. The multiplicity of primordial abnormalities occurring around resegmentation would make it unlikely for a truly bifid dens to be a result of anomalous ossification, which occurs much later.

Clinical significance

Our entire experience of 3 cases suggests that the bifid dens is associated with atlantoaxial instability because the central pivot is hypoplastic when bifid. In our first case, the hypoplastic dens is aggravated by the dislocated ossiculum

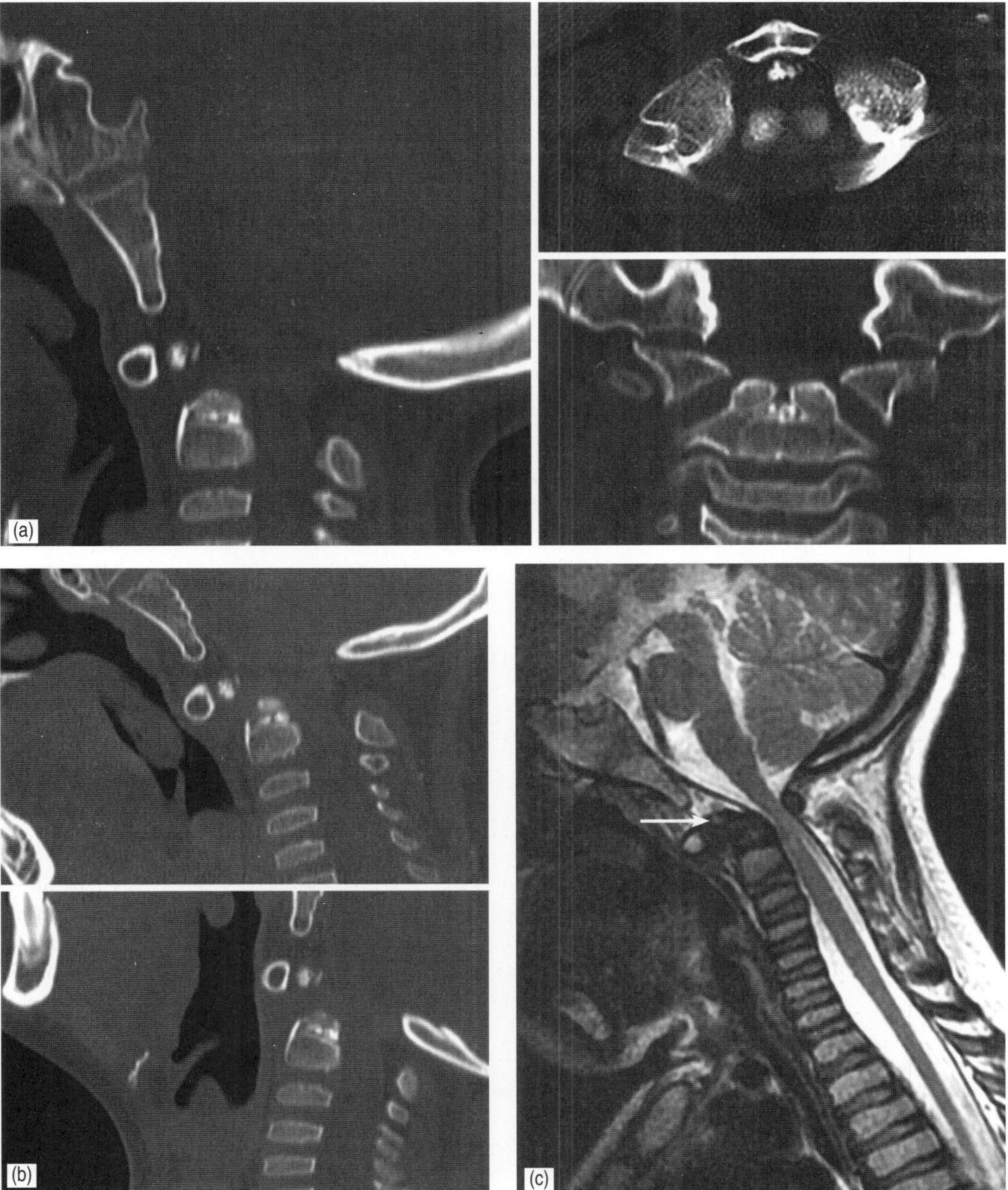

Fig. 22. Completely bifid dens. (a) Note complete lack of midline integration of basal dental segment down to lower dental synchondrosis, and an un-fused and forward dislocated apical dens, suggesting midline integration abnormality interferes with growth and fusion of adjacent upper dental synchondrosis. (b) Flexion–extension CT shows C_1–C_2 instability. (c) Sagittal MR shows severe cord compression with flexion. Arrow points to small ossiculum.

terminale, negating any possibility for TAL anchorage (Figs 22b and c). In our second and third case, the hypermobile 'hemi-os' pops backwards during flexion and accentuates the cord compression (Fig. 23b).

Stabilization for case 1 had to include the occiput into the fusion because of an incomplete posterior arch of C_1. In the other two cases, C_1–C_2 fusion is combined with a transoral, transmandibular resection of both halves of the dens to relieve the anterior compression.

Basilar impression, platybasia and retroflexed dens

Basilar impression is suspected when the dens moves into the plane of the foramen magnum. It has been defined radiographically by the relationship of the tip of the dens with anatomical lines: McGregor's line, the most reliable, is drawn between the hard palate and the lowest point of the occiput and should not be protruded by the dens for >5 mm. Likewise, Chamberlain's line between the hard palate and the opisthion should not be crossed by >2.5 mm, and McRae's line between the basion and opisthion should not be crossed at all (Fig. 24).[46,47] These lines were devised in the pre-magnetic resonance imaging (MRI) era. Today, the sagittal MRI is by far the best way to assess the clinical relevance of basilar impression.

Congenital basilar impression, which is relevant to this chapter, is less a result of upward indentation of the brainstem by the dens, as the word 'impression' implies, than a drop of the

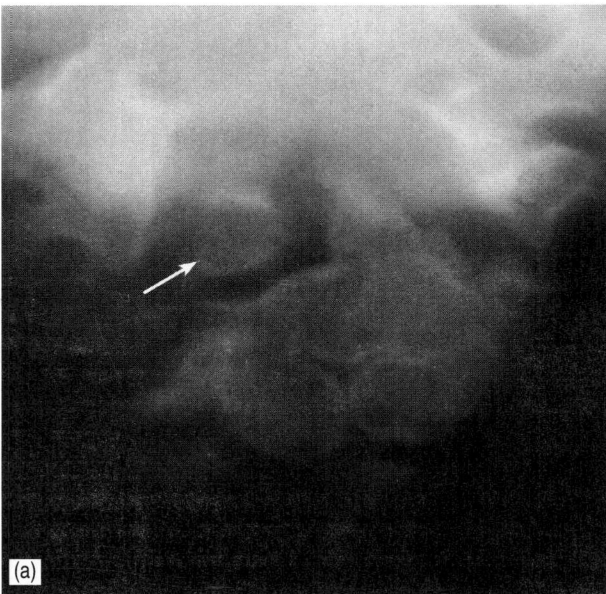

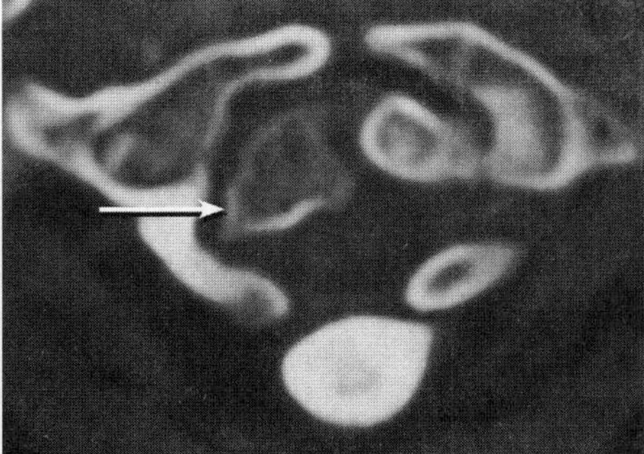

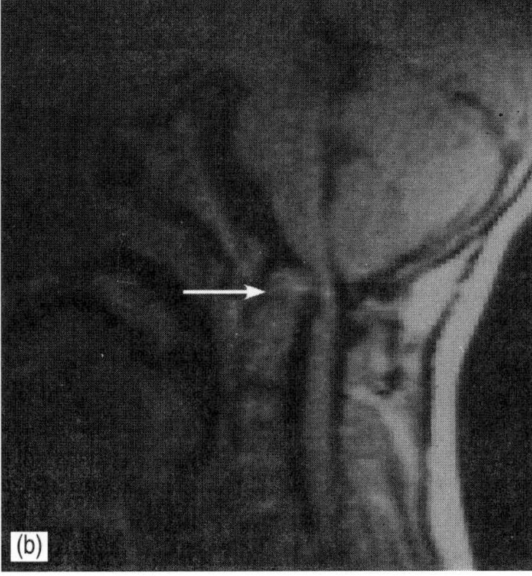

Fig. 23. Absent midline integration of basal dental segment. (a) Non-fusion of right hemi-os to the C_2 centrum suggests interference with adjacent dental synchondrosis fusion. Note bifid C_3 centrum and fusion of C_2 and C_3 centra. (b) Floating hemi-os (arrow) on the axial CT (left) and backward popping of the hemi-os with cord compression on MRI (right).

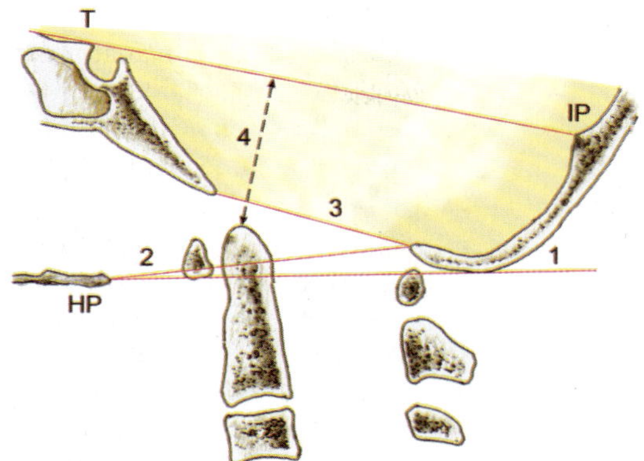

Fig. 24. Radiographic criteria for basilar impression.
1=McGregor's line between hard palate (HP) and the lowest
point of occiput. Basilar impression is present if the dens
protrudes >5 mm above this line. 2=Chamberlain's line
between hard palate and opisthion. Positive diagnosis if dens
protrudes >2.5 mm above line. 3=McRae's line between basion
and opisthion should be above the dens.
4=Klaus index, distance between tip of dens and the
tuberculum—cruciate line between tuberculum (T) and internal
occipital protuberance (IP). This measures depth of the
posterior fossa.

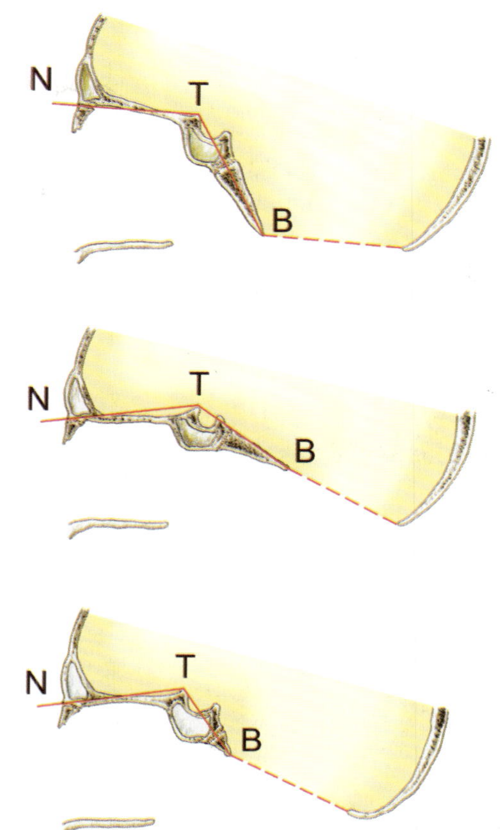

Fig. 25. Normal clival angle (top) measured by the NTB angle
of Welcker joining the nasion (N), tuberculum (T), and basion
(B). The angle should be less than 130°. Platybasia (middle) is
marked by an increased NTB angle. This raises the basion and
forces the foramen magnum plane (dotted line) to tilt upwards.
The same upward tilt of this plane also occurs with a short
clivus (lower).

posterior fossa contents on to the erect dens on
account of a shallow occipital 'box' and flattened
skull base. The causative occipital dysplasia is
caused by deformed growth of all three parts of
the occiput. The basioccipital (pars basilaris) and
the exoccipital (pars lateralis, including the
condyles and the foramen magnum rim), which
expand by endochondral ossification, are hypoplastic; the supraoccipital—the squama, which
expands by membranous ossification and therefore
depends on growth of the chondrocranium—is
obligatorily smaller.

Two types of congenital basilar impression can
be distinguished. Anterior basilar impression is
caused by changes in the basioccipital complex,
which derives from the axial (median) occipital
sclerotomes. The most dramatic change is
platybasia, when the nasion–tubercular–basion
angle (NTB angle of Welcker) is increased and
the sphenoclival block appears severely flattened.
Platybasia is often accompanied by a shortened
basioccipital or clivus, which normally measures

>3.2 cm from the spheno-occipital synchon-
drosis to the basion. The summated effect of a
short and flattened clivus is that the basion,
which normally lies below the nasion– opisthion
line (of Boogaard), is raised way above it and
moves cranially (Fig. 25). This forces the plane of
the foramen magnum to tilt upwards in a lordotic
angle, and with it the planes of the occipital
condyles and of the condyle–atlas articulations
(Fig. 26).

The fusion and chondrification of the

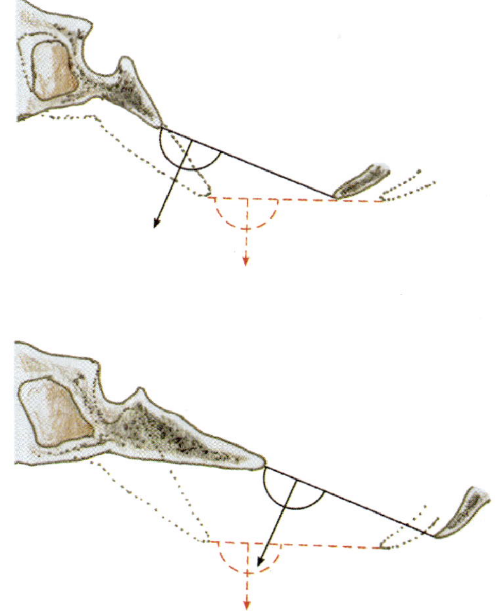

Fig. 26. Severe lordotic tilting of the plane of the occipital condyle in short clivus (upper) and platybasia (lower). Normal clivus and opisthion are represented by dotted outlines; and orientation and plane of the occipital condyle are represented by arrow and semi-circle, respectively; red for normal, and black for abnormal.

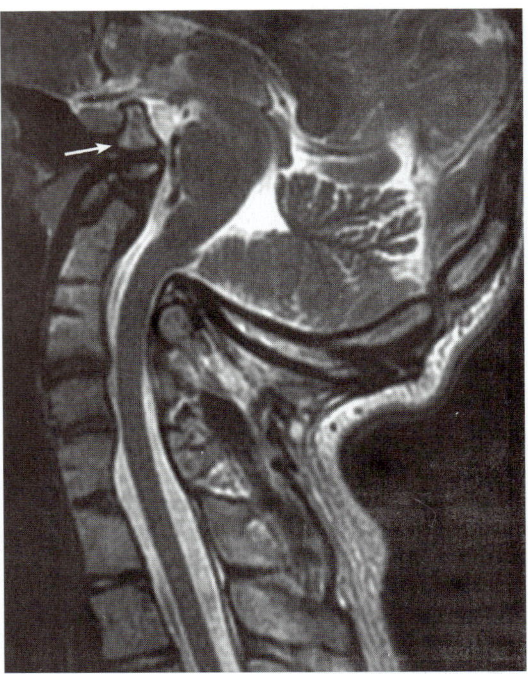

Fig. 27. Exceedingly short (<1 cm) and blunted clivus (arrow) with severe lordotic tilt of the plane of the foramen magnum, leading to a sympathetic lordotic bend of the dental pivot resulting in a retroflexed odontoid and basilar impression.

basioccipital and the exoccipital sclerotomes occur slightly earlier than the resegmentation of the C_1–C_2 sclerotomes. A severely lordotic skull base angle consequently forces the emerging upper cervical sclerotomal column to bend backwards 'in sympathy', especially its centra complex that will ultimately form the dens–axis (Fig. 27). This explains the frequent association of platybasia and short clivus with a retroflexed and lordotic dens that in severe cases points sharply and wickedly backwards into the brainstem in severe anterior basilar impressions (Fig. 28). Clinical studies have indeed shown that patients with basilar impression have a significantly shorter clivus than control groups.[77]

In the posterior form of basilar impression, the exoccipitals, derived from the lateral sclerotomes of the proatlas, rise up towards the foramen magnum, bringing with them the occipital condyles and opisthion. Alternatively, the exoccipital bones may be thin and the condyles flat and hypoplastic. In either case, the dens is secondarily elevated towards the cranial cavity without being lordotic or retroflexed. The opisthion, however, often invaginates into the cranial aperture (basilar invagination).

The upward migration of the anterior and posterior occiput in essence reduces the posterior fossa volume, estimated by the index of Klaus, which measures the distance between the tip of the dens and the tuberculo-cruciate line (between the tuberculum sellae and the internal occipital protuberance) (Fig. 24). This index should exceed 30 mm.[48] With significant reduction to below 25 mm, the developing cerebellum and brainstem are desperately crowded and herniate downwards, accounting for the common association of ectopic cerebellar tonsils (Chiari I

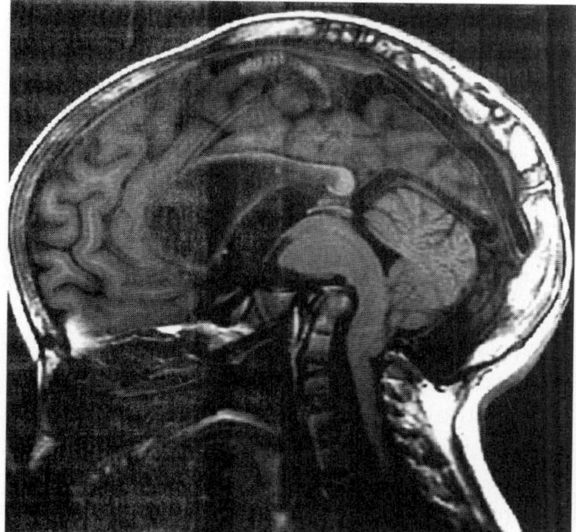

Fig. 28. Extreme platybasia (NTB angle=180°), short clivus (<1.5 cm), and forward folding of the clivus-axis angle of Wackenheim (80°), causing lordotic tilt of the foramen magnum plane and plane of the occipital condyles, resulting in a retroflexed dens and severe basilar impression. Note violation of McGregor's, Chamberlain's, and McRae's lines by the dens and distortion of the brainstem.

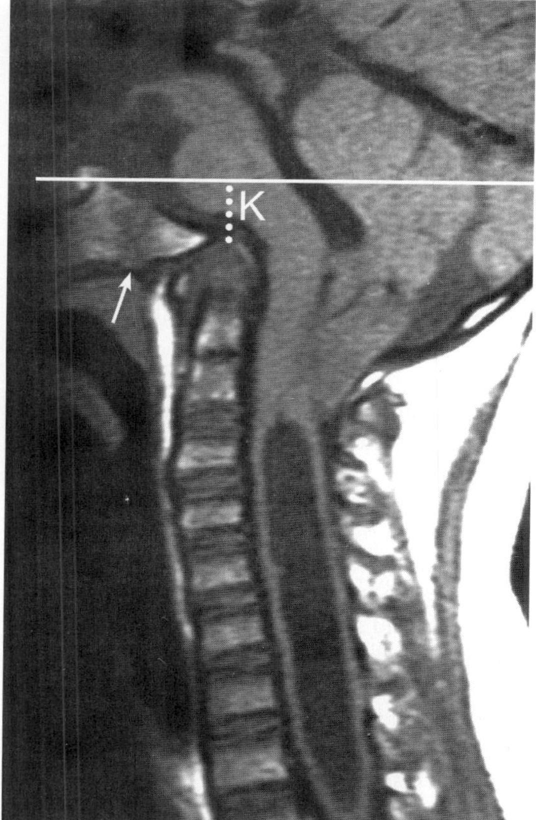

Fig. 29. Platybasia and short clivus (<1.5 cm, with sphenoclival synchondrosis marked by arrow) causing severe basilar impression and mild retroflexed dens. Note shallow posterior fossa with a Klause index (K) of <1.8 cm; and ectopic cerebellar tonsils and cervical syringomyelia.

malformation) with severe basilar impression, platybasia, shortened clivus, and retroflexed dens (Fig. 29). Occasionally, the lower brainstem also lies well below the plane of the foramen magnum ('Chiari 1.5').[78] It is our impression that the truly congenital form of Chiari I malformation often includes skull base dysplasia and the much debated acquired Chiari I malformation consists only of ectopic cerebellar tonsils. Studies have shown that patients with hindbrain herniation and basilar impression have a higher brain to posterior fossa volume ratio than those with just hindbrain herniation, and both groups have higher ratios than controls.[77,79,80]

Clinical significance

Platybasia without basilar impression is asymptomatic. Indentation of the anterior medulla by the dens, however, produces brainstem dysfunction and lower cranial neuropathies more frequently than 'pure' cerebellar ectopia without an anterior compression vector. The brainstem deficits include neurogenic dysphagia,[81,82] nasal or hoarse voice due to paresis of the palatal levator and vocal cords, sleep apnoea, and intermittent or progressive spastic quadriparesis. Tussive headaches, syncope, and gait dyscoordination are also common complaints.

Posterior decompression for Chiari I malformation with coexisting basilar impression carries a much higher late complication rate than for pure cerebellar ectopia. Even if the anterior vector is not initially symptomatic, the slightest amount of postoperative cranial settling after nullification of the posterior tension band will deliver the brainstem straight on to the pointing dens to cause rapid onset of new brainstem signs.[83] In addition, platybasia and a decrease in the clivus–axis angle (of Wackenheim) accentuates the forward bending moment acting on the clivus–dens pivot point, and accelerates the forward 'folding' of the cranio-cervical axis (Figs 30a and b). It is our distinct impression that this type of postoperative instability occurs far more commonly in the associative type of Chiari I malformation. We therefore avoid removing the C_2 lamina during the decompression, if necessary at the expense of resecting the tips of the tonsils.

If symptomatic post-decompression cranial settling does occur despite precautions, skull traction with calipers, with the neck in slight extension should be rendered under muscle relaxation and sedation for a few days, aiming at reversing the kyphotic deformity and telescoping effect at the foramen magnum. Occiput–C_1–C_2 fusion should be done after reduction (Figs 30c and d). If brainstem indentation persists, transoral resection of the dens may be necessary.

Anomalies of the surrounding ring structures

These can be divided into anomalies of the proatlas and of the C_1 sclerotome.

Anomalies of proatlas

Hyperplasia of the proatlas hypochordal bow: Third occiput condyle embryogenesis

The hypochordal bow is an arcual strip of mesenchyme ventral to the axial sclerotome. In humans, only the hypochordal bows of the proatlas and C_1 resegmented sclerotome persist.[25] The hypochordal bow of the proatlas normally forms a small midline osseus tubercle attached to the ventral surface of the basioccipital below the rim of the foramen magnum (Fig. 7). Rarely, it remains as a fully ossified structure distinct from the basioccipital bone. If the entire arc is preserved, it is called a pre-basioccipital arch, which looks like a U-shaped bony valance on the underside of the anterior rim of the foramen magnum (Fig. 31).[42,48,84] If only the paramedian arch persists, two parasagittal spikes project downwards from the clivus, called the basilar processes.[42,48,84] Neither of these bony excrescences encroach on the foramen magnum and are thus harmless. Occasionally, however, the median portion of the proatlas hypochordal bow becomes exuberantly hyperplastic and forms a prominent bone spur that juts obliquely backwards from the basioccipital tip, which does cause neural compression. This median bony process is firmly attached to the basion, and frequently forms true synovial joints with the anterior arch of C_1 and the odontoid apex (Fig. 32).[84] It is thus rather aptly termed a median or third occipital condyle (condylus tertius).[48,84–87] These articulations, though bizarre, are not surprising if one remembers that the anterior arch of C_1 comes from the hypochordal bow of the first cervical sclerotome directly subjacent to the hypochordal bow of the proatlas, and the dental apex develops from the proatlas centrum; joint formation between corresponding components of adjacent sclerotomes is 'normal' in the lower vertebral levels.

Clinical significance

A third occipital condyle may be mistaken for an os avis on radiographs, as both are osseous appendages of the clival tip. However, it is important to distinguish them because of their very different implications of stability. In os avis, the dental pivot has lost its top and becomes perilously hypoplastic, whereas the dental pivot in the case of the third occipital condyle has normal height and therefore remains a solid anchor for the TAL; instability is unlikely.

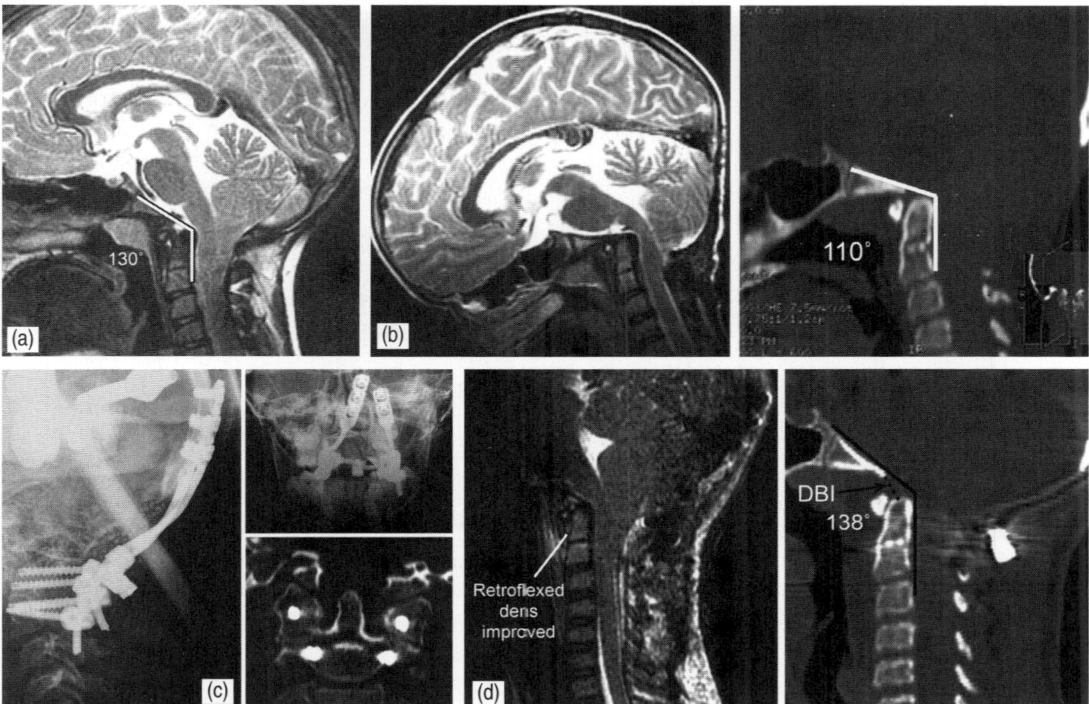

Fig. 30. A 12-year-old girl with retroflexed dens, mild basilar impression and Chiari I malformation. (a) Preoperative clivus-axis angle (Wackenheim) of 130°. (b) Postoperative cranial settling causing forward folding of Wackenheim's angle to 110° and shortening of dens–basion interval (DBI). Note worsened anterior brain stem compression. (c) Caliper traction (left) for 4 days followed by C_1–C_2 Goel-Harm's screw-plate posterior fusion. (d) Post-fusion reversal of Wackenheim's angle to 138° and increase of DBI to 1.8 cm. Note relief of brainstem compression and symptoms.

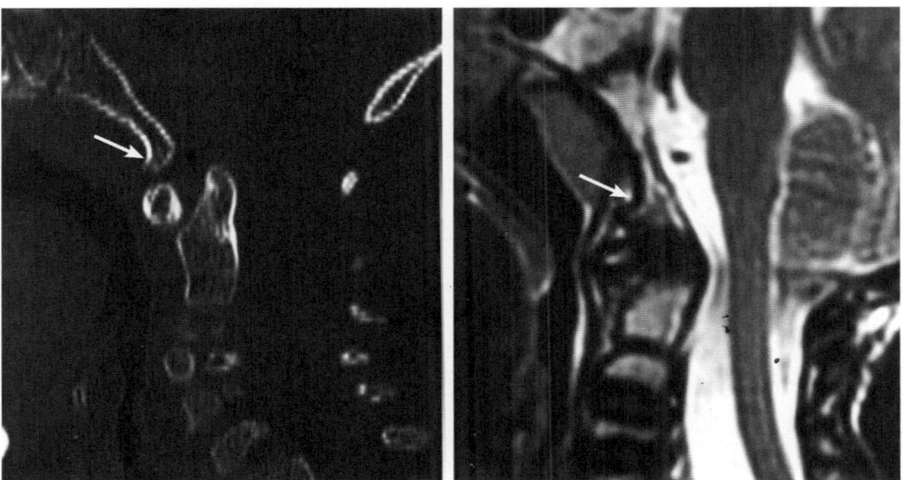

Fig. 31. Pre-basioccipital arch (thin arrows), a U-shaped bony valance on the ventral lip of the anterior foramen magnum rim. This results from complete preservation of the hypochordal bow of the proatlas.

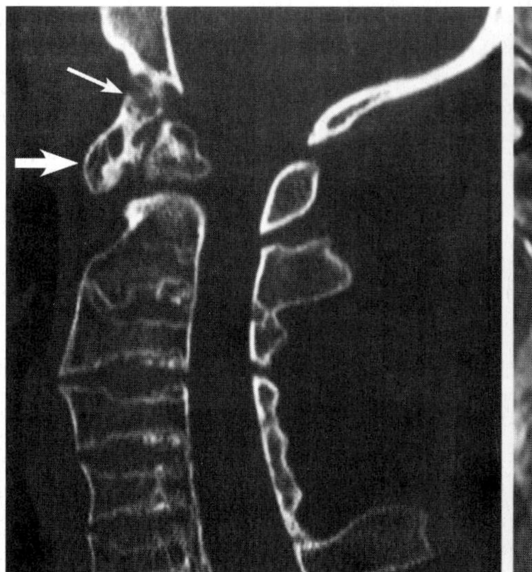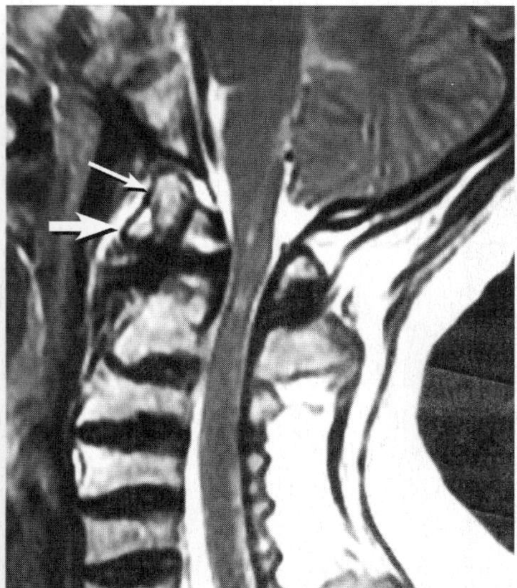

Fig. 32. Third occipital condyle, or condylus tertius (thin arrow) attached to the ventral surface of the clival tip, and fused to the anterior atlantal arch (thick arrow). On MRI, the condyle appears to form a synovial joint with an ossiculum terminale that is un-fused to the basal dens. The third occipital condyle represents midline hyperplasia of the proatlas hypochordal bow.

Although some third condyles are short and protrude along the contour of the clivus or even curl forward away from the brainstem (Fig. 33), others can be enormous backward pointing cantilevers[35,48,85,87] producing serious neurological deficits. Because there is no instability, transoral, transclival resection of the third condyle is adequate treatment.

Hyperplasia of exoccipital sclerotome: Hypertropic occipital condyle

Hyperplasia of the lateral sclerotome of the proatlas, precursor to the exoccipital bone, results in hypertrophy of the lateral and posterior rim of the foramen magnum including a massively gnarled occipital condyle. Bilateral condylar hypertrophy causes pincer-like cervicomedullary compression and early symptoms,[35] but unilateral hypertrophy can also lead to severe lateral distortion of the lower brainstem and slow neurological deterioration (Fig. 34). An uneven atlanto-occipital joint surface and chondromalacia may also produce chronic neck pain and stiffness. Treatment consists of resection of the occipital condyle via the far-lateral approach, followed by occiput (O)-cervical fusion for the expected O–C$_1$ instability.

Assimilation of atlas: Non-resegmentation of the proatlas sclerotome

Congenital fusion of the atlas with the occiput is one of the most common anomalies of the CVJ, with a prevalence rate from 0.08% to 2.8% in the general population.[88–91] Atlantal assimilation or occipitalization ranges from complete incorporation of the atlas into the occiput to discrete osseous bridges between the two. Gholve *et al.*[92] identified three fusion zones. Zone 1 assimilation involves the anterior atlantal arch between the front of the lateral masses (20% in their series); zone 2 assimilation involves primarily the lateral processes (17%); and zone 3 assimilation is fusion at the posterior atlantal arch (13%) (Fig. 35). Combination of zones is seen in >50% of

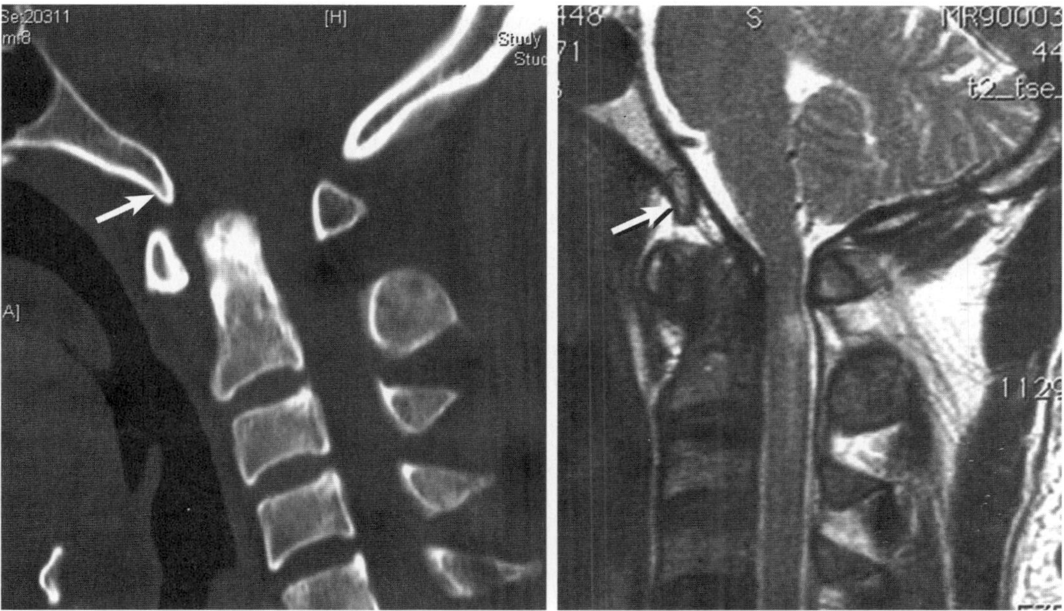

Fig. 33. A short third occipital condyle (arrow) curving forward from the clival tip away from the foramen magnum.

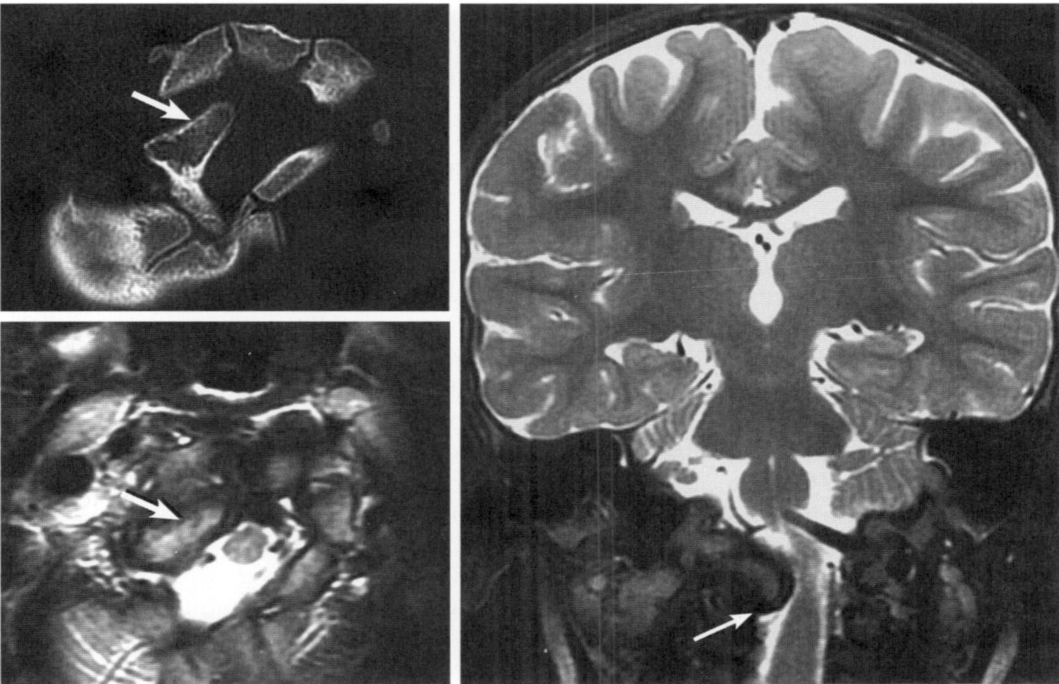

Fig. 34. Unilateral hyperplasia of the occipital condyle (arrow) with cervicomedullary distortion. This represents hyperplasia of the exoccipital (lateral) sclerotome of the proatlas.

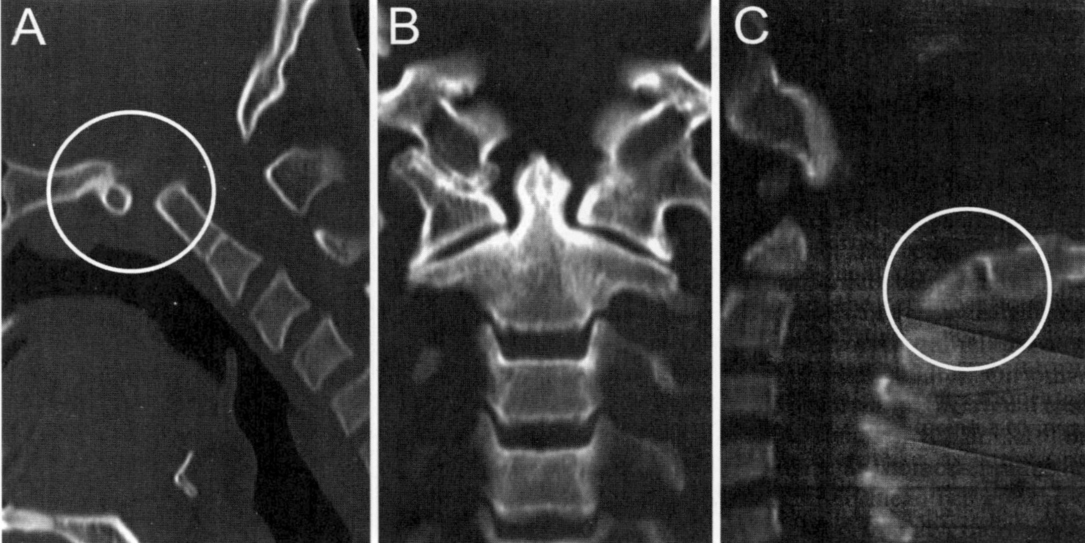

Fig. 35. C_1 assimilation or occipitalization. (A) Assimilation of the anterior atlantal arch (Zone 1 assimilation). (B) Assimilation of the lateral masses (Zone 2 assimilation). (C) Posterior arch (Zone 3) assimilation.

patients.[92] Thirty-seven per cent of Gholve's patients also had associated basilar impression, 20% had Klippel–Feil syndrome, 17% Chiari I malformation, and 37% had cervical stenosis.

embryonic axis, inappropriate repression of *Pax-1* at the proatlas–C_1 sclerotome interphase and other vertebral levels may be involved in associative cases of atlas assimilation.

Embryogenesis

It has already been mentioned that inactivation of *Hox d-3* gene expression in mice results in anterior homeotic transformation at the CVJ, such that the C_1 vertebra takes on an occipital identity and the head–neck transitional zone moves caudally to the C_1–C_2 junction. All mutants have assimilation of C_1 to the basiocciput.[1,54] It is therefore tempting to ascribe human cases of isolated C_1 assimilation to similar mutations of the human *Hox* gene homologues. However, in cases of combined C_1 assimilation and Klippel–Feil syndrome in which multiple levels of cervical fusion are seen below C_2, the *Hox* gene theory will require multiple *Hox* mutations and alterations of multiple *Hox* codes, which is highly improbable. As *Pax-1* expression is involved in resegmentation of all levels of the

Clinical significance

Assimilation of the atlas to the occiput means that the first mobile segment between the skull and spine has been transferred to the C_1–C_2 junction, as are all the motion stresses including that of flexion–extension, normally of restricted range at this level and for which the local joint anatomy is ill-suited. This also means the supporting myoligamentous structures are more likely to suffer 'over-stretch' failure. Almost 60% of Gholve *et al.*'s patients with C_1 assimilation has C_1–C_2 instability defined as an atlantal–dens interval (ADI) >4 mm in adults and >5 mm in children.[92] McRae and von Torklus and Gehle had similar findings.[46,47,93,94] More than half of Gholve *et al.*'s patients with instability also had C_2–C_3 fusion, which adds to the burden of stresses at C_1–C_2.

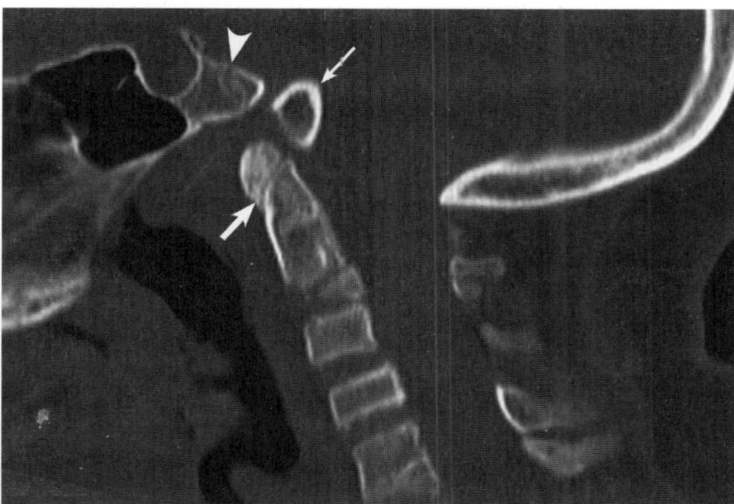

Fig. 36. Un-fused clivus to basioccipital. The clivus, or lower basioccipital segment (thin arrow) is un-fused to the upper basioccipital segment, which is attached to the sphenoid bone at the spheno-occipital synchondrosis (arrow head). The anterior atlantal arch (thick arrow) is fused to the apical dens to form a pseudo centrum for C_1. This may represent posterior homeotic transformation.

The symptoms of C_1–C_2 instability range from persistent neck pain and stiffness to frank myelopathy. Typically, the neurological deficits begin at the 3rd or 4th decade of life[46] and tend to worsen with age.[47] We have also seen concomitant hypertrophy of the posterior arch of C_2, which accentuates the neural compromise. Management for symptomatic cases is stabilization between occiput and C_2–C_3 in concert with treatment for the other associated malformations.

Un-fused occipital condyle and clivus: Posterior homeotic transformation

Unilateral or bilateral non-fusion of the occipital condyle with the skull base has been described.[35] The result is usually an unstable atlanto-occipital articulation and bony distortion around the joint that could indent the brainstem. Occasionally, only the clivus is un-fused and the dens is fused to the anterior atlantal arch as if the atlas is acquiring its own centrum (Fig. 36). These phenotypes are reminiscent of the transgenic murine mutant with disturbance in *Hox d-4* expression and posterior homeotic transforma-

tion of the cranio-vertebral transitional zone, in which the exoccipital region contains un-fused neural arch-like structures resembling the posterior arch of C_1, and C_1 acquires a centrum instead of an anterior arch. Treatment of these rare entities consists of bony resection when necessary, followed by occipital–cervical fusion in case of instability.

Anomalies involving the C_1 re-segmented sclerotome

Aplasia and hypoplasia of the C_1 hypochordal bow: Anomalies of anterior atlantal arch

Aplasia of the hypochordal bow of the C_1 sclerotome leads to complete absence of the anterior atlantal arch. This is an exceedingly rare anomaly; only a few post-mortem cases can be found in the literature, in which the anterior arch was replaced by loose connective tissue.[48,95,96] The centrum primordium of C_1 is often simultaneously affected. Our one example of absent

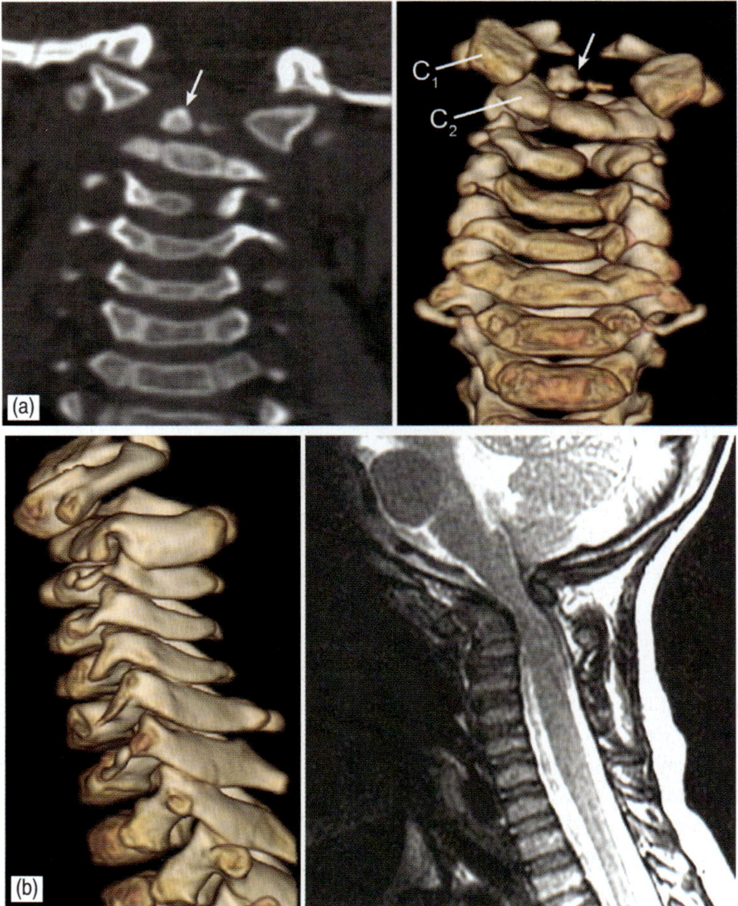

Fig. 37. Complete aplasia of C_1 hypochordal bow-complete aplasia of C_1 anterior arch. (a) CT and 3-D reconstruction shows no anterior atlantal arch or insertion tubercles for the TAL. The 2 anterior stunted dental hemi-os (arrow) are un-fused to the C_2 centrum. Posterior arch of C_1 is also un-fused. (b) Extreme C_1–C_2 flexion instability and severe cord compression.

anterior C_1 arch is clinically unstable because the basal dental segment is un-integrated in the midline, and the two 'hemi-os' are stunted. The insertion tubercles of the TAL are either greatly attenuated or non-existent, and the TAL itself may also be absent, as it is derived from mesenchyme adjacent to that of the hypochordal bow and centrum. It is not visualized on MRI in our case (Fig. 37a). The result is severe anterior subluxation of C_1 on C_2 with cord compression (Fig. 37b).

When blighted development of the hypochordal bow is accompanied by complete aplasia of the primordium of the C_1 centrum, the result is an extremely unstable C_1–C_2 complex. Our example shows a match-head sized remnant of the C_1 anterior arch in front of an axial body without any dental pivot (Fig. 38). The child presented with quadriparesis.

Because the atlas in these cases is usually reduced, deformed, and feeble, posterior instrument fusion needs to incorporate the

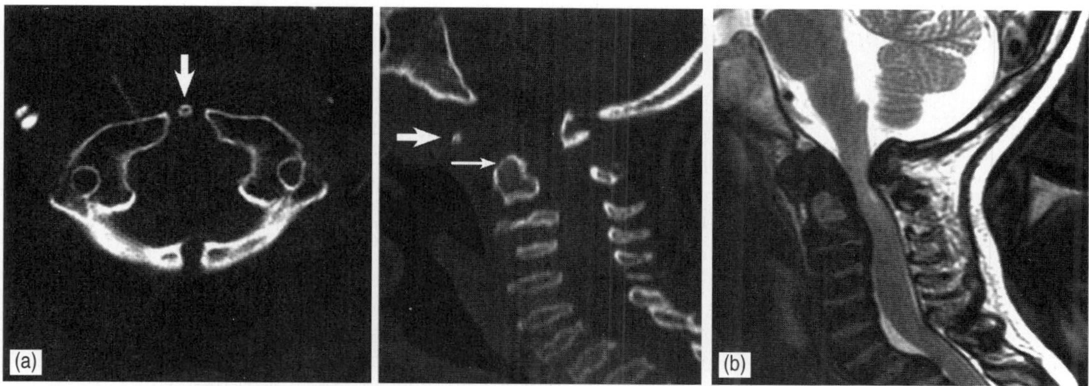

Fig. 38. Severe hypoplasia of C_1 hypochordal bow-small anterior C_1 arch. (a) Match-head size anterior C_1 arch (thick arrow) associated with complete agenesis of the dens (thin arrow), a result of concomitant C_1 centrum aplasia. (b) C_1–C_2 instability with cord compression.

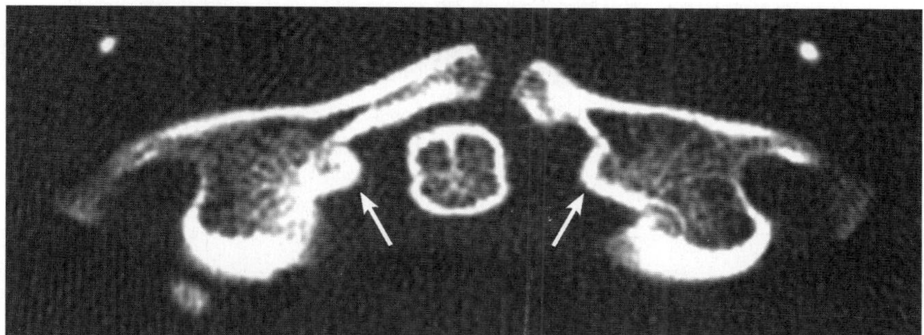

Fig. 39. Complete agenesis of posterior atlantal arch and bifid anterior atlantal arch. Normal TAL insertion tubercles (arrows). There is no C_1–C_2 instability.

occiput and often has to be extended down to C_3 or C_4 to distribute the stresses on the upright plates. If the child is very young (<3 years old) with a large head and puny nuchal musculature, postoperative halo is recommended.

Aplasia and hypoplasia of the lateral C_1 sclerotome: Anomalies of posterior atlantal arch

Varying degrees of aplasia of the lateral sclerotome of C_1 result in partial or complete agenesis of the posterior atlantal arch. Posterior atlantal arch deficiencies are 10 times more common than anterior arch defects.[46,47,97] Von Torklus and Gehle[94] documented six subtypes,

the rarest being total agenesis. The example of total agenesis given here has no bony arch posterior to the lateral masses, and the anterior arch is bifid (Fig. 39). Partial agenesis can be unilateral or bilateral, with preservation of all or portions of the posterior tubercle, which appears floating without bony attachment to the rest of the C_1 vertebra (Figs 40A and B). MRI seems to indicate presence of cartilage in the scaffolding of the incomplete ring, but rather ample tilting of the lateral masses away from the remaining posterior tubercle during flexion (Fig. 40C) suggests that the cartilaginous mould was never formed, and the developmental error probably occurred at the mesenchymal (membranous) stage.[98–100]

Unlike with aplasia of the hypochordal bow and

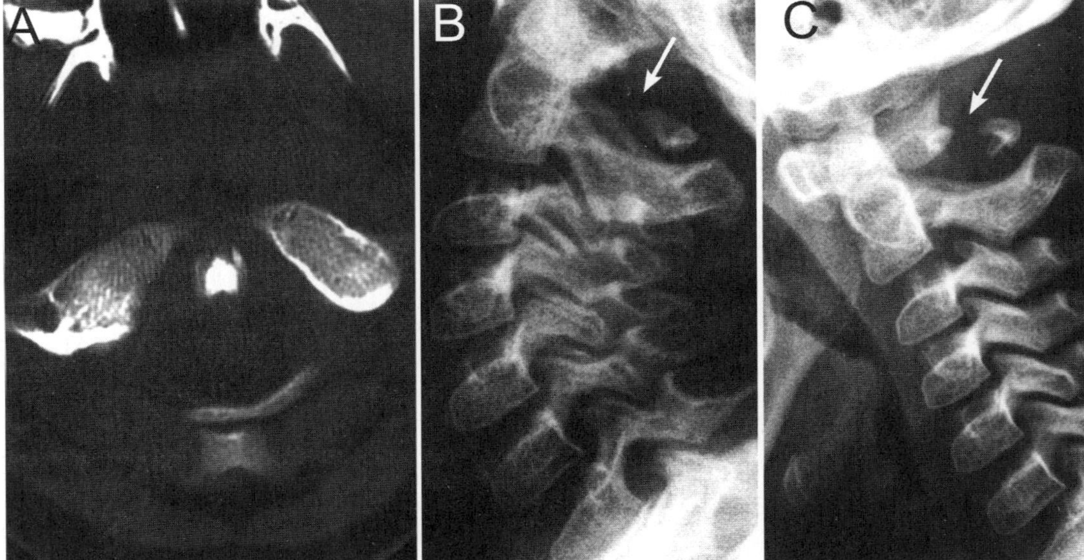

Fig. 40. Partial agenesis of posterior atlantal arch. (A) The posterior tubercle and arch remnant appear floating and unconnected to the lateral masses. (B and C) Flexion and extension shows ample tilting of the lateral masses away from the posterior tubercle (arrows), suggesting absence of a cartilaginous mould. In spite of this tilting, there is no translational instability.

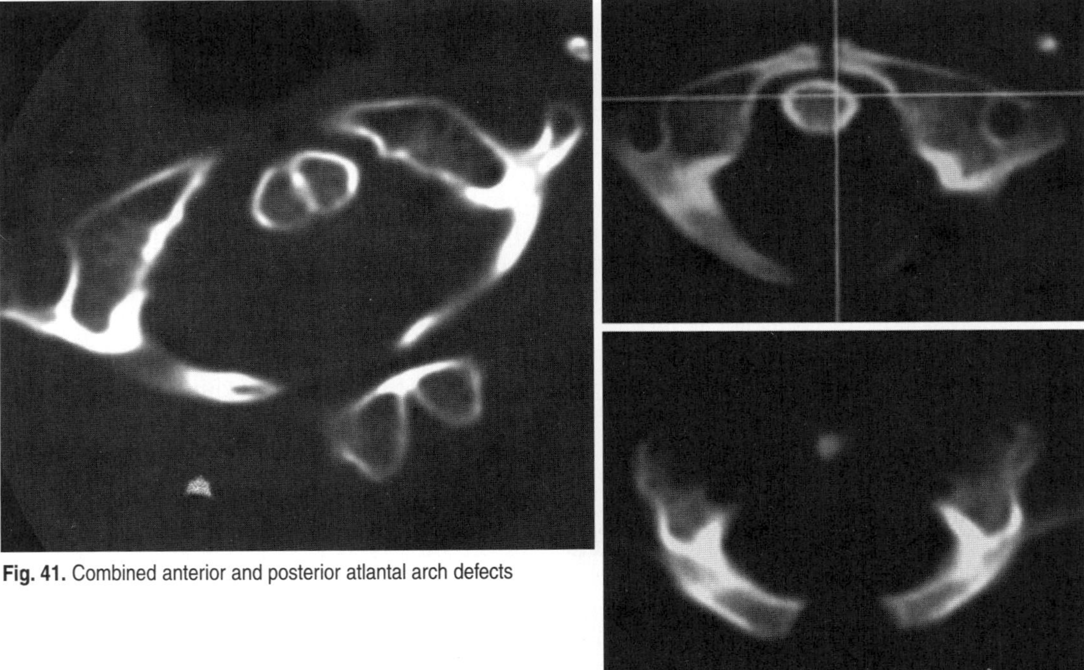

Fig. 41. Combined anterior and posterior atlantal arch defects

Fig. 42. Bifid anterior and posterior atlantal arches

anterior arch defects, the centrum sclerotome of C_1 is not affected in posterior arch defects. The dental pivot and TAL anchorage are thus normal (Fig. 39). The C_1–C_2 complex in patients with posterior arch defects is usually stable, in spite of the intimidating appearance of the radiographs. None of our patients required fusion.

Combined dysplasia of the hypochordal bow and lateral sclerotome of C_1-combined anterior and posterior atlantal arch defects

Simultaneous hypoplasia of the hypochordal bow and lateral sclerotome of C_1 leads to combined anterior and posterior atlantal defects. The anterior arcual defect is usually incomplete and the insertion tubercles and TAL are mostly intact, thereby maintaining stability against translation. However, because the two lateral masses are essentially loose bones connected by incompetent soft tissues, axial loading forces can split them apart, similar to the mechanism of a Jefferson fracture (Fig. 41).

Bifid anterior and posterior atlantal arches

Midline gaps in the posterior atlantal tubercle are common incidental findings. Anterior bifid C_1 arch is less common but probably just as innocuous. Combined anterior and posterior C_1 bifidity is uncommon (Fig. 42). The examples we have seen are all stable entities, although the gaps never close with age. Rare cases with in-curling of the free-ends of the un-fused posterior arches have been known to compress the spinal cord[97] and require surgical decompression.

References

1. Dietrich S, Kessel M. The vertebral column. In: Thorogood P (ed). In: Embryos, genes, birth defects. Chichester: John Wiley and Sons; 1997:281–302.
2. Davis GK, Jaramillo CA, Patel NH. Pax group III genes and the evolution of insect pair-rule patterning. *Development* 2001;**128**:3445–58.
3. Davis GK, Patel NH. The origin and evolution of segmentation. *Trends Cell Biol* 1999;**9**:M68–M72.
4. Pourquié O. Vertebrate somitogenesis: A novel paradigm for animal segmentation? *Int J Dev Biol* 2003;**47**:597–603.
5. Keynes RJ, Stern CD. Mechanisms of vertebrate segmentation. *Development* 1988;**103**:413–29.
6. Bellairs R. The segmentation of somites in the chick embryo. *Boll Zool* 1980;**47**:245–2.
7. Stern CD, Keynes RJ. Interactions between somite cells; the formation and maintenance of segment boundaries in the chick embryo. *Development* 1987;**99**:261–72.
8. Huang R, Zhi Q, Ordahl CP, *et al.* The fate of the first avian somite. *Anat embryol (Berl)* 1997;**195**:435–49.
9. Pourquié O. The segmentation clock: Converting embryonic time into spatial pattern. *Science* 2003;**301**:328–30.
10. Forsberg H, Crozet F, Brown NA. Waves of mouse Lunatic fringe expression, in four-hour cycles at two-hour intervals, precede somite boundary formation. *Curr Biol* 1998;**8**:1027–30.
11. McGrew MJ, Dale JK, Fraboulet S, *et al.* The lunatic fringe gene is a target of the molecular clock linked to somite segmentation in avian embryos. *Curr Biol* 1998;**8**:979–82.
12. Sawada A, Shinya M, Jiang YJ, *et al.* Fgf/MAPK signaling is a crucial positional cue in somite boundary formation. *Development* 2001;**128**:4873–80.
13. Dubrulle J, McGrew MJ, Pourquié O. FGF signaling controls somite boundary position and regulates segmentation clock control of spatiotemporal Hox gene activation. *Cell* 2001;**106**:219–32.
14. Palmeirim I, Henrique D, Ish-Horowicz D, *et al.* Avian hairy gene expression identifies a molecular clock linked to vertebrate segmentation and somitogenesis. *Cell* 1997;**91**:639–48.
15. Christ B, Wilting J. From somites to vertebral column. *Annals of Anatomy* 1992;**174**:23–32.
16. Christ B, Jacob HJ, Jacob M. On the formation of the myotomes in avian embryos. An experimental and scanning electron microscope study. *Experientia* 1978;**34**:514–16.
17. Aoyoma H, Asamoto K. Determination of somite cells: Independence of cell differentiation and morphogenesis. *Development* 1988;**104**:15–28.
18. Jacob M, Christ B, Jacob HJ. Über die regionale Determination des paraxialen Mesoderms junger Hühnerembryonen. *Verh Anat Ges* 1975;**69**:263–9.

19. Kieny M, Mauger A, Sengel P. Early regionalization of the somitic mesoderm as studied by the development of the axial skeleton of the chick embryo. *Dev Biol* 1972;**28**:42–161.

20. Koseki H, Wallin J, Wilting J, *et al.* A role for *Pax-1* as a mediator of notochordal signals during the dorsoventral specification of vertebrae. *Development* 19993;**119**:649–60.

21. Dalgleish AE. A study of the development of thoracic vertebrae in the mouse assisted by autoradiography. *Acta Anatomica* 1985;**122**:91–8.

22. Remak R. Untersuchungen über die Entwicklung der Wirbeltiere. Berlin: Reimer; 1855.

23. Ebner von E. Urwirbel und Neugliederung der Wirbelsäule. Wien: Sitzungsber Akad Wiss 1888;**III/97**:194–206.

24. Christ B, Jacob HJ, Seifert R. Über die Entwicklung der Zervikookzipitalen Übergangsregion. In: Hohmann D, Kügelgen B, Liebig K (eds). *Neuro-orthopädie*. Berlin, Heidelberg: Springer; 1988;**4**:13–22.

25. Müller F, O'Rahilly R. Segmentation in staged human embryos: The occipitocervical region revisited. *J Anat* 2003;**203**:297–15.

26. Dietrich S, Gruss P. Undulated Phenotypes suggest a role of Pax-1 for the development of vertebral and extravertebral structures. *Dev Biol* 1995;**167**:529–48.

27. Bagnall KM. The migration and distribution of somite cells after labelling with the carbocyanine dye, DiI: The relationship of this distribution to segmentation in the vertebrate body. *Anat Embryol* 1992;**185**:317–24.

28. Bagnall KM, Sanders EJ. The binding pattern of peanut lectin associated with sclerotome migration and the formation of the vertebral axis in the chick embryo. *Anat Embryol* 1989;**180**:505–13.

29. David KM, Crockard A. Congenital malformations of the base of the skull, atlas and dens. In: Benzel EC (ed). *The cervical spine*. 4th ed. Philadelphia: Lippincott Williams and Wilkins; 2005:415–26.

30. Couly GF, Coltey PM, Le Douarin NM. The triple origin of skull in higher vertebrates: A study in quail-chick chimeras. *Development* 1993;**117**:409–29.

31. Reiter A. Die Frühentwicklung der menschlichen Wirbelsäule. II. Mitteilung: Die Entwicklung der Occipitalsegmente und der Halswirbelsäule. *Z Anat Entwickl* 1944;**113**:66–104.

32. Wilting J, Ebensperger C, Müller TS, *et al. Pax-1* in the development of the cervico-occipital transitional zone. *Anat Embryo* 1995;**192**:221–7.

33. Lufkin T, Mark M, Hart CP, *et al.* Homeotic transformation of the occipital bones of the skull by ectopic expression of a homeobox gene. *Lett Nature* 1992;**359**:835–41.

34. Menezes AH. Embryology, development and classification of disorders of the craniovertebral junction. In. Dickman CA, Sonntag VKH, Spetzler RF (eds). *Surgery of the craniovertebral junction.* New York: Thieme; 1998:3–12.

35. Menezes AH, Fenoy KA. Remnants of occipital vertebrae: Proatlas segmentation abnormalities. *Neurosurgery* 2009;**64**:945–53.

36. Müller F, O'Rahilly R. Occipitocervical segmentation in staged human embryos. *J Anat* 1994;**185**:251–8.

37. Cattell JS, Filtzer DL. Pseudosubluxation and other normal variations in the cervical spine in children. *J Bone Joint Surg* 1965;**47A**:1295–309.

38. Cave AJE. The morphological constitution of the odontoid process. *J Anat* 1938;**72**:621.

39. Hensinger RN, Fielding JW, Hawkins RJ. Congenital anomalies of the odontoid process. *Orthop Clin North Am* 1978;**9**:901–12.

40. Sensing EC. The development of the occipital and cervical segments and their associated structures in human embryos. *Contributions to embryology* 1957;**36**:152–61.

41. Pendergrass EP, Schaeffer JP, Hodes PJ. *The head and neck in roentgen diagnosis.* 2nd ed. Springfield, Illinois: Charles C. Thomas; 1956:1529–30.

42. Prescher A. The craniocervical junction in man, the osseous variations, their significance and differential diagnosis. *Annals of Anatomy* 1997;**179**:1–19.

43. Torklus von D, Gehle W. *Die Obere Halswirbelsäule.* Vol. 2. Stuttgart: Aufl. Thieme; 1975.

44. Wollin DG. The OS odontoideum: Separate odontoid process. *J Bone Joint Surg Am* 1963;**45**:1459–84.

45. Markuske H. Untersuchungen zur Static und Dynamik der kindlichen Halswirbelsäule: Der Aussagewert seitlicher Röntgenaufnahmen. In: Die Wirbelsäule in Forschung und Praxis 50. Hippokrates, Stuttgart, 1978.

46. McRae DL. Bony abnormalities in the region of the foramen magnum; correlation of the anatomic and neurologic findings. *Acta Radiol* 1953;**40**:335–54.

47. McRae DL. The significance of abnormalities of the cervical spine. *Am J Roentgenol* 1960;**84**:3–25.

48. Torklus von D, Gehle W. Anomalies and malformations. In: von Torklus D, Gehle W (eds). *The upper cervical spine*. Stuttgart: Thieme; 1972:14–53.

49. Wadia NH. Myelopathy complicating congenital atlantoaxial dislocation (a study of 28 cases). *Brain* 1967;**90**:449–72.

50. Müller F, O'Rahilly R. The human chondrocranium at the end of the embryonic period, proper, with particular reference to the nervous system. *American Journal of Anatomy* 1980;**159**:33–58.

51. Kessel M. Respecification of vertebral identities by retinoic acid. *Development* 1992;**115**:487–501.

52. Kessel M, Gruss P. Homeotic transformation of murine vertebrae and concomitant alteration of Hox codes induced by retinoic acid. *Cell* 1991;**67**:1–20.

53. Haack H, Kessel M. Homeobox genes and skeletal patterning. In: Hall BK (ed). *Bone*. Vol 9. CRC Press, Boca Raton; 1994:119–44.

54. Condie B, Capecchi MR. Mice homozygous for a targeted disruption of *Hox d-3* (*Hox-4.1*) exhibit anterior transformations of the first and second cervical vertebrae, the atlas and axis. *Development* 1993;**119**:579–95.

55. Wallin J, Mizutani Y, Imai K, *et al*. A new Pax gene, *Pax-9*, maps to mouse chromosome 12. *Mammal Genome* 1993;**4**:354–8.

56. Smith CA, Tuan RS. Human PAX gene expression and development of the vertebral column. *Clinical Orthopaedics and Related Research* 1994;**302**:241–50

57. Jones FS, Georges C, Guss P, *et al*. Activation of the cytotactin promoter by the homeobox-containing gene Evx-1. *Proc Natl Acad Sci USA* 1991;**89**:2091.

58. Jones FS, Prediger EA, Dennis BA, *et al*. Cell adhesion molecules as targets for Hox genes: Neural cell adhesion molecule promoter activity is modulated by cotransfection with *Hox 2.5* and *2.4*. *Proc Natl Acad Sci USA* 1991;**89**:2091.

59. Musil L, Goodenough D. Gap junctional intercellular communication and the regulation of connexin expression and function. *Curr Opin Cell Biol* 1990;**2**: 875.

60. Dietrich S, Schubert FR, Gruss P. Altered Pax gene expression in notochord mutants of the mouse: The notochord is required for the dorsoventral patterning of the somite. *Mech Dev* 1993;**44**:189–207.

61. Wallin J, Wilting J, Koseki H, *et al*. The role of *Pax-1* in axial skeleton development. *Development* 1994;**120**:1109–21.

62. Stapleton P, Weith A, Urbanek P, *et al*. Chromosomal localization of seven PAX genes and cloning of a novel family member, *PAX-9*. *Natural Genetics* 1993;**3**:292.

63. Crockard H, Stevens M. Craniovertebral junction anomalies in inherited disorder: Part of the syndrome or caused by the disorder? *Euro J Pediatr* 1995;**154**:504–12.

64. Hawkins RJ, Fielding JW, Thompson WJ. Os odontoideum: Congenital or acquired. *J Bone Joint Surg* 1976;**38-A**:413–14.

65. Hensinger RN: Osseous anomalies of the craniovertebral junction. *Spine* 1986;**11**:323–33.

66. Menezes AH. Congenital and acquired abnormalities of the craniovertebral junction. In: Youmans JR (ed). *Neurological surgery*. 4th ed. Philadelphia: WB Saunders, 1996:1035–89.

67. Menezes AH, Ryken TC. Craniovertebral abnormalities in Down's syndrome. *Pediatric Neurosurgery* 1992;**18**:24–33.

68. Kirlew KA, Hathout GM, Reiter SD, *et al*. Os odontoideum in identical twins: Perspectives on etiology. *Skeletal Radiol* 1993;**22**:525–7.

69. Morgan MK, Onofrio BM, Bender CE. Familial os odontoideum: Case report. *J Neurosurg* 1989;**70**: 636–9.

70. David KM, Thorogood PV, Stevens JM, *et al*. The dysmorphic cervical spine in Klippel-Feil syndrome: Interpretations from developmental biology. *Neurosurg Focus* 1999;**6**:Article 1.

71. David KM, Thorogood P, Stevens JM, *et al*. The one bone spine: A failure of notochord/sclerotome signaling? *Clinical Dysmorphology* 1997;**6**:303–14.

72. Prescher A, Brors D, Adam G. Anatomic and radiologic appearance of several variants of the craniocervical junction. *Skull Base Surg* 1996a;**6**: 83–94.

73. George AW. A method for more accurate study of injuries to the atlas and axis. *N Engl J Med Surg* 1919;**181**:395–8.

74. Giacomini C. Sull' esistenza dell' 'osodontoideum: nell' uomo. *Gior d R Accad Di Med Di Torino* 1886; **49**:24-8.

75. Jenkins Jr FA. The evolution and development of the dens of the mammalian axis. *Anat Rec* 1969;**164**: 173–84.

76. Starck D. Das Skelettsystem. In: Starck D (ed). *Vergleichende Anatomie der Wirbeltiere*. vol. 2. New York, Berlin, Heidelberg: Springer; 1979:44–95.

77. Nishikawa M, SakamotoH, Hakuba A, *et al*. Pathogenesis of Chiari malformation: A morphometric study of the posterior cranial fossa. *J Neurosurg* 1997; **86**:40–7.

78. Tubbs RS, Iskandar BJ, Bartolucci AA, *et al*. A critical analysis of the Chiari 1.5 malformation. *J Neurosurg* 2004;**101**:179–83.

79. Stover LJ, Bergan U, Nilsen G, *et al*. Posterior cranial fossa dimensions in the Chiari I malformation; relation to pathogenesis and clinical presentation. *Neuroradiology* 1993;**35**:113–18.

80. Vega A, Quintana F, Berciano J. Basichondro-cranium anomalies in adult Chiari type I malformation: A morphometric study. *J Neurol Sci* 1990;**99**:137–45.

81. Pollack I, Pang D, Albright LA, *et al.* Outcome following hind brain decompression of symptomatic Chiari malformations in children previously shunted with myelomeningoceles. *J Neurosurg* 1992;**77**:881–8.

82. Pollack IF, Pang D, Kocoshis S, *et al.* Neurogenic dysphagia resulting from Chiari malformations. *Neurosurg* 1992;**30**:709–19.

83. Grabb PA, Mapstone TB, Oakes WJ. Ventral brainstem compression in pediatric and young adult patients with Chiari I malformations. *Neurosurgery* 1999;**44**:520–8.

84. Ludinghausen von M, Schindler G, Kageyama I, *et al.* The third occipital condyle, a constituent part of a median occipito-atlanto-odontoid joint: A case report. *Surg Radiol Anat* 2002;**24**:71–6.

85. Kotil D, Kalayci M. Ventral cervicomedullary junction compression secondary to condylus occipitalis (median occipital condyle), a rare entity. *Spinal Disord Tech* 2005;**18.4**:382–5.

86. Prescher A. The differential diagnosis of isolated ossicles in the region of the dens axis. *Gegenbaurs Morphol Jahrb* 1990;**136**:139–54.

87. Rao P. Median (third) occipital condyle. *Clinical Anatomy* 2002;**15**:148–51.

88. Burwood RJ. The cranio-cervical junction. Thesis Anatomy University of Bristol; 1970.

89. Chevrel JP. [Occipitalization of the atlas]. *Arch Anat Pathol (Paris)* 1965;**13**:104–8.

90. Macalister A. Notes on the development and variations of the atlas. *J Anat Physiol* 1893;**27**:519–42.

91. Tramontano-Guerritore G. Die atlanto-occipital union. *Anat Anz* 1927;**64**:173–84.

92. Gholve PA, Hosalkar HS, Ricchetti ET, *et al.* Occipitalization of the atlas in children, morphologic classification, associations, and clinical relevance. *J Bone Joint Surg* 2007;**89A**:571–8.

93. McRae DL, Barnum AS. Occipitalization of the atlas. *Am J Roentgenol Radium Ther Nucl Med* 1953;**70**:23–46.

94. Torklus von D, Gehle W. Neue Perspektiven der Entwicklungsstörungen der oberen Halswirlbelsäule. *Z Orthop* 1969;**105**:78.

95. Geipel P. Zur Kenntnis der Spaltbildungen des Atlas und Epistropheus, *Teil IV. Zbl, Path* 1955;**94**:19.

96. Le Double AF. Traité des variations des os du crane de l'homme et de leur signification au point de vue de l'Anthropologie zoologique. Paris: Vigot Frères;, Paris 1903 u. 1912.

97. Devi BI, Shenoy SN, Panigrahi MK, *et al.* Arch of atlas-a rare cause of symptomatic canal stenosis in children. *Pediatric Neurosurgery* 1997;**26**:214–18.

99. Chigira M, Kaneko K, Mashio D, *et al.* Congenital hypoplasia of the arch of the atlas with abnormal segmentation of the cervical spine. *Arch Orthop Trauma Surg* 1994;**113**:110–12.

99. Logan WW, Stuard ID. Absence of posterior arch of the atlas. *AJR* 1973;**118**:431–4.

100. Schulze P, Buurman R. Absence of the posterior arch of the atlas. *AJR* 1980;**134**:178–80.

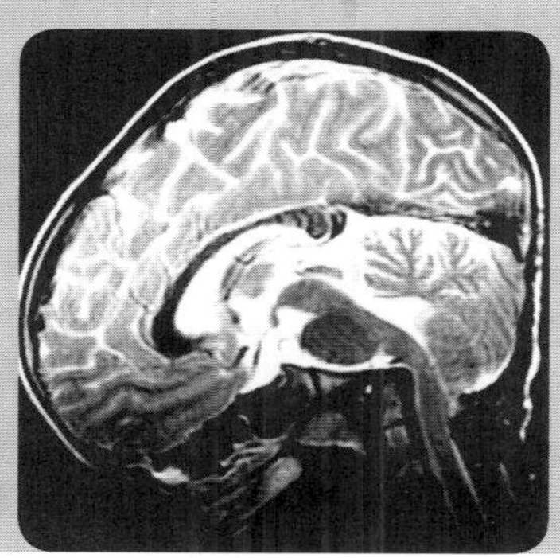

Vascular neurosurgery

5

Skull base approaches to aneurysms

R.N. BHATTACHARYA, S.K. MISHRA, M. PRASAD

Introduction

A conventional pterional approach provides access to most simple anterior circulation aneurysms. Skull base approaches are required for complex anterior and posterior circulation aneurysms. In such cases, conventional exposure can lead to inadequate visualization due to bony and/or neurovascular obstruction. To achieve adequate exposure, intolerable sustained retraction of neurovascular structures is required, which may lead to increased morbidity and mortality.

Discussion

Skull base approaches can be (i) anterolateral, (ii) lateral, (iii) posterolateral, (iv) suboccipital, and (v) transfacial/transoral.

Anterolateral approaches

These provide a low obtuse angle to work with, unlike an acute high angle as obtained by standard exposures, thereby reducing brain retraction.

- Frontozygomatic approach
- Orbitozygomatic approach
- Extended orbitozygomatic approach
- Supraorbital approach

Frontozygomatic approach

- Involves osteotomy of the zygoma
- Shortens the operative depth by 2–3 cm
- Provides exposure and access to the medial end of the sphenoid wing and floor of the middle fossa
- Structures between the anterior clinoid process and tentorial hiatus become visible
- Provides access to basilar bifurcation aneurysms.

Orbitozygomatic approach (Fig. 1)

- *Modification of the frontozygomatic approach*; includes removal of the orbital rim
- Improves access in the vertical dimension
- Provides increased freedom to manipulate in the coronal plane

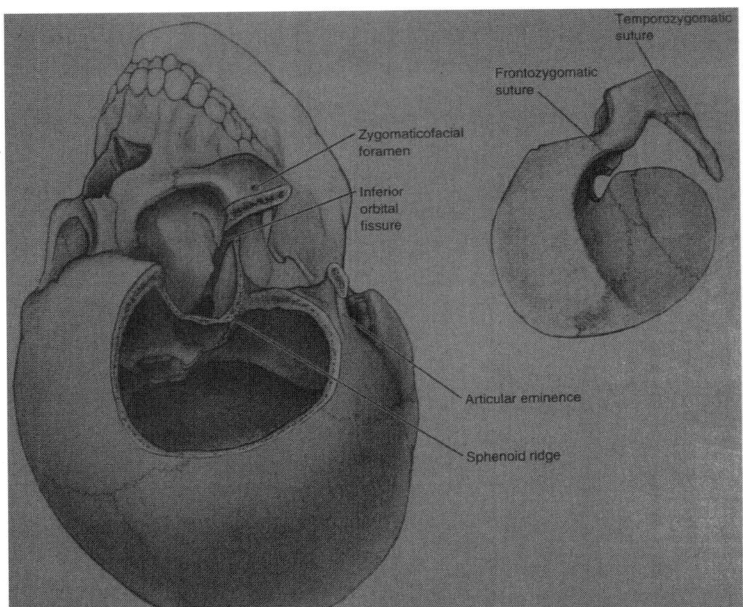

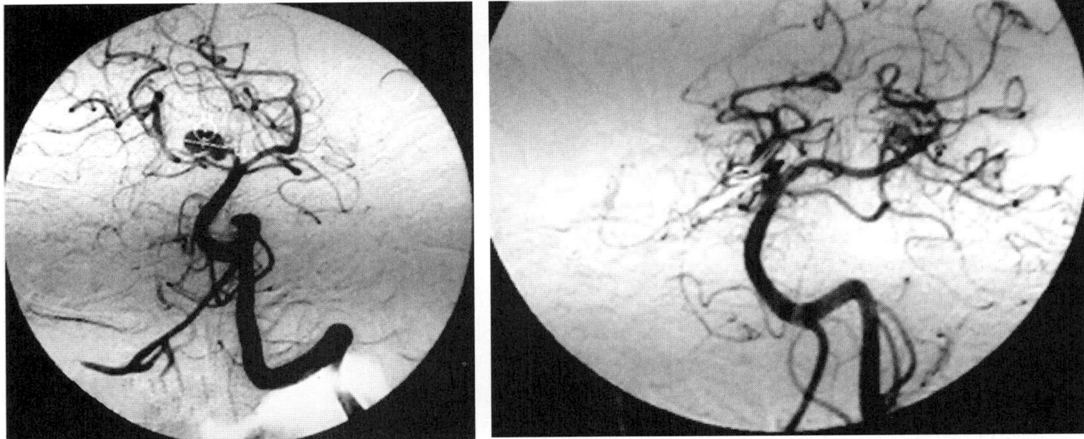

Fig. 1. Pre- and postoperative digital subtraction angiography (DSA) of a large posterior carotid artery (PCA) aneurysm clipped through the orbitozygomatic approach

- By removal of the superior orbital rim and orbital roof, a 10° angle increases, thus offering a wide angle of exposure of the basilar apex and reducing the need for brain retraction.

craniotomy, the anterior clinoid process and upper clivus are removed. This approach is particularly useful for low-lying basilar apex aneurysms.

Extended orbitozygomatic approach[1]

In addition to standard orbitozygomatic

Supraorbital keyhole approach (Figs 2 and 3)

Cosmetic advantage: Most simple anterior

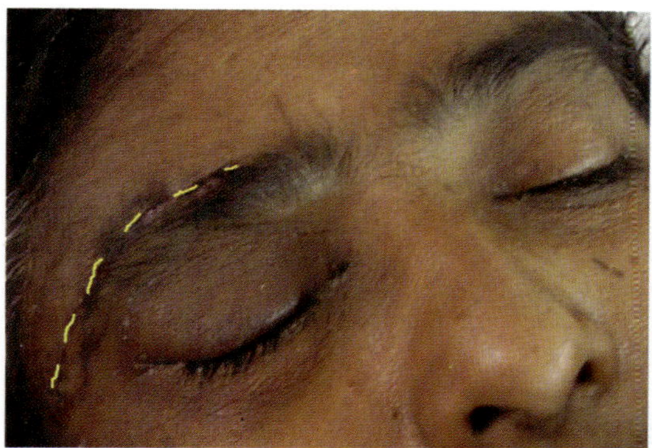

Fig. 2. Incision for the supraorbital keyhole approach

circulation aneurysms can be accessed. However, proximal control of the aneurysm as well as large aneurysms are problematic.

Lateral approaches

These involve resection of the petrous bone and are divided into anterior and posterior petrosectomy.

Anterior petrosectomy (Kawase)[2]

This is an extended middle fossa approach used for the middle basilar artery (BA). Removal of the petrous bone within the Kawase triangle (actually a rhomboid) is called anterior petrosectomy. Its boundaries are

- Mandibular nerve (V3) (anterior)
- Greater superficial petrosal nerve (GSPN) (lateral)
- Arcuate eminence (posterior)
- Inferior carotid artery (ICA) (inferior)
- Superior petrosal sinus (medial)

The disadvantage is that it provides a narrow operative corridor.

Posterior petrosectomy

- Retrolabyrinthine trans-sigmoid approach[3]

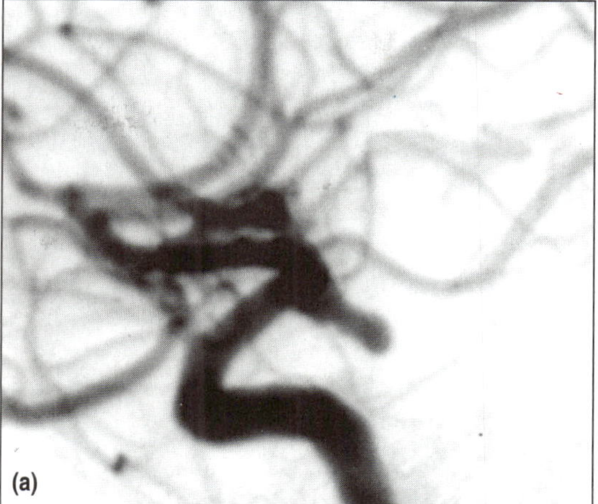

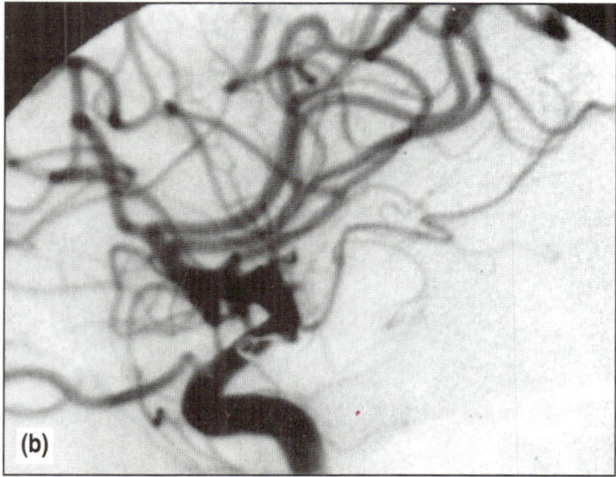

Fig. 3. Preoperative (a) and postoperative DSA (b) showing a paraposterior communicating artery aneurysm (parapcom) clipped through the supraorbital keyhole approach

- Retrolabyrinthine presigmoid approach (Fig. 4)
- Transcochlear approach
- Translabyrinthine approach

The retrolabyrinthine trans-sigmoid approach is indicated for the BA–anterior inferior cerebellar artery (AICA) junction, and lower BA and vertebral artery (VA)–BA junction. A complete mastoidectomy with skeletonization of the pre- and retrosigmoid dura and posterior semicircular canal is done, followed by division of the sigmoid sinus. This approach is not suitable for giant aneurysms or when the sigmoid sinus cannot be sacrificed.

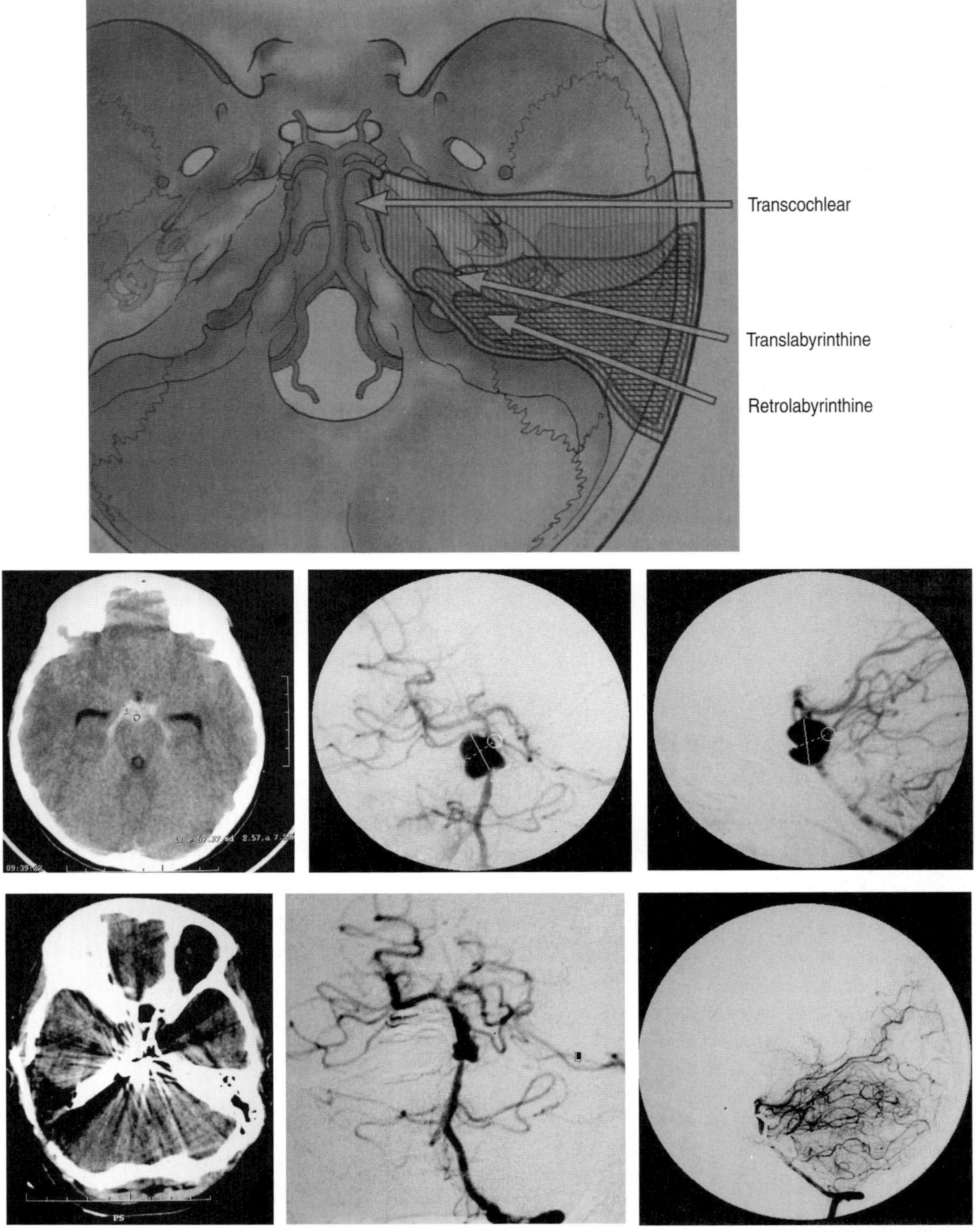

Fig. 4. Pre- and postoperative DSA showing clipping through the retrolabyrinthine presigmoid approach for a midbasilar aneurysm

The retrolabyrinthine presigmoid approach is used when the sigmoid sinus cannot be sacrificed. Transcochlear and translabyrinthine approaches damage hearing and are rarely used.

Posterolateral approaches

- Combined supra- and infratentorial approaches
- Lateral suboccipital approach
- Extreme lateral transcondylar approach

Combined supra- and infratentorial approaches

These are used to access the middle third of the BA, VA–BA junction and AICA. Despite doing such an extensive exposure, the surgical corridor is still confined and retraction of the brainstem, temporal lobe or both may be required.

Lateral suboccipital approach

This approach is used to access the proximal posterior inferior cerebellar artery (PICA) (anterior and lateral medullary segments) and proximal VA (Figs 5a and 5b).

Extreme lateral transcondylar approach[4]

This approach is used for the distal VA. It is relatively contraindicated when there is instability at the cranio-vertebral junction.

Suboccipital approach

- Midline suboccipital—Distal PICA
- Paramedian suboccipital—PICA–VA junction, proximal VA

Transfacial/transoral approaches

These approaches are uncommonly used. They can be used for the middle third of the BA and VA–BA junction as either a transoral transclival approach alone, or combined with Leforte 1 maxillotomy.[5] These are advantageous in obviating brain retraction.

The disadvantages are

- limited width of exposure
- very deep operative field
- operating through a field colonized by bacteria.

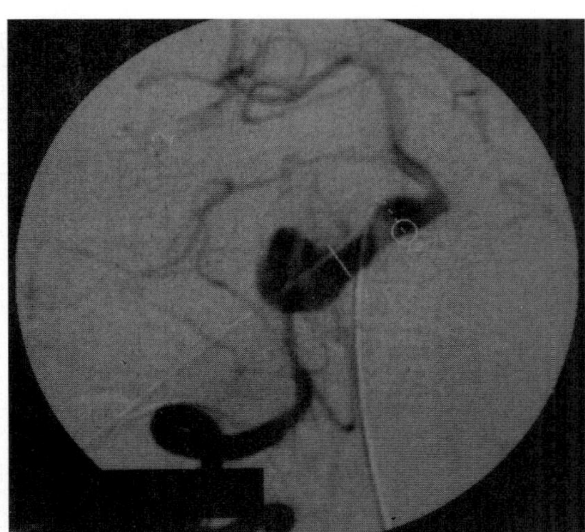

Fig. 5a. Preoperative DSA showing a giant VA dissecting aneurysm

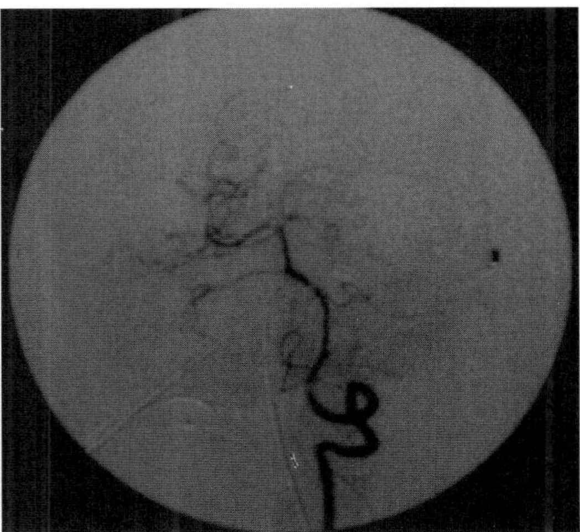

Fig. 5b. Postoperative DSA showing an excised giant VA dissecting aneurysm

Conclusion

Skull base approaches should be tailored to provide the optimal space required for accessing and obliterating aneurysms that cannot be clipped successfully by conventional approaches.

References

1. Bernardo A, Stieg PE. Orbitozygomatic approach for upper basilar aneurysms. In: Macdonald RL (ed). *Vascular neurosurgery*. New York: Thieme; 2008: 70–6.

2. Kawase T, Bertalanffy H, Otani M, *et al.* Surgical approaches for vertebrobasilar trunk aneurysms. *Acta Neurochir (Wien)* 1996;**138**:402–10.

3. Giannotta SL, Marceri DR. Retrolabyrinthine transsigmoid approach to basilar trunk and vertebrobasilar junction aneurysms. *J Neurosurg* 1988;**69**:461–6.

4. Giannotta SL. Surgical treatment of basilar trunk aneurysms. In: Le Roux PD, Winn HR, Newell DW (eds). *Management of cerebral aneurysms*. Philadelphia: Saunders; 2004:829–3.

5. Uttley D, Moore AJ. Skull base approaches for aneurysm occlusion. In: Le Roux PD, Winn HR, Newell DW (eds). *Management of cerebral aneurysms*. Philadelphia: Saunders; 2004:643–58.

6

Giant aneurysm—Quo vadis

ANIL NANDA, VIJAYAKUMAR JAVALKAR, LISSA BAIRD,
ANIRBAN DEEP BANERJEE

Introduction

Surgical clipping of a giant intracranial aneurysm is technically challenging due to the size, calcification, and direct involvement of parent and collateral branches.[1] Surgical clipping may require additional procedures such as a bypass. Endovascular treatment is favoured at many centres due to its low morbidity. Recent advances such as intracranial stents and compliant balloons have facilitated treatment of wide-necked intracranial aneurysms.[2–4] In this chapter, we review the operative experience of the primary author (AN). We also review recently published papers concerning the management of giant intracranial aneurysms.

Materials and methods

The study was approved by the Institutional Review Board of the Louisiana State University Health Sciences Center, Shreveport. The database maintained at the department of Neurosurgery, the LSUHSC-S was searched for giant intracranial aneurysms operated by the primary author (AN), which underwent surgical clipping from 2000 to 2009. Medical charts, operative reports, imaging studies and clinical follow-up evaluations were reviewed retrospectively for all the patients with giant intracranial aneurysms (≥25 mm).

Patients

Over this period we could identify 36 patients with giant intracranial aneurysms. All patients underwent surgical clipping. The size, shape, configuration of the aneurysms was assessed using cerebral angiography. In addition, MRI, MRA and CT angiography were employed for some patients. The LSUHSC-S has a fully equipped endovascular suite for the past 3 years and the feasibility of coiling/clipping was assessed by the primary author (AN) and the endovascular team.

Results

The mean age of the patients was 51 years (range 29–69 years). Females were predominant (25:11).

In 9 patients multiple aneurysms were noted. In our series giant aneurysms were most commonly located at ophthalmic internal carotid artery (ICA) (50%). Headache as a presenting symptom was noted in 70%. Seizure as a presenting symptom was noted in only 8% of the patients. Cranial nerve deficits were noted in 33%. Only 22% of the patients presented with subarachnoid haemorrhage.

Surgical approaches

Pterional craniotomy was employed in the majority (72%) followed by the orbitozygomatic (19%) and far lateral approach in 6% only.

Complications

Intraoperative complications

Intraoperative rupture was encountered in 4 cases. We observed carotid compromise in one patient and hence saphenous grafting was attempted. The other intraoperative complications were tear and occlusion of the carotid (repaired) in one case and MCA spasm in another case. In one case we observed delayed occlusion of the ICA.

Postoperative complications

We observed motor weakness in 5 cases and cranial nerve deficits in 3 cases. Postoperative CSF fistula was noted in one patient. One patient developed postoperative hydrocephalus.

Operative outcome

Glasgow Outcome Scale (GOS) was used to assess the clinical outcome. A GOS score of 5 represents an excellent outcome, 4 represents a good outcome with moderate disability, 3 represents a fair outcome with severe disability, 2 represents a poor outcome (vegetative), and 1 is dead. At the time of discharge, 61% had GOS 5, 14% had GOS 4, 8% had GOS 3 and 11% had GOS 1. Figures 1–3 elucidate the representative cases in our series.

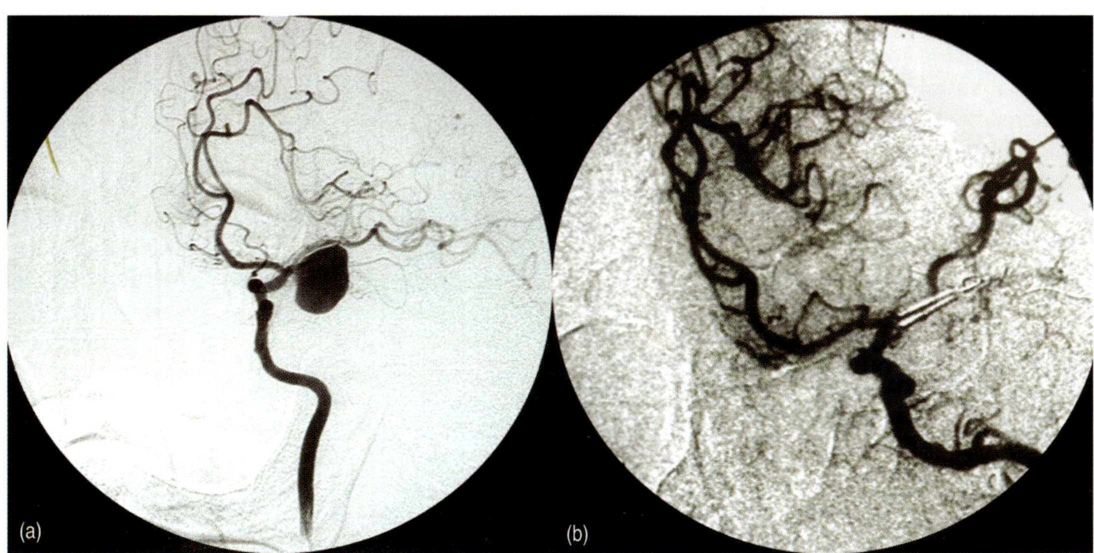

Fig. 1. Pre- (a) and post-clipping (b) images of a giant MCA aneurysm

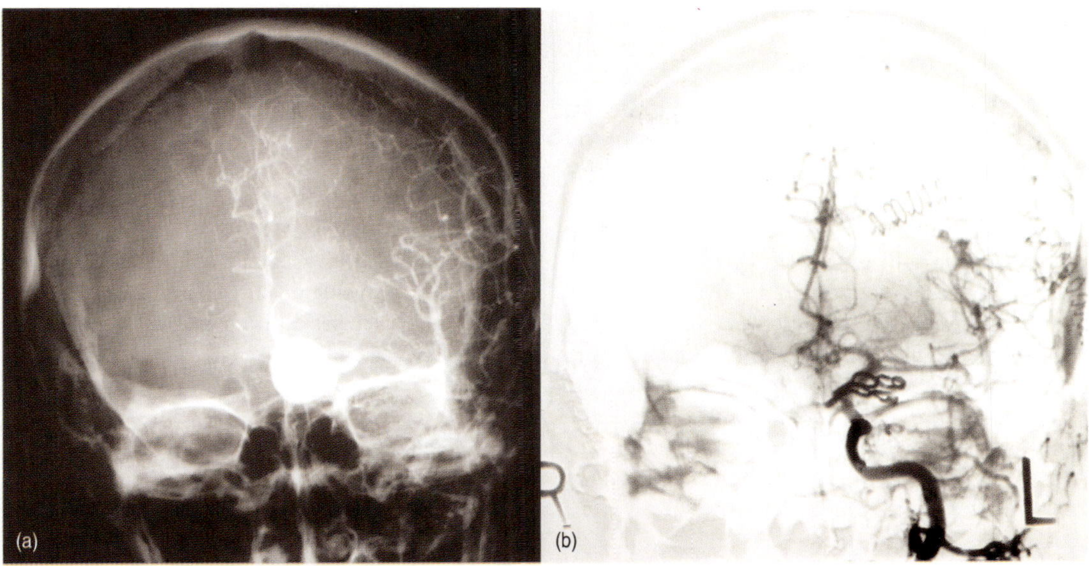

Fig. 2. Pre- (a) and post-clipping (b) images of a giant ophthalmic ICA aneurysm

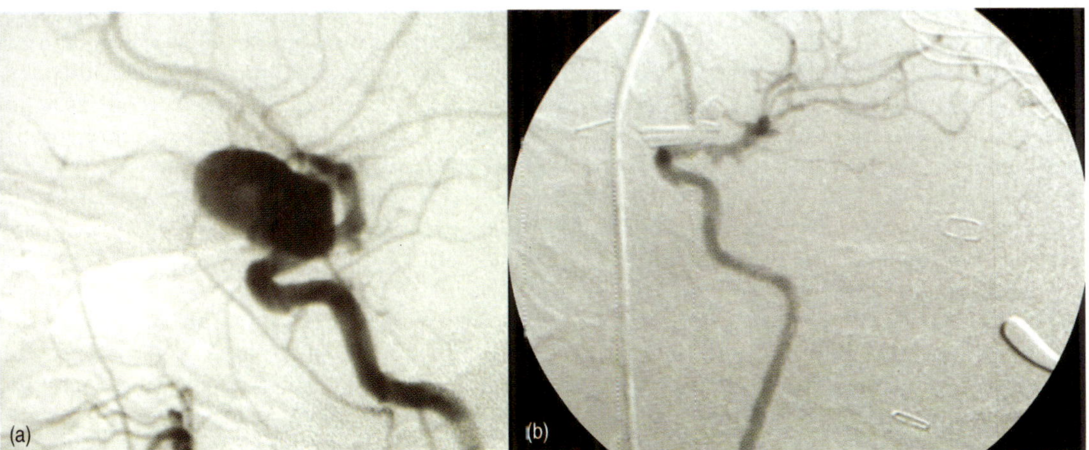

Fig. 3. Pre- (a) and post-clipping (b) images of a giant ophthalmic ICA aneurysm

Discussion

To clip or coil an aneurysm? The largest prospective randomized trial to date comparing the outcomes in coiling versus clipping was the ISAT study (International Subarachnoid Aneurysm Trial). The ISAT study, which published its report in 2002, showed that for patients with ruptured intracranial aneurysms for which endovascular and neurosurgical clipping are treatment options, the outcome in terms of survival free of disability was significantly better with endovascular coiling at one year.[5] The same group in 2005 showed that in subjects with ruptured intracranial aneurysms suitable for both treatment modalities (endovascular, clipping), endovascular coiling is more likely to result in independent survival at 1 year than clipping and the survival benefit continues for at least 7 years.[6] In 2009, it published the data regarding the risk of recurrent subarachnoid haemorrhage, death or dependence, and standardized mortality rates after clipping or coiling.[7] The study showed that there was an increased risk of rebleeding from coiled aneurysms when compared with clipped aneurysms. Twenty-four rebleeds occurred more than 1 year after treatment. Of these, 13 were from treated aneurysms (10 in the coiling group and 3 in the clipping group; log rank p=0.06 by intention-to-treat analysis).[7] The aneurysm size in the ISAT study was stratified into ≤5 mm, 6–10 mm and ≥11 mm, and there was no classification of aneurysms as 'giant' in the ISAT study.[5]

Endovascular management of giant intracranial aneurysms

Parkinson et al.[8] critically reviewed the treatment strategies for giant intracranial aneurysms by endovascular treatment (after 1994). Overall, in their analysis, 316 patients underwent treatment by endovascular means (coiling, parent vessel occlusion, onyx, stenting with or without coil/onyx). Mean complete occlusion rate or cure was achieved in only 57% of the patients with a mortality rate of 7.7%. Their critical review suggests that the results of endovascular treatment with preservation of the parent vessel are not encouraging with the current technology.[8]

Van Rooij et al.[9] reviewed their clinical experience of endovascular treatment of 232 very large and giant aneurysms. They concluded that parent vessel occlusion, when tolerated, is the endovascular therapy of choice for all large and giant aneurysms. They proposed that coiling is a low-risk alternative in patients when parent vessel occlusion is not tolerated.[9] They also concluded that selective aneurysm occlusion with onyx offers no advantage when compared with selective coiling.[9]

Jahromi et al.[10] reported long-term clinical and radiological outcome from a series of 39 giant intracranial aneurysms treated with endovascular repair in 38 patients. Ninety-five per cent or higher occlusion rates were documented in 64% of the aneurysms and a 100% occlusion rate was documented in only 36% of the aneurysms. Parent vessel preservation was maintained in only 74%. The mortality rate was 29%. The authors conclude that endovascular therapy can provide a useful alternative to an open surgical procedure when the surgical risk is high and in patients with systemic comorbidities.[10]

Surgical management of giant intracranial aneurysms

Cantore et al.[1] reviewed their operative experience of giant intracranial aneurysms treated with surgical clipping or high flow extracranial–intracranial (EC–IC) bypass. A total of 99 patients were treated by surgery; of these, 58 underwent surgical clipping and 41 underwent EC–IC bypass followed by aneurysm trapping. The mortality rate with surgical clipping was 6.9% whereas it was 9.8% with EC–IC bypass. The graft patency rate was 93%. The choice of treatment plan (direct clipping vs high flow EC–IC bypass plus trapping) for supraclinoid aneurysms depends on the surgeon's experience and other factors such as the size of the neck, calcification and fusiform dilatations.[1] These authors believe that the reference standard for giant intracranial aneurysm is direct surgical clipping.

Sharma et al.[11] reviewed their operative experience with 181 giant aneurysms (177 patients) of which 107 aneurysms (103 patients) underwent direct surgical clipping. Forty-six patients with good collateral circulation were treated by gradual occlusion and ligation of the ICA in the neck. Nine patients with good collateral circulation, but persisting symptoms after ICA ligation, required trapping for obliteration of the aneurysm. Eleven patients with poor collateral circulation required EC–IC bypass before proximal ICA ligation. The total treatment mortality rate was 9%. Overall, the outcome was excellent in 131 (74.0%), good in 22 (12.4%), and poor in 8 (4.5%) patients. These authors believe that direct surgical clipping is safe and effective, and needs to be considered as a first line of treatment.

Hauck *et al.*[12] reviewed their operative experience of 62 patients with unruptured large or giant intracranial aneurysms. Complete aneurysm occlusion (100%) was achieved in 90% of patients and the surgical risk in patients less than 50 years of age was 8%. They conclude that surgical clipping is the treatment of choice in patients less than 50 years of age. When the giant aneurysms incorporate branches or the presence of intraluminal thrombus, calcification can be managed with a team approach by employing coil embolization after surgical bypass.[13]

Conclusion

Even with the advances in endovascular coiling and the evolution of surgical strategies, it is still not very clear what the optimal strategy for managing these aneurysms should be. Each and every aneurysm is a different case and the strategy to manage these lesions should be based on the experience of the surgeon and the characteristics of the aneurysm. A combined team approach would be an optimal strategy for the management of these lesions.

References

1. Cantore G, Santoro A, Guidetti G, *et al.* Surgical treatment of giant intracranial aneurysms: Current viewpoint. *Neurosurgery* 2008;**63**:279–89; discussion 289–90.
2. Kessler IM, Mounayer C, Piotin M, *et al.* The use of balloon-expandable stents in the management of intracranial arterial diseases: A 5-year single-center experience. *AJNR Am J Neuroradiol* 2005;**26**:2342–3.
3. Kis B, Weber W, Berlit P, *et al.* Elective treatment of saccular and broad-necked intracranial aneurysms using a closed-cell nitinol stent (Leo). *Neurosurgery* 2006;**58**:443–50; discussion 443–50.
4. Sluzewski M, van Rooij WJ, Beute GN, *et al.* Balloon-assisted coil embolization of intracranial aneurysms: Incidence, complications, and angiography results. *J Neurosurg* 2006;**105**:396–9.
5. Molyneux A, Kerr R, Stratton I, *et al.* International Subarachnoid Aneurysm Trial (ISAT) of neurosurgical clipping versus endovascular coiling in 2143 patients with ruptured intracranial aneurysms: A randomised trial. *Lancet* 2002;**360**:1267–74.
6. Molyneux AJ, Kerr RS, Yu LM, *et al.* International subarachnoid aneurysm trial (ISAT) of neurosurgical clipping versus endovascular coiling in 2143 patients with ruptured intracranial aneurysms: A randomised comparison of effects on survival, dependency, seizures, rebleeding, subgroups, and aneurysm occlusion. *Lancet* 2005;**366**:809–17.
7. Molyneux AJ, Kerr RS, Birks J, *et al.* Risk of recurrent subarachnoid haemorrhage, death, or dependence and standardised mortality ratios after clipping or coiling of an intracranial aneurysm in the International Subarachnoid Aneurysm Trial (ISAT): Long-term follow-up. *Lancet Neurol* 2009;**8**:427–33.
8. Parkinson RJ, Eddleman CS, Batjer HH, *et al.* Giant intracranial aneurysms: Endovascular challenges. *Neurosurgery* 2008;**62**:1336–45.
9. van Rooij WJ, Sluzewski M. Endovascular treatment of large and giant aneurysms. *AJNR Am J Neuroradiol* 2009;**30**:12–18.
10. Jahromi BS, Mocco J, Bang JA, *et al.* Clinical and angiographic outcome after endovascular management of giant intracranial aneurysms. *Neurosurgery* 2008;**63**:662–74; discussion 674–5.
11. Sharma BS, Gupta A, Ahmad FU, *et al.* Surgical management of giant intracranial aneurysms. *Clin Neurol Neurosurg* 2008;**110**:674–81.
12. Hauck EF, Wohlfeld B, Welch BG, *et al.* Clipping of very large or giant unruptured intracranial aneurysms in the anterior circulation: An outcome study. *J Neurosurg* 2008;**109**:1012–18.
13. Shi ZS, Ziegler J, Duckwiler GR, *et al.* Management of giant middle cerebral artery aneurysms with incorporated branches: Partial endovascular coiling or combined extracranial–intracranial bypass—a team approach. *Neurosurgery* 2009;**65**:121–29; discussion 129–31.

7

Intracranial dural arteriovenous fistulae

ARVIND NANDA, HARSH RASTOGI

Introduction

Intracranial dural arteriovenous fistulae (DAVF) are uncommon lesions. Their true incidence is unknown. DAVF are abnormal arteriovenous connections within the dura and are usually located within the walls of the dural sinus or an adjacent cortical vein. DAVF tend to present later in life than arteriovenous malformations (AVMs).

DAVF were first described by Sachs and Tonnis (Aminoff, 1973),[1] and are defined as abnormal connections between the arterial and venous side of the vascular tree located on the surface of the dura mater. Arterial supply is provided by the meningeal branches, and either the dural sinuses or meningeal or subarachnoid veins drain the lesion. Occasionally, as a fistula grows or becomes more diffuse, pial recruitment from parenchymal vessels can occur.

DAVF comprise 10%–15% of all intracranial AVMs (Newton and Cronqvist, 1969). There is a female preponderance with symptoms usually developing during middle to late adulthood. The initiating events which lead to the development of a DAVF are not clear, but there are many papers reporting an association with trauma, infection, recent surgery and dural sinus thrombosis. On the other hand, in many patients with this disorder, none of the stated causative factors can be probed from the patient's history. The causative factors listed above are common but DAVF are rare lesions. Lasjaunias and Berenstein[2] have suggested 'an underlying dural weakness' facilitating dural shunts in some individuals, while other people faced with the same insults do not develop DAVF.

Aetiology and pathogenesis

DAVF are relatively rare lesions. Originally, these were thought to be congenital. However, many DAVF have been proved to be acquired. It is hypothesized that DAVF develop either by the opening of existing microshunts within the dura or by angiogenesis, leading to the development of new shunts.

The triggering factor for the development of DAVF is thought to be a change of the normal arteriovenous pressure gradient within the dura. Either elevation of the arterial pressure (arterial hypertension) or increase in the venous pressure (venous hypertension) may dilate existing arteriovenous communications leading to haemodynamically significant shunts.

While the predisposing factor for the development of a permanent DAVF remains unknown, several events may increase the venous pressure and serve as a trigger. These include developmental anomalies of the venous system, venous thrombosis, and head trauma or transcranial surgery.

It is presumed that head trauma caused by the either surgery or injury may induce venous thrombosis or at least alteration of the venous outflow, subsequently resulting in changes in the arteriovenous pressure gradient (Lasjaunias and Berenstein, 1987).[2] The frequent coincidence of DAVF with previous major surgery (other than transcranial) and child delivery suggests that increased systemic thrombotic activity may also serve as a trigger. DAVF occurring in association with pregnancy and the menopausal period suggests that hormonal changes may play a role, potentially by inducing increased angiogenesis (Djindjan and Merland, 1978).[3]

The natural course of DAVF is variable with some cases regressing spontaneously, as in some angiographically documented cases of carotid–cavernous fistulas. Other DAVF may progress to aggressive lesions leading to severe clinical abnormalities with recruitment of arterial supply from additional vessels and hypertrophy of existing ones. Sometimes partial or incomplete treatment of benign lesions can convert DAVF to aggressive lesions.

Over the years, the angioarchitecture of DAVF was documented more precisely and many cases were followed up over time. It was stated by many authors that DAVF were 'venous' lesions, meaning that the natural history, symptomatology as well as prognosis of the disease were dependent on venous features.

Symptoms and signs

Intracranial DAVF are rare in infancy and childhood. The most common symptoms are headache, pulsatile tinnitus and/or bruit, cranial nerve palsies, ocular symptoms including proptosis and chemosis ('red eye'), optic nerve atrophy, papilloedema, nausea/vomiting as signs of raised intracranial tension, epileptic seizures and focal neurological deficit. Some cases with an aggressive clinical course may present with signs of raised intracranial pressure due to intracranial haemorrhage or infarction. High-flow fistulae that typically present in infants and children may lead to heart failure.

Potential pathomechanisms include venous congestion, perfusion deficit due to venous hypertension, mass effect and arterial steal phenomenon. DAVF in the anterior cranial fossa frequently present with intradural bleeding.

Cavernous sinus DAVF present with proptosis, chemosis, ocular movement disorder due to VI/III nerve palsy (due to mass effect) leading to diplopia, retinal haemorrhage, reduced vision, pulsatile tinnitus and bruit. Transverse and sigmoid sinus DAVF present with pulsatile bruit.

DAVF involving the confluence of sinuses tend to be large with exceedingly high flow and with reflux into the straight and superior sagittal sinuses producing haemorrhagic and non-haemorrhagic neurological complications.

DAVF located on the tentorium frequently bleed. Lesions in the posterior fossa and particularly those of the clivus and foramen magnum may drain into the spinal medullary veins that typically produce spinal venous hypertension, resulting in myelopathy and neurological deficit.

DAVF of the superior sagittal sinus produce a complex neurological picture due to raised intracranial tension. They present as headache and papilloedema, visual disturbances, progressive dementia, neurological deficits and seizures.

Classification

There have been many attempts to classify DAVF, and presently two main classification schemes have gained acceptance. One classification is according to the venous drainage pattern, which has many important implications for prognosis, and another one classifies DAVF according to location, which is more practical and used more frequently in daily practice.

The venous drainage pattern of DAVF is very important. As the high arteriovenous shunting in DAVF continues, there is progressive pathology on the venous side. A high-flow vascular malformation drains into the intracranial veins and dural sinuses, especially in the presence of additional disturbing factors such as venous occlusion and reflux into the cortical veins. This results in intracranial venous hypertension, which is a crucial factor predisposing to an aggressive disease course. The two commonly used classification systems are shown in Tables 1 and 2. There are only 3 subtypes in the Borden classification. However, the Cognard classification

Table 1. The Borden classification system

Type 1	DAVF drainage into a dural venous sinus or meningeal vein with normal antegrade flow; usually benign clinical behaviour
Type II	Antegrade drainage into a dural venous sinus and onwards but retrograde flow occurs in the cortical veins; may present with haemorrhage
Type III	Direct retrograde flow of blood from the fistula into the cortical veins causing venous hypertension with a risk of haemorrhage

Table 2. The Cognard classification system

Type 1	Normal antegrade flow into a dural venous sinus
Type IIa	Drainage into a sinus with retrograde flow within the sinus
Type IIb	Drainage into a sinus with retrograde flow into cortical vein(s)
Type IIa+b	Drainage into a sinus with retrograde flow within the sinus and cortical vein(s)
Type III	Direct drainage into a cortical vein without venous ectasia
Type IV	Direct drainage into a cortical vein with ectasia >5 mm and 3x larger than the diameter of the draining vein
Type V	Direct drainage into spinal perimedullary veins

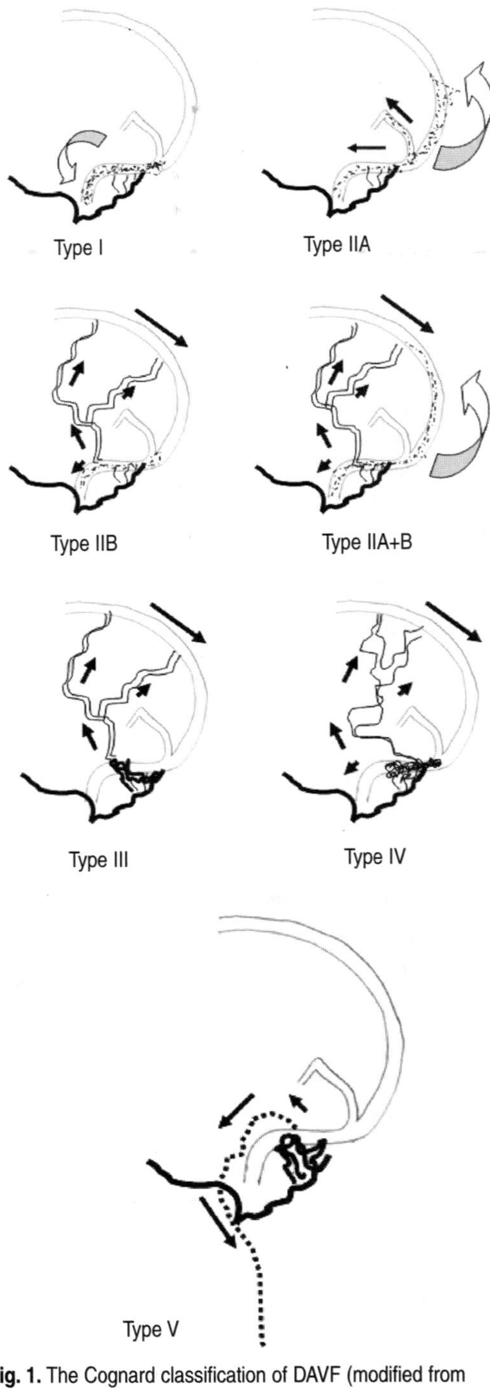

Fig. 1. The Cognard classification of DAVF (modified from Cognard C)

is more detailed and elaborates on the direction of flow, whether normal (antegrade) or retro-grade, and the presence or absence of cortical venous recruitment. In addition, spinal perimedullary venous drainage is specifically recognized.

Classification according to location

When classified according to location, transverse sigmoid sinus DAVF make up the majority of DAVF. Cavernous sinus DAVF (10%–16%), tentorial DAVF (8%–12%), superior sagittal sinus DAVF (8%) and anterior cranial fossa DAVF (5%) and rare locations (torcula, foramen magnum, and deep venous fistula) are other types of DAVF (Table 3).

Imaging

CT, MRI and angiography all have roles to play in the investigation of patients with a possible

Table 3. Venous drainage pathways of intracranial DAVF in different locations

Location	Potential venous drainage pathway
Anterior fossa	Olfactory vein, frontal veins
Cavernous sinus	Contralateral cavernous sinus, ophthalmic veins, inferior petrosal sinus, temporal veins
Transverse sigmoid sinus	Sigmoid sinus, jugular vein, straight sinus, superior sagittal sinus
Confluence of sinuses	Superior sagittal sinus, transverse sinus, straight sinus, occipital veins, temporal veins
Tentorium	Superior petrosal sinus, petrous vein, tentorial veins, vein of Rosenthal, lateral mesencephalic vein, spinal perimedullary veins
Foramen magnum	Clival venous plexus, spinal perimedullary veins

DAVF. Because the clinical and imaging features can be non-specific, the diagnosis of a DAVF is often delayed or missed. Occasionally, plain films can demonstrate grooving within the skull vault due to chronic compression from enlarged middle meningeal vessels.

If haemorrhage is suspected, non-enhanced CT is a prerequisite. Venous congestion may appear as an area of low density on CT. In most institutions CT is more readily available and cheaper than MRI and so becomes the first-line investigation for patients presenting with tinnitus, headache or other vague neurological symptoms. Multi-detector CT angiography (MDCTA) can now provide high-resolution detail of the vascular anatomy.

T_2-weighted MRI is more sensitive to white matter changes due to venous congestion or infarction when compared with CT. It has the drawback of being less sensitive to the changes of acute haemorrhage. If dilated cortical veins are present they may be seen on conventional spin echo sequences and visualized using MR angiographic techniques such as phase-contrast venography or contrast-enhanced MR angio-graphy.

Benign disease, without cortical venous reflux, can be missed using both CT and MRI. Conventional catheter angiography therefore remains the investigation of choice if there is a strong clinical suspicion of a fistula.

Treatment

Currently available therapeutic options include no treatment, conservative treatment, palliative or definitive endovascular treatment, and surgery and radiosurgery. The natural history of DAVF may vary, from spontaneous cure to fatal haemorrhage. With this large spectrum, it is not the diagnosis but rather the expected prognosis of the disease which should indicate treatment. This makes proper classification of patients by angiography mandatory.

Conservative treatment

This option is offered to patients with Borden type 1 fistula who most often have a lesion on the cavernous sinus or on the transverse/sigmoid sinuses. It has two components: manual compression is used to facilitate spontaneous closure of the fistula. Medical treatment is used to control ocular symptoms if present. Treatment is dependent on the clinical picture and the grade of fistula. A multidisciplinary approach involving a neurosurgeon and a neuroradiologist is required.

In case of benign transverse sinus fistulae, the pulsating occipital artery can be compressed over the mastoid by the patient for up to 30 minutes per treatment. This may reduce flow and induce spontaneous thrombosis.

Patients who have DAVF in the cavernous sinus can be treated with compression of common carotid artery–jugular vein complex on the side of the fistula and is called the 'Matas manoeuvre'. As this manipulation carries some risk, patients with atherosclerotic carotid disease should not be so treated. Patients are instructed to compress with their contralateral hand, so that if cerebral ischaemia occurs resulting in motor weakness it will automatically interrupt the procedure. The suspected mechanism is simultaneous decrease of arterial and increase of venous pressure, prompting thrombosis of the arteriovenous connection.

In cavernous sinus DAVF the ocular symptoms require ophthalmological and medical therapy, including control of the intraocular pressure and protective treatment of the conjunctiva in cases of extensive chemosis. Mild diuresis using furosemide (Lasix) 5–10 mg/day provides significant relief from the external ocular symptoms. Visual acuity, the fundus and intraocular pressure should be periodically checked in patients on conservative treatment.

Endovascular treatment

The goal of aggressive treatment of a DAVF can be as follows:

- cure of the lesion
- conversion of a high-risk fistula to a low-risk one
- palliation of symptoms caused by a low-risk lesion.

The pathological entity of DAVF seems to be located within the wall of the dural sinuses, veins or leptomeningeal veins. The pathophysiological effect of the shunt is exercised on the venous system. Complete and permanent cure can be achieved only by closing all pathological connections between the arterial and venous side of the lesion. This can be achieved by following techniques:

- Transarterial route using particles, glue, coils. Onyx, a liquid embolic agent, has become the agent of choice in a majority of DAVF.
- Transvenous route using coils; glue is less commonly used
- Surgical route
- Combined endovascular and surgical routes are used in complex cases.
- Stereotactic radiation is rarely used.

Summary

DAVF can present in a variety of ways and their diagnosis can be missed on conventional cross-sectional imaging. Conventional catheter angiography remains the investigation of choice if the diagnosis is clinically suspected. A spectrum of pathology exists ranging from the benign to the life-threatening. Treatment is indicated in aggressive disease. This is characterized by cortical venous reflux on angiographic investigations. A multidisciplinary approach is required before considering treatment, which can be surgical, endovascular or occasionally radio-surgical. Endovascular treatment is being increasingly used to achieve complete cure of complex DAVF.

References

1. Sachs E. *The diagnosis and treatment of brain tumors.* St Louis, Mo: Mosby; 1931:168–71.
2. Lasjaunias P, Berenstein A. *Surgical neuroangiography, Vol 2, Endovascular treatment of craniofacial lesions.* Berlin, Heidelberg, New York: Springer; 1987:273–315.
3. Djindjan R, Merland JJ, Theron J. *Superselective arteriography of external carotid artery.* New York: Springer Verlag; 1978:606–28.

Suggested reading

1. Szikora I. Dural arteriovenous malformations. In: Frosting M (ed). *Intracranial vascular malformations and aneurysms.* Springer-Verlag; 2006:101–42.
2. William E, Whitefield. Intracranial dural arteriovenous fistulae. *ACNR* Vol. 7, No. 3, 10–12.
3. Newton TH, Cronqvist S. Involvement of dural arteries in intracranial arteriovenous malformations. *Radiology* 1969;**93**:1071–8.
4. Kirist SA. Intracranial dural arteriovenous fistulas: A brief review on classification and general features. *Turkish Neurosurgery* 2006;**16**:57–64.

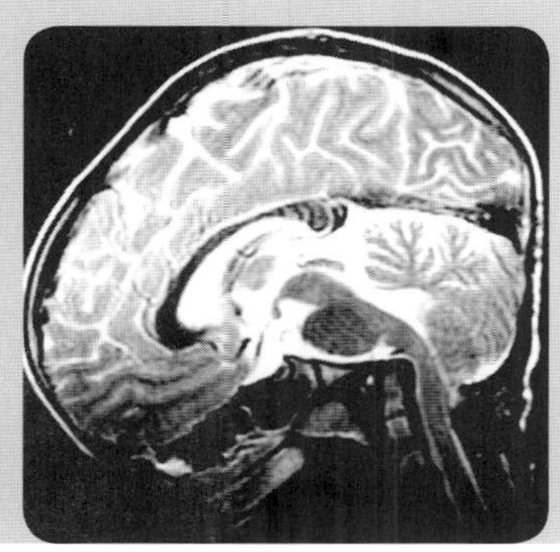

Skull base surgery

8

Evolution and future of skull base surgery: The paradigm of skull base meningiomas

SALVATORE DI MAIO, MANUEL FERRIERA, D. RAMANATHAN,
R. GARCIA-LOPEZ, MICHAEL H. ROCHA, LALIGAM N. SEKHAR

ABSTRACT

Skull base meningiomas represent the paradigm for the evolution of skull base surgery within the past 50 years into a distinct neurosurgical subspecialty. The evolution of surgical approaches to skull base meningiomas is reviewed, together with the current issues regarding radiation therapy, management of cavernous sinus tumour, oncological management of atypical and malignant sub-types, and molecular genetics and future therapeutic options.

Up to as recently as the 1970s, the diagnosis of a cranial base meningioma implied for the majority of patients a dismal prognosis, leading to severe functional impairment or death, either from natural progression or futile surgical efforts. The evolution of skull base surgery as a neurosurgical subspecialty, with refinement of circumferential skull base approaches and micro-surgical techniques have since revolutionized outcomes for these patients. The management of skull base meningiomas has further evolved from a purely surgical endeavour to one comp-lemented by advanced imaging techniques and neuronavigation, preoperative embolization, radiotherapy and radiosurgery techniques, and more recently, experimental drug therapy, advances in genetic profiling, and overall oncological management. Skull base meningiomas are thus the paradigm for the evolution of skull base surgery into a distinct and fascinating subspecialty. This chapter outlines the history and development of skull base surgery as a separate subspecialty, the particular issues surrounding the management of skull base meningiomas, the introduction of radiation therapy techniques, the use of the endoscope, and future trends in the management of skull base meningiomas.

History of meningioma surgery

The history of meningioma surgery has been eloquently described previously by Al-Rodhan and Laws in 1990.[1] After documented failed attempts by Heister in 1743 and others,[2] Professor Zanobi Pecchioli in Siena, Italy, resected an ulcerated tumour from the right sinciput in July 1835.[3] He was discharged 4 months later, and remained recurrence-free for 30 months.[4] Similarly, William Williams Keen performed the first successful removal of an intracranial meningioma in the USA in December 1887.[5]

The first successful operation for a cranial base meningioma was performed by Francesco Durante in Rome in 1884, which he reported in *The Lancet*.[6] Durante, originally from Sicily, localized an olfactory groove tumour in a 35-year-old woman based on a history of anosmia, memory and cognitive impairment and a subtle displacement of the left globe. He performed an osteoplastic craniotomy of multiple bone flap fragments using a scalpel and mallet and, after a fairly uneventful tumour resection, a drainage tube was temporarily left from the resection cavity to the 'left nasal fossa' through the ethmoid sinus, followed by nasal packing in the form of an iodoform tampon. The entire operation lasted 'about an hour', and the patient made an excellent recovery with prolonged (>10 years) survival.[7] William Macewen at the Royal Infirmary in Glasgow, Scotland, concurrently resected an olfactory groove meningioma in a 14-year-old girl using an antiseptic trephining technique.[8]

Harvey Cushing is pre-eminent in the history of meningioma surgery. Having first coined the term 'meningioma' in 1922[9] and published his famous text, *Meningiomas, their classification, regional behaviour, life history, and surgical end results*, in 1938.[10] Following his inaugural utilization of William Bovie's electorsurgical unit in 1926, surgical morbidity and mortality during meningioma surgery was dramatically reduced.[11] Numerous other pioneering developments, including progress in anaesthesia and neuro-anaesthesia,[12] of which Cushing's legacy is again celebrated (the ether charts, blood pressure measurement during anaesthesia, and employment of the first neuroanaesthetist[13]), the transition from trephine to the 'modern neurosurgical engine',[14] neuroradiology,[15] incorporation of the operating microscope,[16] all formed the basis of neurosurgery as it is performed today and the cradle for the eventual evolution of modern skull base neurosurgery.

Epidemiology and natural history of skull base meningiomas

Meningiomas occur with an annual population incidence of 6.0 per 100,000 person-years,[17] and have recently surpassed gliomas as the most common primary brain and central nervous system tumour in the USA, accounting for 33.8% of all tumours.[18] Meningiomas of the cranial base account for approximately 25% of all meningiomas,[19] with a reported ratio of calvarial to skull base distribution of 2.3:1.[20] From the anterior to posterior skull base, typical tumour locations are subject to various terminologies but include: olfactory groove; planum sphenoidale and tuberculum sellae; optic nerve sheath; sphenocavernous; hyperostosing sphenoorbital; cavernous sinus; tentorial; petroclival and clival; cerebellopontine angle (petrous ridge); jugular foramen; and lower clival and foramen magnum.

A number of studies have examined the natural history of untreated and residual meningiomas,[21–31] including a systematic review of the literature.[32] Composite data, the majority of which is from convexity, falx and parasagittal meningiomas, demonstrated that 51% of asymptomatic meningiomas with an initial diameter ≤2.5 cm did not demonstrate growth on serial imaging over a median follow-up of 4.6 years;[32] however, natural history was substantially affected by meningioma location. For instance, in one series of primarily observed petroclival meningiomas, serial growth was demonstrated in 76% of 21 patients over a mean follow-up of 82 months.[26] The definition of growth, both in natural history and treatment (typically radiation therapy) studies is variable and sometimes insensitive; for example, growth defined as an increase ≥2 mm in any one axis. Volumetric assessment has been shown to be more accurate and sensitive, particularly given the often irregular morphology of many cranial base tumours.[21]

As a group, they are challenging lesions to achieve a grade 0 or 1 resection, and are thus associated with a higher recurrence rate relative to non-skull base meningiomas.[33] Furthermore, their generally histologically benign nature demands a well-conceived long-term treatment plan minimizing treatment morbidity to preserve quality of life.[34]

Development of skull base surgery

Skull base surgery developed as a specialty in late 1980s, and, despite detractors, gained considerable acceptance and popularity in the 1990s. Among the key elements of skull base surgery pertinent to meningiomas include: the extension of traditional cranial exposures to include the skull base to minimize brain injury, and provide enhanced exposure; the use of tumour resection techniques that minimize brain resection or retraction, cranial nerve or vascular injury, and, for benign or locally aggressive pathology, to provide gross total tumour resection; reconstructive techniques to overcome vascular (and to a lesser degree cranial nerve) injuries, in the form of bypasses; reconstructive and closure techniques to eliminate CSF leaks or infection, and to promote a good cosmetic and functional outcome; postoperative and follow-up care to optimize recovery; and interdisciplinary collaboration (for example, preoperative embolization, adjuvant radiation therapy) as needed. A selected list from the many contributions to the development of modern skull base approaches is shown in Table 1 and can be also found elsewhere both for skull base[35,36] and endoscopic neurosurgery.[37,38]

Goals of meningioma surgery

Regardless of meningioma location, treatment objectives for cranial base meningiomas can been

Table 1. Selected key contributions in the evolution of modern skull base surgery

Author and year	Comment
Ketcham (1963)[130]	Craniofacial resection for anterior skull base malignancy
House (1964)[131]	Translabyrinthine approach to acoustic tumours
Parkinson (1965)[83] and Dolenc (1989)[85]	Anatomy and surgical approaches to the cavernous sinus
Fisch (1978, 1982)[132,133]	Infratemporal fossa approach
	Classificiation and surgery for glomus jugulare tumours
Jane (1982)[134]	Supraorbital approach
Yasargil (1984)[135]	Pterional approach
Malis (1985)[136]	Combined subtemporal suboccipital approach
Hakuba (1986)[137]	Orbitozygomatic approach
Sekhar and Schramm (1987)[138]	Preauricular subtemporal–infratemporal approach
	First comprehensive skull base surgery programme in North America
Samii (1988)[139]	Supra-infratentorial pre-sigmoid approach
Al-Mefty (1988)[140]	Posterior transpetrosal approach
Kawase (1991)[141]	Anterior transpetrosal–transtentorial approach
Crockard (1985)[142]	Transoral approach to the lower clivus and upper cervical spine
Sen and Sekhar (1990)[143] and Sekhar (1994)[144]	Extreme lateral transcondylar approach

summarized in the following manner:

1. *Complete tumour resection*
   Extent of resection has been demonstrated to be the primary prognostic factor of long-term freedom from recurrence.[39–41] Simpson grade I removal is associated with 4%–15% long-term recurrence.[42] With seemingly aggressive resection, delayed recurrences are known to occur.[43] For convexity meningiomas, gross total resection, including a generous tumour-free dural margin,[44] can be curative, particularly for WHO grade I benign lesions. Although the value of gross total resection for meningiomas in various subsets of the cranial base has not been systematically analysed, a number of series have indirectly demonstrated the value of maximal removal on long-term recurrence.[19,45–49] Furthermore, cranial base meningiomas appear to be histologically distinct from non-skull base tumours, as a greater proportion of these tumours are benign (WHO grade 1) with lower MIB-1 labelling indices.[30,51] Maximal resection would thus be more likely to spare the patient from requiring postoperative irradiation, in addition to reducing the recurrence rate. The likelihood of achieving a gross total resection of skull base meningiomas is related to a number of factors[52] such as prior radiation therapy, multiple cranial fossa involvement, vessel encasement, and preoperative cranial nerve deficits, in addition to differences in local expertise in skull base techniques.

2. *Preservation of patient's function and quality of life*
   Patients with cranial base meningiomas frequently present with minimal functional impairment, for which surgery or other therapies can at best aim to preserve. All patients prefer a recovery to full function, and any attempts to achieve a gross total resection should be tempered by the potential consequences to this goal. Critical appraisal of outcomes should be location specific and ideally include appropriate ophthalmological, endocrine, cosmetic and cognitive evaluations as well as return to work and preoperative level of activity. In addition, there has been recent scientific focus on measuring and reporting more subjective outcomes such as level of satisfaction with care and quality of life following treatment for skull base malignancies, including meningiomas,[53] although the literature on this topic remains sparse compared to other histologies and disciplines.[34,54–56] Interestingly, extent of resection was identified in multivariate regression to predict health-related quality of life following meningioma surgery.[57]

3. When this is not possible, a reasonable goal would be at least independence for daily living (KPS ≥70)

4. *Adjuvant or alternative treatment*
   When complete tumour resection is not possible due to 2, or 3 above, adjuvant or alternative treatment, typically in the form of fractionated radiotherapy or stereotactic radiosurgery, should be implemented, with the intended objective of preserving goals 1 to 3.

Radiotherapy and radiosurgery

Conformal radiation therapy techniques have been particularly useful for skull base meningiomas, where sparing of critical structures such as cranial nerves, pituitary gland and the brainstem are relevant. Fractionated techniques offer the advantage of relative sparing of radio-sensitive structures such as the optic apparatus, as well as treatment of tumours larger than the approximate radiosurgery threshold of 3 cm.

Stereotactic radiosurgery was first innovated in 1951 by Lars Leksell and Borje Larsson;[58] the first Gamma Knife unit was subsequently developed by Leksell in 1968, with which he initially treated two patients with intractable pain.[59] By 1971, the first meningioma was treated using the gamma knife by Backlund.[60] Following contributions by Steiner and Lunsford, gamma knife units have since been popularized all over the world, and the new generation PerfeXion gamma knife (AB Elekta, Stockholm, Sweden) should prove to advance cranial radiosurgery further.[61] Currently an extensive literature of various radiation techniques for cranial base meningiomas has been published, including Gamma Knife, Linear Accelerator-based systems, and the robotically operated Cyberknife both as primary treatment and as adjuvant therapy following subtotal surgical resection.[62,63] General considerations of stereotactic radiosurgery techniques over fractionated radiotherapy include availability, convenience of single versus fractionated treatments, smaller tumour size (up to 3 cm), limited extent of brainstem effacement, and adequate distance from the optic apparatus >3–5 mm. In these situations, fractionated streotactic radiotherapy represents a viable option with comparable tumour control rates and acceptable toxicity profile.

Outcomes of primary and adjunctive radiation therapy for cranial base meningiomas

'Tumour control', frequently defined as the ability of a therapeutic modality to prevent radiological or clinical progression, should be assessed taking into account the pre-treatment behaviour of the lesion, given the frequently indolent nature of smaller, particularly asymptomatic meningiomas without treatment. Unfortunately, in many radiation therapy series, history of tumour growth before treatment is not documented. Multiple therapeutic modalities, whether radiation therapy is primary or adjuvant, modifications in delivery planning and variable long-term follow-up contribute to the difficulty of interpreting outcomes. With these limitations in mind, the following results can be gleaned from the literature. For fractionated photon and proton radiotherapy, 10-year tumour control rates range from 88% to 96%, with late toxicity (usually grade 1–2) and new cranial neuropathy rates ranging from 8.2% to 16%.[64–66] Actual tumour volume reduction rates vary based on

definitions used, for example >50% volume reduction, and range from 14% to 22.7%. Radiosurgery series for skull base meningiomas are more numerous, and 7–10-year follow-up data reveal tumour control rates from 82.3% to 94.7%.[67–76] Any decrease in tumour volume was documented in 13.9%–51% of patients. Permanent late toxicity ranged from 3% to 22.5%. Retreatment the form of surgery or further radiation therapy is infrequently reported but in one series was 12.9%.[68]

Cognitive deficits are a known complication following therapeutic cranial radiation, including for meningiomas, and is particularly related to larger therapeutic volumes and higher doses.[77–79] The incidence of cognitive decline following radiation therapy for skull base meningiomas is not well reported, although in one series fractionated radiation therapy did not appear to produce cognitive decline at least in the short-term.[80] This is primarily because the patients are not carefully studied for such problems and the true incidence is likely underreported.[81] Clearly, with survivable, largely benign lesions such as meningiomas, long-term data are required to document the delayed incidence of cognitive impairment following radiation therapy. Very long-term follow-up of irradiated meningiomas also indicates that most of them recur, and there is a much higher mortality rate.[19]

Management of cavernous sinus invasion

The natural history specific to meningiomas involving the cavernous is largely unknown, and is further complicated by histological grade, the presence of symptoms, and whether the meningioma is purely within the confines of the cavernous sinus, is an extension of a larger spheno- or petro-cavernous tumour, or is affecting only the lateral dural wall of the cavernous sinus.[82] Aggressive resection of cavernous sinus portions of meningiomas was practised and popularized in the 1980s and 1990s, after the pioneering efforts of Parkinson[83,84] and Dolenc,[85] as well as developments by Sekhar[86] and Al-Mefty.[87] Surgical extirpation of cavernous sinus meningiomas has remained controversial, however, secondary to cranial nerve and potential vascular morbidity, often at the expense of incomplete resection. Although techniques for cavernous carotid resection and bypass with total tumour removal have been described,[88] microscopic gross total resection may be hindered by tumour remnants along cranial nerves along the sinus.[89,90]

Medium-term series of fractionated radiotherapy and Gamma Knife and linear accelerator-based radiosurgery to cavernous sinus meningiomas have reported comparable outcomes,[91–94] with improvement in cranial nerve related symptoms in 50%–67%, and new morbidity in 6%. The highest reported rate of optic neuropathy was 2%. The retreatment rate was as high as 12%. Progression-free survival ranged from 84% to 100% at 5 years, however the majority of studies do not report documented tumour growth prior to radiation, or patients with growing residual are mixed with those irradiated at initial presentation. Long-term data are awaited.

The optimal management strategy for cavernous sinus meningiomas has evolved.[82,95,96] It has become normal practice at surgery for larger tumours secondarily involving the cavernous sinus to perform subtotal resection and irradiate cavernous sinus residual if indicated, for example in the case of known preoperative growth or histologically atypical or malignant lesions. Irradiation of benign and/or radiologically stable cavernous sinus meningiomas should likely be avoided, given that, in the long-term, these tumours can recur,[97] at which point therapeutic options become limited and they are more difficult to treat surgically. When indicated, stereotactic radiosurgical techniques have proved to be a valuable adjunct in treating meningiomas in this difficult location. However, surgical resection of the tumours is still the principal therapeutic option for tumours involving only the outer dural wall of the cavernous sinus, as well as for post-irradiation or recurrent tumours, if necessary, with a carotid artery bypass.

Enter the endoscope

Since the introduction of the endoscope in pituitary neurosurgery in a sustained manner by Jho and Carrau in 1997,[98] endoscopic techniques have been reported in preliminary fashion for certain cranial base meningiomas, specifically planum sphenoidale, olfactory groove, tuberculum sellae, clival, and some posterior fossa tumours.[99–102]

A number of limitations have been well-recognized using these techniques, most notably a high rate of postoperative CSF rhinorrhea, a limited rate of gross total tumour resection with negative dural margins, and most importantly, an unknown long-term recurrence rate. The question remains whether endoscopic techniques can achieve complete skull base meningioma resection with minimal morbidity. One of the major issues with respect to meningiomas is that the margins of the tumour are not adequately delineated by preoperative MRI imaging, and standard skull base techniques permit wide resection of such margins, while transnasal enoscopic techniques do not. Micro-dissection techniques using the endoscopic-type surgical corridors have thus far been impeded by current trigger-type instrumentation, and it remains cumbersome to perform true sharp-dissection when required during endoscopic operations without injury to neurovascular structures, which are notoriously difficult to repair endoscopically. When the tumour involves arteries (especially encasement), endoscopic dissection may be difficult, and management of any vascular injury is very difficult. Furthermore, patients selected for purely endoscopic resection of meningiomas (a narrow base of attachment, limited bony involvement, an obvious arachnoid plane on preoperative MRI, and smaller tumour size) often have features for which standard skull base microsurgical resection techniques have demonstrable excellent long-term outcome. Notwithstanding, there are a number of potential advantages to endoscopic instrumentation, which include: the ability to introduce the viewing instrument directly over the region of interest, including potential 'blind spots' during endocranial approaches, sharper image and higher contrast afforded by digital endoscopes with 3-CCD (charged coupled device) sensors,[103] and a natural endonasal corridor to the midline skull base without brain retraction. To aid with depth perception, 3D endoscopes may be available soon. To date, no comparative studies between endoscopic and open approaches for skull base meningiomas have been published, and long-term data on current endoscopic series are still pending. Data specific to the primary 4 goals of meningioma surgery outlined above should be addressed, as well as operative time and cost should be reported. In the end, the endoscope is simply another tool within the skull base surgeon's armamentarium for viewing the tumour, and to assist in its resection.[104] Endoscope-assisted microsurgery is an option which may gain wider acceptance by neurosurgeons for meningioma surgery. It has the ability to extend the reach of the surgical microscope. However, further technical developments are needed.

Current paradigmme of cranial base meningioma surgery

(Harborview Medical Center, University of Washington, 2010)

From 2005 to present, 182 cranial base meningiomas have been operated by the senior author (LNS) at Harborview Medical Center. These include 15 foramen magnum, 46 petroclival, 28 sphenocavernous or clinoidal, often with vascular encasement, 40 tuberculum sellae or planum sphenoidale, 22 tentorial or medial temporal meningiomas, and 31 meningiomas in other skull base locations.

Evaluation for surgical resection of cranial base meningiomas begins with a thorough history and physical and neurological examination. Prior surgery to the tumour and/or radiation therapy, patient's age, medical condition/co-morbidities, functional status, support structure, and neurological complaints and findings are documented. When indicated, formal ophthalmological, cognitive and endocrine evaluations are sought.

Preoperative studies include magnetic resonance imaging as well as computed tomography with bone algorithms. A number of features are examined as part of a preoperative evaluation of risk to functional outcome and likelihood of complete tumour removal. Factors such as tumour size, number of involved fossae, and relationship to cranial nerves, brainstem, and/or pituitary gland are assessed, as well as vascular encasement and sinus (in particular cavernous sinus) invasion. Arachnoid planes on T_2-weighted imaging are assessed as present, partially present, or absent. Occipito-cervical instability from the tumour and/or resulting from the planned surgical approach should be clinically and radiologically evaluated when appropriate.

For small- to medium-sized tumours, magnetic resonance angiography and/or venography is performed to evaluate the relationship of the tumour to major intracranial vessels, as well as dominance and status of major venous sinuses. For giant tumours, we prefer preoperative angiography to evaluate the above features, as well as to interrogate the tumour's blood supply and potentially embolize feeding vessels.

The preoperative angiogram provides a map of the intracranial arterial and venous vascular tree. In many cases, this information is not available by other imaging. Arterial supply (internal or external supply), dominance of the venous anatomy and in some cases safe targets for embolization are readily apparent with this study. The morbidity of an angiogram and/or embolization is exceedingly low in our institution. The safe embolization of large skull base

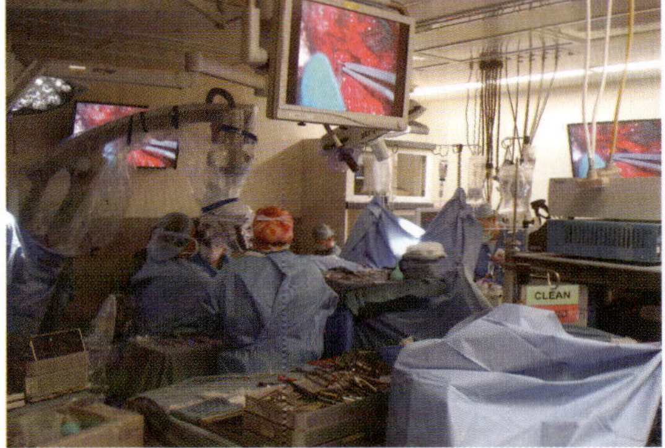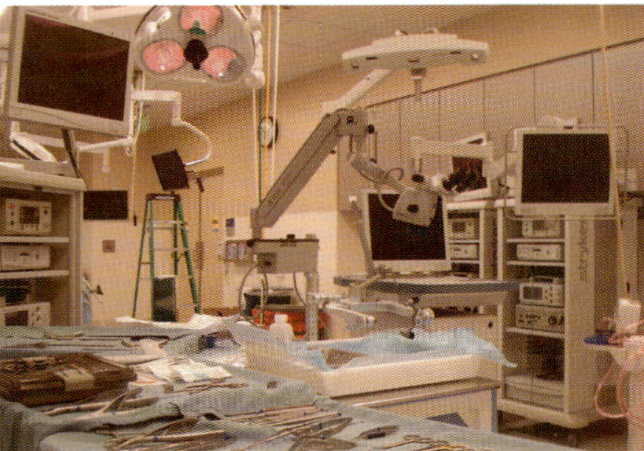

Fig. 1. Left: Photograph of operating room setup with surgeon and assistant comfortably seated, and high definition displays projecting microscope video, preoperative imaging and neuronavigation display. **Right:** Our cadaver laboratory provides trainees with the opportunity to learn skull base approaches.

tumours, where the blood supply is not reached until the end of the operation, can potentially effect intra-operative blood loss and the need for blood transfusion, length of the operation, extent of resection and neurological sequelae (when the tumour is easily suckable from the surrounding neurovascular structures). It is not presently clear whether the presence of necrosis in embolized tumours has an impact on the grading of these tumours or if those tumours are more or less likely to reoccur.

The operating room team consists of a neuroanaesthesiologist, nurse and scrub technician, and surgical team with experienced surgeon, and good assistant(s). Total intravenous anaesthesia, usually using propofol and remifentanyl, is implemented for its compatibility with intra-operative monitoring and maximizing brain relaxation. Potential for blood loss, arterial and/or venous sinus injury, and air embolism are communicated and preparations are made accordingly. Neuronavigation equipment for small- and medium-sized tumours is typically implemented. Intra-operative monitoring is used in virtually all cases. Baseline monitoring includes long tract motor evoked potentials and somatosensory evoked potentials. When indicated, we use brainstem auditory evoked responses, cranial nerve monitoring in the form of free-running and locally evoked responses for III, V, VI, VII, IX, X, XI and XII, and electrical

transcortically evoked stimulation of CN VII motor-evoked potentials.

We are equipped with a large dedicated operating room with multiple screens for viewing preoperative images, neuronavigation, and to display high definition video from the microscope with the capability for 3D recording (Fig. 1, left). Routine equipment includes reciprocating saw, Sonopet bone and soft tissue aspirators, CO_2 contact laser, endoscope for intra-operative inspection during and after tumour removal, microsurgical instruments for tumour dissection, resection, as well as for vascular/neural anastamosis.

The University of Washington Institute for Simulation and Interprofessional Studies (ISIS; www.isis.washington.edu) at Harborview Medical Center provides for cadaver-based surgical simulation and training. This has been useful for training residents and fellows, who can study and perform the approach in preparation for the index operation. Surgeons may also practice new or unusual operative approaches (Fig. 1, right). This, in conjunction with recorded operative videos has been extremely useful for education.

Atypical and malignant meningiomas

Following revisions in the WHO diagnostic criteria for atypical meningioma in 2000,[105] in which the threshold for the designation of atypical meningioma was lowered by the addition of necrosis as a diagnostic criteria, the incidence of atypical meningioma increased disproportionately. In one series,[106] the annual percentage of atypical meningiomas rose from 4.4% in 1999–2000 to 32.7%–35.5% in 2004–2006, following publication of the updated diagnostic criteria.

Using the 2000 WHO criteria, Durand *et al.* reported 5- and 10-year overall survival for atypical meningiomas of 78.4% and 53.3%, respectively, and progression-free survival of 48.4% at 5 years and 22.6% at 10 years.[107] For malignant meningiomas, 5- and 10-year overall survival was 44.0% and 14.2%, and progression-free survival was 8.4% and 0% at 5 and 10 years, respectively.

There is reason to believe that atypical tumours are not as common at the skull base as other cranial locations.[51] The reason for this is unclear but may be related to the site of origin, progression in other cranial locations or skull base tumours reaching clinical attention earlier. Regardless, this entity is seen relatively commonly at large volume centres. The presence of bony involvement suggests more aggressive tumours.[108] It is, however, unknown if the resection of this tumour-infiltrated bone or targeting of this area with postoperative radiation changes the natural history of the disease.

The high recurrence rate of atypical meningiomas was reflected in a retrospective review of 108 patients who had undergone Simpson grade 1 resection, of which 30 patients (28%) recurred during a mean period of 36 months.[109] Interestingly, no recurrence was seen in 8 patients who also received postoperative adjuvant radiation, although this difference in radiographic recurrence did not reach statistical significance. This retrospective study has become the basis of prospective randomized trials within the Radiation Therapy Oncology Group (RTOG) and the European Organization for Research and Treatment of Cancer group (EORTC).

The optimum oncological management of atypical and malignant meningiomas remains controversial. Prior to a treatment plan, in patients with recurrent atypical or malignant meningiomas, staging of the disease must be performed. These tumours tend to metastize to the lung and liver via the venous sinus system. The use of MRI, PET CT and octreotide scans can be useful. It is generally agreed that malignant meningiomas, regardless of extent of surgical resection, should receive postoperative focal radiation therapy given their aggressive natural history.[110,111] For atypical meningiomas, the role of adjuvant radiation therapy is less clear,[112] specifically whether to irradiate postoperatively irrespective of the extent of resection or only in the context of residual tumour.[113] Currently a multi-centre retrospective study in which all atypical and malignant meningiomas were referred for external beam radiation therapy did not find significant differences in progression-free or overall survival based on the extent of resection;[114] however, this may be due to referral bias. Prospective comparative trials should help further elucidate optimum management.

Meningioma molecular genetics

The current WHO histological grading system is less than ideal to predict (i) progression-free survival and (ii) response to therapy (surgery, surgery adjuvant radiation or chemotherapy) of meningiomas. Many are familiar with cases of WHO grade 1 meningiomas that underwent a Simpson grade 1 resection only to go on and quickly re-occur. The grading system is very useful in predicting aggressive behaviour in WHO grade 2 and 3 meningiomas. Greater ambiguity regarding expected behaviour and management occurs in cases of grade 1 meningiomas with 1 or 2 atypical criteria that nonetheless do not satisfy WHO grade 2 criteria.

Cytogenetic markers in cancer have become extremely important for predicting outcomes and response to therapy. Clinically important markers have been developed for gastrointestinal stromal tumours (GIST), melanoma, CML and certain lung cancers. In the field of neuro-oncology, the only marker that has had a clinical impact is the absence of 1p19q in oligo-dendrogliomas, with its resultant effect on survival and chemo-sensitivity. The molecular genetics of meningiomas and meningioma progression, as well as discussions of future treatments, have been the subject of several extensive reviews.[33,115–117] Loss of heterozygosity at chromosome 22 with inactivation of the NF-2 gene, a member of the Protein 4.1 family, is the earliest and best characterized genetic change associated with meningiomas,[118] and is affected in the majority of NF-2 related tumours and over 50% of sporadic meningiomas.[119] Other homologue genes within the protein 4.1 family have been studied but candidate genes, such as DAL-1 on chromosome 18p, which have been found in the majority of atypical and malignant meningioma specimens;[120] however, alterations in this gene have failed to produce tumours in animal models.[121]

While the NF-2 gene mutation, although common, is not felt to be a marker of meningioma progression but rather an early genetic event in meningioma formation,[116] deletions in chromosomes 1p and 14q appear to correlate in several studies with a higher histological grade and/or rate of recurrence.[122–125] The expression of autocrine factors, including platelet-derived growth factor, epidermal growth factor and insulin-like growth factor and their respective receptors has been demonstrated in meningiomas as well.[116] Progression to atypical meningioma is associated with telomerase activation, rare in benign meningioma but present in a substantial fraction of more aggressive meningiomas,[116] and loss of progesterone receptor expression.[126]

Molecular genetic alterations isolated to cranial base meningiomas are less known. Cranial base meningiomas are more frequently meningo-thelial,[127,128] more frequently lower grade at initial resection,[50] more frequently demonstrate retention of heterozygosity at chromosome 22 (i.e. NF-2 gene intact), at least in the anterior skull base,[127] and have a lower histological grade and lower MIB-1 at recurrence[51] compared to non-skull base meningiomas. The accumulation of progression–association chromosomal alterations and presence of a complex cytogenetic profile may help explain tumour invasiveness despite their 'benign' histological appearance.[129] However, despite an increased understanding of the molecular genetics of meningiomas, there has yet to be an advance which aids in grading, predicts clinical behaviour, guides management, or serves as an efficacious therapeutic target.

Future treatment of meningiomas

The world of cancer research has grown exponentially, while the advancement of treatments for brain tumours has been poor. Despite efforts in the field of gliomas, the outcome and prognosis for those patients has not changed significantly. The study of meningiomas has never been popular within the research community. The reason for this could be due to the misconception of these tumours being curative and benign. The neurosurgeon, and specifically, the skull base neurosurgeon knows this to be false. The meningioma comes in many different shades, ranging from totally benign to frankly malignant. Furthermore, even the benign tumours that occur at the skull base prove challenging to remove safely. Second-look surgeries are always more difficult and thus the initial surgery is the patient's best opportunity for long-term survival.

After surgery, what is the goal of therapy? Is it to prevent disease recurrence? Is it to halt progression of residual disease? These questions must guide our advancement of therapies. The role of radiotherapy, in the form of conventional fractionated therapy, gamma-knife irradiation for the treatment of WHO 1, 2 and grade 3 tumours needs to be better defined. The afore-mentioned prospective randomized multi-centre trials will provide much needed guidance here.

The need for cytogenetic markers (chromosomal loss or gain, or mutations) for the guidance of adjuvant therapy is much-needed in the treatment of these difficult tumours. With the resolution of SNP arrays and whole-genome wide sequencing, the day is near for targeted therapies.

Conclusion

As little as 50 years ago, the majority of skull base meningiomas were still considered unapproachable. The evolution of skull base surgery as a distinct subspecialty is a reflection in part of immense innovations in surgical approaches and techniques to render these lesions resectable. Opponents who disparage skull base surgery would argue that skull base meningiomas can be removed by 'simple approaches' such as the subfrontal or retrosigmoid routes, for example, and follow with radiation therapy for residual when appropriate. Approaches such as the transorbital transpetrosal and partial transcondylar are perhaps unnecessary, create more morbidity and are a waste of time. There are certainly specific situations where this approach is appropriate, for example older patients. However, proponents would argue that appropriately selected skull base approaches minimize cranial nerve and brain morbidity, and facilitate maximal removal of tumour. Patients with skull base meningiomas are expected to have near-normal life expectancies in the majority of cases; therefore treatment should encompass a 10-, 20- or even 30-year plan. Options for 'recurrences' following radiation therapy for subtotally resected meningiomas are very limited. Randomized comparative studies are unlikely to answer these questions definitively, and one needs to go back to the goals of skull base meningioma removal for comparison.

References

1. al-Rodhan NR, Laws ER Jr. Meningioma: A historical study of the tumor and its surgical management. *Neurosurgery* 1990;**26**:832–46; discussion 846–7.

2. Okonkwo DO, Laws ER Jr. Meningiomas: Historical perspectives. In: Lee JH (ed). *Meningiomas: Diagnosis, treatment and outcome*. London: Springer; 2008:3–10.

3. Giuffre R. Successful radical removal of an intracranial meningioma in 1835 by Professor Pecchioli of Siena. *J Neurosurg* 1984;**60**:47–51.

4. Wang H, Lanzino G, Laws ER Jr. Meningioma, the soul of neurosurgery: Historical review. *Semin Neurosurg* 2003;**14**:163–8.

5. Bingham WF. W.W. Keen and the dawn of American neurosurgery. *J Neurosurg* 1986;**64**:705–12.

6. Durante F. Contribution to endocranial surgery. *Lancet* 1887;**2**:654–55.

7. Tomasello F, Germano A. Francesco Durante: The history of intracranial meningiomas and beyond. *Neurosurgery* 2006;**59**:389–96; discussion 389–96.

8. Macewen W. Intra-cranial lesions, illustrating some points in connexion with the localization of cerebral affections and the advantages of antiseptic trephining. *Lancet* 1881;**2**:581–2.

9. Cushing H. The meningiomas (dural endotheliomas): Their source, and favoured seats of origin. *Brain* 1922;**45**:282–316.

10. Cushing H, Eisenhardt L. *Meningiomas, their classification, regional behaviour, life history, and surgical end results*. Springfield, IL: Charles C. Thomas; 1938.

11. Cushing H, Bovie WT. Electrosurgery as an aid to the removal of intracranial tumors. *Surg Gynecol Obstet* 1928;**47**:751–84.

12. Samuels SI. History of neuroanesthesia: A contemporary review. *Int Anesthesiol Clin Fall* 1996;**34**:1–20.

13. Molnar C, Nemes C, Szabo S, *et al*. Harvey Cushing, a pioneer of neuroanesthesia. *J Anesth* 2008;**22**:483–6.

14. Pait TG, Dennis MW, Laws ER Jr, *et al*. The history of the neurosurgical engine. *Neurosurgery* 1991;**28**:111–28; discussion 128–119.

15. Houser OW. Neuroradiology: A historical perspective. *Radiology* 1995;**196**:1–2.

16. Lougheed WM, Tom M. A method of introducing blood into the subarachnoid space in the region of the circle of Willis in dogs. *Can J Surg* 1961;**4**:329–37.

17. Porter KR, McCarthy BJ, Freels S, *et al*. Prevalence estimates for primary brain tumors in the United States by age, gender, behavior, and histology. *Neuro Oncol* 2010;**12**:520–7.

18. CBTRUS. *CBTRUS Statistical Report: Primary Brain and Central Nervous System Tumors Diagnosed in the United States in 2004–2006*. 2010; www.cbtrus.org.

19. Mathiesen T, Lindquist C, Kihlstrom L, *et al.* Recurrence of cranial base meningiomas. *Neurosurgery* 1996;**39**:2–7; discussion 8–9.

20. Park BJ, Kim HK, Sade B, *et al.* Epidemiology. In: Lee JH (ed). *Meningiomas: Diagnosis, treatment, and outcome*. London: Springer; 2008:11.

21. Hashiba T, Hashimoto N, Izumoto S, *et al.* Serial volumetric assessment of the natural history and growth pattern of incidentally discovered meningiomas. *J Neurosurg* 2009;**110**:675–84.

22. Herscovici Z, Rappaport Z, Sulkes J, *et al.* Natural history of conservatively treated meningiomas. *Neurology* 2004;**63**:1133–4.

23. Nakamura M, Roser F, Michel J, *et al.* The natural history of incidental meningiomas. *Neurosurgery* 2003;**53**:62–70; discussion 70–61.

24. Nakamura M, Roser F, Michel J, *et al.* Volumetric analysis of the growth rate of incompletely resected intracranial meningiomas. *Zentralbl Neurochir* 2005; **66**:17–23.

25. Bindal R, Goodman JM, Kawasaki A, *et al.* The natural history of untreated skull base meningiomas. *Surg Neurol* 2003;**59**:87–92; discussion 92.

26. Van Havenbergh T, Carvalho G, Tatagiba M, *et al.* Natural history of petroclival meningiomas. *Neurosurgery* 2003;**52**:55–62; discussion 62–54.

27. Egan RA, Lessell S. A contribution to the natural history of optic nerve sheath meningiomas. *Arch Ophthalmol* 2002;**120**:1505–8.

28. Niiro M, Yatsushiro K, Nakamura K, *et al.* Natural history of elderly patients with asymptomatic meningiomas. *J Neurol Neurosurg Psychiatry* 2000; **68**:25-8.

29. Go RS, Taylor BV, Kimmel DW. The natural history of asymptomatic meningiomas in Olmsted County, Minnesota. *Neurology* 1998;**51**:1718–20.

30. Olivero WC, Lister JR, Elwood PW. The natural history and growth rate of asymptomatic meningiomas: A review of 60 patients. *J Neurosurg* 1995;**83**:222–4.

31. Kuratsu J, Kochi M, Ushio Y. Incidence and clinical features of asymptomatic meningiomas. *J Neurosurg* 2000;**92**:766–70.

32. Sughrue ME, Rutkowski MJ, Aranda D, *et al.* Treatment decision-making based on the published natural history and growth rate of small meningiomas. *J Neurosurg* 2010;**113**:1036–42.

33. Johnson MD, Sade B, Milano MT, *et al.* New prospects for management and treatment of inoperable and recurrent skull base meningiomas. *J Neurooncol* 2008;**86**:109–22.

34. Akagami R, Napolitano M, Sekhar LN. Patient-evaluated outcome after surgery for basal meningiomas. *Neurosurgery* 2002;**50**:941–8; discussion 948–9.

35. Donald PJ. History of skull base surgery. In: Donald PJ (ed). *Surgery of the skull base*. Philadelphia: Lippincott-Raven; 1998:3–13.

36. Goodrich JT. A millennium review of skull base surgery. *Childs Nerv Syst* 2000;**16**:669–85.

37. Maroon JC. Skull base surgery: Past, present, and future trends. *Neurosurg Focus* 2005;**19**:E1.

38. Prevedello DM, Doglietto F, Jane JA Jr, *et al.* History of endoscopic skull base surgery: Its evolution and current reality. *J Neurosurg* 2007;**107**:206–13.

39. Simpson D. Recurrence of intracranial meningiomas after surgical treatment. *J Neurol Neurosurg Psychiatry* 1957;**20**:22–39.

40. Mirimanoff RO, Dosoretz DE, Linggood RM, *et al.* Meningioma: Analysis of recurrence and progression following neurosurgical resection. *J Neurosurg* 1985; **62**:18–24.

41. Adegbite AB, Khan MI, Paine KW, *et al.* The recurrence of intracranial meningiomas after surgical treatment. *J Neurosurg* 1983;**58**:51–6.

42. Yamasaki F, Yoshioka H, Hama S, *et al.* Recurrence of meningiomas. *Cancer* 2000;**89**:1102–10.

43. Jaaskelainen J. Seemingly complete removal of histologically benign intracranial meningioma: Late recurrence rate and factors predicting recurrence in 657 patients. A multivariate analysis. *Surg Neurol* 1986;**26**:461–9.

44. Kinjo T, al-Mefty O, Kanaan I. Grade zero removal of supratentorial convexity meningiomas. *Neurosurgery* 1993;**33**:394–99; discussion 399.

45. Obeid F, Al-Mefty O. Recurrence of olfactory groove meningiomas. *Neurosurgery* 2003;**53**:534–42; discussion 542–33.

46. Jung HW, Yoo H, Paek SH, *et al.* Long-term outcome and growth rate of subtotally resected petroclival meningiomas: Experience with 38 cases. *Neurosurgery* 2000;**46**:567–74; discussion 574–65.

47. Kano T, Kawase T, Horiguchi T, *et al.* Meningiomas of the ventral foramen magnum and lower clivus: Factors influencing surgical morbidity, the extent of tumour resection, and tumour recurrence. *Acta Neurochir (Wien)* 2010;**152**:79–86; discussion 86.

48. Mirone G, Chibbaro S, Schiabello L, *et al.* En plaque sphenoid wing meningiomas: Recurrence factors and surgical strategy in a series of 71 patients. *Neurosurgery* 2009;**65**(6 Suppl):100–8; discussion 108–9.

49. Natarajan SK, Sekhar LN, Schessel D, *et al.* Petroclival meningiomas: Multimodality treatment and outcomes at long-term follow-up. *Neurosurgery* 2007;**60**:965–79; discussion 979–81.

50. Sade B, Chahlavi A, Krishnaney A, *et al.* World Health Organization Grades II and III meningiomas are rare in the cranial base and spine. *Neurosurgery* 2007;**61**:1194–8; discussion 1198.

51. McGovern SL, Aldape KD, Munsell MF, *et al.* A comparison of World Health Organization tumor grades at recurrence in patients with non-skull base and skull base meningiomas. *J Neurosurg* 2010;**112**: 925–33.

52. Levine ZT, Buchanan RI, Sekhar LN, *et al.* Proposed grading system to predict the extent of resection and outcomes for cranial base meningiomas. *Neurosurgery* 1999;**45**:221–30.

53. Gil Z. Quality of life in patients with skull base tumors. *Skull Base* 2010;**20**:1.

54. Kalkanis SN, Quinones-Hinojosa A, Buzney E, *et al.* Quality of life following surgery for intracranial meningiomas at Brigham and Women's Hospital: A study of 164 patients using a modification of the functional assessment of cancer therapy–brain questionnaire. *J Neuro-Oncol* 2000;**48**:233–41.

55. Mohsenipour I, Deusch E, Gabl M, *et al.* Quality of life in patients after meningioma resection. *Acta Neurochirurgica* 2001;**143**:547–53.

56. Schiestel C, Ryan D. Quality of life in patients with meningiomas: The true meaning of 'benign'. *Frontiers in Bioscience* 2009;**1**:488–93.

57. Miao Y, Lu X, Qiu Y, *et al.* A multivariate analysis of prognostic factors for health-related quality of life in patients with surgically managed meningioma. *J Clin Neurosci* 2010;**17**:446–9.

58. Leksell L. The stereotaxic method and radiosurgery of the brain. *Acta Chir Scand* 1951;**102**:316–19.

59. Leksell L. Cerebral radiosurgery I: Gammathalamotomy in two cases of intractable pain. *Acta Chir Scand* 1968;**134**:585–95.

60. Szeifert GT, Kondziolka D, Atteberry DS, *et al.* Radiosurgical pathology of brain tumors: Metastases, schwannomas, meningiomas, astrocytomas, hemangioblastomas. *Prog Neurol Surg* 2007;**20**: 91–105.

61. Regis J, Tamura M, Guillot C, *et al.* Radiosurgery with the world's first fully robotized Leksell Gamma Knife PerfeXion in clinical use: A 200-patient prospective, randomized, controlled comparison with the Gamma Knife 4C. *Neurosurgery* 2009;**64**: 346–55; discussion 355–46.

62. Minniti G, Amichetti M, Enrici RM. Radiotherapy and radiosurgery for benign skull base meningiomas. *Radiat Oncol* 2009;**4**:42.

63. McGregor JM, Sarkar A. Stereotactic radiosurgery and stereotactic radiotherapy in the treatment of skull base meningiomas. *Otolaryngol Clin North Am* 2009;**42**:677–88.

64. Debus J, Wuendrich M, Pirzkall A, *et al.* High efficacy of fractionated stereotactic radiotherapy of large base-of-skull meningiomas: Long-term results. *J Clin Oncol* 2001;**19**:3547–53.

65. Milker-Zabel S, Zabel A, Schulz-Ertner D, *et al.* Fractionated stereotactic radiotherapy in patients with benign or atypical intracranial meningioma: Long-term experience and prognostic factors. *Int J Radiat Oncol Biol Phys* 2005;**61**:809–16.

66. Wenkel E, Thornton AF, Finkelstein D, *et al.* Benign meningioma: Partially resected, biopsied, and recurrent intracranial tumors treated with combined proton and photon radiotherapy. *Int J Radiat Oncol Biol Phys* 2000;**48**:1363–70.

67. Iwai Y, Yamanaka K, Ikeda H. Gamma Knife radiosurgery for skull base meningioma: Long-term results of low-dose treatment. *J Neurosurg* 2008;**109**: 804–10.

68. Kondziolka D, Mathieu D, Lunsford LD, *et al.* Radiosurgery as definitive management of intracranial meningiomas. *Neurosurgery* 2008;**62**:53–58; discussion 58–60.

69. Davidson L, Fishback D, Russin JJ, *et al.* Postoperative GammaKnife surgery for benign meningiomas of the cranial base. *Neurosurgery* 2007;**23**:E6.

70. Hasegawa T, Kida Y, Yoshimoto M, *et al.* Long-term outcomes of Gamma Knife surgery for cavernous sinus meningioma. *J Neurosurg* 2007;**107**:745–51.

71. Kreil W, Luggin J, Fuchs I, *et al.* Long-term experience of gamma knife radiosurgery for benign skull base meningiomas. *J Neurol Neurosurg Psychiatry* 2005;**76**:1425–30.

72. Pollock BE, Stafford SL. Results of stereotactic radiosurgery for patients with imaging defined cavernous sinus meningiomas. *Int J Radiat Oncol Biol Phys* 2005;**62**:1427–31.

73. Lee JY, Niranjan A, McInerney J, *et al.* Stereotactic

radiosurgery providing long-term tumor control of cavernous sinus meningiomas. *J Neurosurg* 2002;**97**: 65–72.

74. Spiegelmann R, Nissim O, Menhel J, *et al.* Linear accelerator radiosurgery for meningiomas in and around the cavernous sinus. *Neurosurgery* 2002;**51**: 1373–9; discussion 1379–80.

75. Shin M, Kurita H, Sasaki T, *et al.* Analysis of treatment outcome after stereotactic radiosurgery for cavernous sinus meningiomas. *J Neurosurg* 2001; **95**:435–9.

76. Kobayashi T, Kida Y, Mori Y. Long-term results of stereotactic gamma radiosurgery of meningiomas. *Surg Neurol* 2001;**55**:325–31.

77. Maire JP, Caudry M, Guerin J, *et al.* Fractionated radiation therapy in the treatment of intracranial meningiomas: Local control, functional efficacy, and tolerance in 91 patients. *Int J Radiat Oncol Biol Phys* 1995;**33**:315–21.

78. Maguire PD, Clough R, Friedman AH, *et al.* Fractionated external-beam radiation therapy for meningiomas of the cavernous sinus. *Int J Radiat Oncol Biol Phys* 1999;**44**:75–9.

79. Dufour H, Muracciole X, Metellus P, *et al.* Long-term tumor control and functional outcome in patients with cavernous sinus meningiomas treated by radiotherapy with or without previous surgery: Is there an alternative to aggressive tumor removal? *Neurosurgery* 2001;**48**:285–94; discussion 294–86.

80. Steinvorth S, Welzel G, Fuss M, *et al.* Neuropsychological outcome after fractionated stereotactic radiotherapy (FSRT) for base of skull meningiomas: A prospective 1-year follow-up. *Radiotherapy Oncology* 2003;**69**:177–82.

81. al-Mefty O, Kersh JE, Routh A, *et al.* The long-term side-effects of radiation therapy for benign brain tumors in adults. *J Neurosurg* 1990;**73**:502–12.

82. Pichierri A, Santoro A, Raco A, *et al.* Cavernous sinus meningiomas: Retrospective analysis and proposal of a treatment algorithm. *Neurosurgery* 2009;**64**:1090–99; discussion 1099–101.

83. Parkinson D. A surgical approach to the cavernous portion of the carotid artery. Anatomical studies and case report. *J Neurosurg* 1965;**23**:474–83.

84. Parkinson D. Collateral circulation of cavernous carotid artery: Anatomy. *Can J Surg* 1964;**7**:251–68.

85. Dolenc VV. *Anatomy and surgery of the cavernous sinus.* Vienna: Springer-Verlag; 1989.

86. Sekhar LN, Moller AR. Operative management of tumors involving the cavernous sinus. *J Neurosurg* 1986;**64**:879–89.

87. Al-Mefty O, Smith RR. Surgery of tumors invading the cavernous sinus. *Surg Neurol* 1988;**30**:370–81.

88. De Jesus O, Sekhar LN, Parikh HK, *et al.* Long-term follow-up of patients with meningiomas involving the cavernous sinus: Recurrence, progression, and quality of life. *Neurosurgery* 1996;**39**:915–9; discussion 919–20.

89. Larson JJ, van Loveren HR, Balko MG, *et al.* Evidence of meningioma infiltration into cranial nerves: Clinical implications for cavernous sinus meningiomas. *J Neurosurg* 1995;**83**:596–9.

90. Sen C, Hague K. Meningiomas involving the cavernous sinus: Histological factors affecting the degree of resection. *J Neurosurg* 1997;**87**:535–43.

91. Litre CF, Colin P, Noudel R, *et al.* Fractionated stereotactic radiotherapy treatment of cavernous sinus meningiomas: A study of 100 cases. *Int J Radiat Oncol Biol Phys* 2009;**74**:1012–17.

92. Skeie BS, Enger PO, Skeie GO, *et al.* Gamma knife surgery of meningiomas involving the cavernous sinus: Long-term follow-up of 100 patients. *Neurosurgery* 2010;**66**:661–8; discussion 668–9.

93. Kimball MM, Friedman WA, Foote KD, *et al.* Linear accelerator radiosurgery for cavernous sinus meningiomas. *Stereotact Funct Neurosurg* 2009;**87**: 120–7.

94. Milker-Zabel S, Zabel-du Bois A, Huber P, *et al.* Fractionated stereotactic radiation therapy in the management of benign cavernous sinus meningiomas: Long-term experience and review of the literature. *Strahlenther Onkol* 2006;**182**:635–40.

95. Walsh MT, Couldwell WT. Management options for cavernous sinus meningiomas. *J Neurooncol* 2009;**92**: 307–16.

96. Long DM. The treatment of meningiomas in the region of the cavernous sinus. *Childs Nerv Syst* 2001; **17**:168–72.

97. Couldwell WT, Cole CD, Al-Mefty O. Patterns of skull base meningioma progression after failed radiosurgery. *J Neurosurg* 2007;**106**:30–5.

98. Jho HD, Carrau RL. Endoscopic endonasal transsphenoidal surgery: Experience with 50 patients. *J Neurosurg* 1997;**87**:44–51.

99. de Divitiis E, Esposito F, Cappabianca P, *et al.* Tuberculum sellae meningiomas: High route or low route? A series of 51 consecutive cases. *Neurosurgery* 2008;**62**:556–63; discussion 556–63.

100. de Divitiis E, Esposito F, Cappabianca P, *et al.* Endoscopic transnasal resection of anterior cranial fossa meningiomas. *Neurosurg Focus* 2008;**25**:E8.

101. Schwartz TH, Fraser JF, Brown S, *et al.* Endoscopic

cranial base surgery: Classification of operative approaches. *Neurosurgery* 2008;**62**:991–1002; discussion 1002–5.

102. Gardner PA, Kassam AB, Thomas A, *et al.* Endoscopic endonasal resection of anterior cranial base meningiomas. *Neurosurgery* 2008;**63**:36–52; discussion 52–34.

103. Cappabianca P, Cavallo LM, Esposito F, *et al.* Endoscopy in meningioma surgery: Basic principles, applications, and indications. In: Lee JH (ed). *Meningiomas: Diagnosis, treatment, and outcome.* London: Springer; 2008:225.

104. Samii M. *Endoscope assisted microsurgery.* Paper presented at International Neurosurgery Congress; July 23, 2010; Hannover, Germany.

105. Louis DN, Scheithauer BW, Budka H, *et al.* Meningiomas. In: Kleihues P, Cavenee WK (eds). *WHO classification of tumours: Pathology and genetics of tumours of the nervous system.* Lyon: IARC Press; 2000.

106. Pearson BE, Markert JM, Fisher WS, *et al.* Hitting a moving target: Evolution of a treatment paradigm for atypical meningiomas amid changing diagnostic criteria. *Neurosurg Focus* 2008;**24**:E3.

107. Durand A, Labrousse F, Jouvet A, *et al.* WHO grade II and III meningiomas: A study of prognostic factors. *J Neurooncol* 2009;**95**:367–75.

108. Gabeau-Lacet D, Aghi M, Betensky RA, *et al.* Bone involvement predicts poor outcome in atypical meningioma. *J Neurosurg* 2009;**111**:464–71.

109. Aghi MK, Carter BS, Cosgrove GR, *et al.* Long-term recurrence rates of atypical meningiomas after gross total resection with or without postoperative adjuvant radiation. *Neurosurgery* 2009;**64**:56–60; discussion 60.

110. Dziuk TW, Woo S, Butler EB, *et al.* Malignant meningioma: An indication for initial aggressive surgery and adjuvant radiotherapy. *J Neurooncol* 1998;**37**:177–88.

111. Sughrue ME, Sanai N, Shangari G, *et al.* Outcome and survival following primary and repeat surgery for World Health Organization Grade III meningiomas. *J Neurosurg* 2010;**113**:202–9.

112. Jo K, Park HJ, Nam DH, *et al.* Treatment of atypical meningioma. *J Clin Neurosci* 2010;**17**:1362–6.

113. Rogers L, Gilbert M, Vogelbaum MA. Intracranial meningiomas of atypical (WHO grade II) histology. *J Neurooncol* 2010;**99**:393–405.

114. Pasquier D, Bijmolt S, Veninga T, *et al.* Atypical and malignant meningioma: Outcome and prognostic factors in 119 irradiated patients. A multicenter, retrospective study of the Rare Cancer Network. *Int J Radiat Oncol Biol Phys* 2008;**71**:1388–93.

115. Riemenschneider MJ, Perry A, Reifenberger G. Histological classification and molecular genetics of meningiomas. *Lancet Neurol* 2006;**5**:1045–54.

116. Simon M, Bostrom JP, Hartmann C. Molecular genetics of meningiomas: From basic research to potential clinical applications. *Neurosurgery* 2007;**60**:787–98; discussion 787–98.

117. Norden AD, Drappatz J, Wen PY. Targeted drug therapy for meningiomas. *Neurosurg Focus* 2007;**23**:E12.

118. Perry A, Gutmann DH, Reifenberger G. Molecular pathogenesis of meningiomas. *J Neurooncol* 2004;**70**:183–202.

119. Harada T, Irving RM, Xuereb JH, *et al.* Molecular genetic investigation of the neurofibromatosis type 2 tumor suppressor gene in sporadic meningioma. *J Neurosurg* 1996;**84**:847–51.

120. Perry A, Cai DX, Scheithauer BW, *et al.* Merlin, DAL-1, and progesterone receptor expression in clinicopathologic subsets of meningioma: A correlative immunohistochemical study of 175 cases. *J Neuropathol Exp Neurol* 2000;**59**:872–9.

121. Yi C, McCarty JH, Troutman SA, *et al.* Loss of the putative tumor suppressor band 4.1B/Dal1 gene is dispensable for normal development and does not predispose to cancer. *Mol Cell Biol* 2005;**25**:10052–9.

122. Zang KD. Meningioma: A cytogenetic model of a complex benign human tumor, including data on 394 karyotyped cases. *Cytogenet Cell Genet* 2001;**93**:207–20.

123. Cai DX, Banerjee R, Scheithauer BW, *et al.* Chromosome 1p and 14q FISH analysis in clinicopathologic subsets of meningioma: Diagnostic and prognostic implications. *J Neuropathol Exp Neurol* 2001;**60**:628–36.

124. Lopez-Gines C, Cerda-Nicolas M, Gil-Benso R, *et al.* Loss of 1p in recurrent meningiomas. A comparative study in successive recurrences by cytogenetics and fluorescence *in situ* hybridization. *Cancer Genet Cytogenet* 2001;**125**:119–24.

125. Muller P, Henn W, Niedermayer I, *et al.* Deletion of chromosome 1p and loss of expression of alkaline phosphatase indicate progression of meningiomas. *Clin Cancer Res* 1999;**5**:3569–77.

126. Wen PY, Drappatz J. Novel therapies for meningiomas. *Expert Rev Neurother* 2006;**6**:1447–64.

127. Kros J, de Greve K, van Tilborg A, *et al.* NF2 status of meningiomas is associated with tumour localization and histology. *J Pathol* 2001;**194**:367–72.

128. Lee JH, Sade B, Choi E, *et al.* Meningothelioma as the predominant histological subtype of midline skull base and spinal meningioma. *J Neurosurg* 2006; **105**:60–4.

129. Korshunov A, Cherekaev V, Bekyashev A, *et al.* Recurrent cytogenetic aberrations in histologically benign, invasive meningiomas of the sphenoid region. *J Neurooncol* 2007;**81**:131–7.

130. Ketcham AS, Wilkins RH, Vanburen JM, *et al.* A combined intracranial facial approach to the paranasal sinuses. *Am J Surg* 1963;**106**:698–703.

131. House WF, Hitselberger WE. Transtemporal bone microsurgical removal of acoustic neuromas. Total versus subtotal removal of acoustic tumors. *Arch Otolaryngol* 1964;**80**:751–2.

132. Fisch U. Infratemporal fossa approach to tumours of the temporal bone and base of the skull. *J Laryngol Otol* 1978;**92**:949–67.

133. Fisch U. Infratemporal fossa approach for glomus tumors of the temporal bone. *Ann Otol Rhinol Laryngol* 1982;**91**:474-9.

134. Jane JA, Park TS, Pobereskin LH, *et al.* The supra-orbital approach: Technical note. *Neurosurgery* 1982; **11**:537–42.

135. Yasargil MG. *Microneurosurgery.* Vol I. Stuttgart: Georg Thieme Verlag; 1984.

136. Malis LI. Surgical resection of tumors of the skull base. In: Wilkins RH, Rengachary SS (eds). *Neurosurgery.* Vol. I. New York: McGraw-Hill; 1985:1011–21.

137. Hakuba A, Liu S, Nishimura S. The orbitozygomatic infratemporal approach: A new surgical technique. *Surg Neurol* 1986;**26**:271–6.

138. Sekhar LN, Schramm VL Jr, Jones NF. Subtemporal-preauricular infratemporal fossa approach to large lateral and posterior cranial base neoplasms. *J Neurosurg* 1987;**67**:488–99.

139. Samii M, Ammirati M. The combined supra-infratentorial pre-sigmoid sinus avenue to the petro-clival region. Surgical technique and clinical applications. *Acta Neurochir (Wien)* 1988;**95**:6–12.

140. Al-Mefty O, Fox JL, Smith RR. Petrosal approach for petroclival meningiomas. *Neurosurgery* 1988;**22**: 510–17.

141. Kawase T, Shiobara R, Toya S. Anterior trans-petrosal-transtentorial approach for sphenopetro-clival meningiomas: Surgical method and results in 10 patients. *Neurosurgery* 1991;**28**: 869–75; discussion 875–66.

142. Crockard HA, Essigman WK, Stevens JM, *et al.* Surgical treatment of cervical cord compression in rheumatoid arthritis. *Ann Rheum Dis* 1985;**44**: 809–16.

143. Sen CN, Sekhar LN. An extreme lateral approach to intradural lesions of the cervical spine and foramen magnum. *Neurosurgery* 1990;**27**:197–204.

144. Babu RP, Sekhar LN, Wright DC. Extreme lateral transcondylar approach: Technical improvements and lessons learned. *J Neurosurg* 1994;**81**:49–59.

9

Cavernous sinus: In and around

ASHISH SURI, SHASHWAT MISHRA, AJAY GARG

The cavernous sinus (CS) has been the most intriguing and forbidding region of the skull base for neurosurgeons. Approaches to the CS or through this region were considered impractical by earlier generations of neurosurgeons, considering the risk of injury to the traversing carotid artery and life-threatening haemorrhage. However, with advancement in micro-anatomical knowledge and surgical techniques, introduction of the operating microscope and better instrumentation, safe surgery in and around the CS became a possibility. Browder[1] and Parkinson[2] were the first to attempt a direct surgical exploration of carotid–cavernous fistulas. Pioneering work by Umansky,[3] Taptas[4] and Dolenc[5] was responsible for establishing the traditional approaches to the CS.

With the development of endovascular techniques and stereotactic radiosurgery, surgical approaches to the CS are less frequently required. Nevertheless, a clear understanding of the microsurgical anatomy and safe operative corridors provide the neurosurgeon additional confidence and skill in handling lesions in and around this region.

Surgical anatomy

Winslow (1732) initially recognized the resemblance of the parasellar venous spaces to the corpora cavernosa of the penis. The term 'cavernous sinus' has been used ever since. Till the middle of the 19th century, the CS was understood to be a venous lake surrounding the intracavernous internal carotid artery (ICA). However, detailed anatomical studies[3,4,6–8] revealed that the CS was much more complex than what was imagined.

Osseous and dural relationships

The bilateral cavernous sinuses are located in the centre of the skull base on both sides of the sella, sphenoid sinus and pituitary gland. They are most easily understood to be boat shaped[9] with medial, posterior, lateral walls and a roof. The narrow 'keel' of this boat is located along the superior orbital fissure (SOF), which marks the anterior boundary of the CS. The posterior wall or the 'bow' rests in the space lateral to the dorsum sellae above the petrous apex. Posteriorly, the cavernous sinuses communicate with the basilar sinus through the posterior wall. The two layers of the dura (endosteal layer facing the cranium and meningeal layer towards the brain) are tightly adherent to each other in the lateral portion of the middle cranial fossa. However, medially, as the dura sweeps over the upper two divisions of the trigeminal nerve, the endosteal layer splits to enclose the venous space of the CS. The lateral wall of the CS is thus double layered consisting of the outer meningeal layer and an inner layer composed of the outer endosteal layer. The fusion of the meningeal layers at the SOF forms the antero-inferior boundary or the 'keel' of the CS. The 'roof' of the CS is formed by the dural reflections stretching between the anterior clinoid process (ACP), posterior clinoid processes and the petrous apex. The sinus is thus triangular in cross-section. Posteriorly, the cavernous sinuses communicate with the basilar sinus through the posterior wall.

The consistent dural landmarks in and around the CS are indispensable for safe surgical approach to this region. Important dural structures include the carotid collar, the upper and lower dural rings and the triangles in the roof of CS.[9,10]

Upper and lower dural rings

The dural reflections from the upper and lower surface of the ACP form the upper and lower dural rings, respectively. The rings are separate anteriorly but fuse posteriorly. Resection of the ACP gives access to a triangular space, 'the clinoidal triangle' with its apex directed posteriorly and base towards the ACP. The clinoidal segment of the extracavernous ICA lies within this space. The space is bounded superiorly by the upper dural ring and inferiorly by the lower dural ring or the carotico-oculomotor membrane (due to its intimate relationship with the III nerve in the roof of the

CS). This space is thus separated from the CS sinus proper by the carotid–oculomotor membrane (COM), but is still considered to constitute the anterior half of the roof of the CS. The COM also turns upward in the clinoidal space to form the carotid collar.

The posterior half of the roof of the CS is constituted by the oculomotor triangle bounded by the anterior petroclinoid, posterior petro-clinoid and interclinoid folds of the dura. The oculomotor nerve pierces the roof of the CS through the oculomotor triangle after travelling through a short cistern, the oculomotor cistern.[11]

The roof of the CS thus consists of the clinoidal triangle anteriorly and the oculomotor triangle posteriorly, both of them constituted by dural folds. Conversely, on the lateral surface of the CS, the triangles are described in relation to the cranial nerves.

Lateral wall of the CS

The triangles revealed on the lateral wall of the CS when the outer meningeal layer is peeled off to reveal the translucent inner endosteal layer, are the supratrochlear and infratrochlear (Parkinsons's) triangles. The supratrochlear triangle is very narrow, bounded superiorly by the oculomotor, inferiorly by the trochlear and posteriorly by the dural entry points of the III and IV cranial nerves. The Parkinson's triangle is relatively wider and is located between the IV nerve and first division of the trigeminal nerve (Figs 1A, B).

Four additional triangles are described in the middle cranial fossa floor in relation to the CS. The anteromedial triangle is described between the ophthalmic and maxillary divisions of the trigeminal nerve. Similarly, the anterolateral triangle is located between the maxillary and mandibular divisions. Of particular importance are the posterolateral (Glasscock's) and the posteromedial (Kawase's) triangle (Fig. 1B).

The posterolateral triangle opens laterally and is bounded anterolaterally by the mandibular

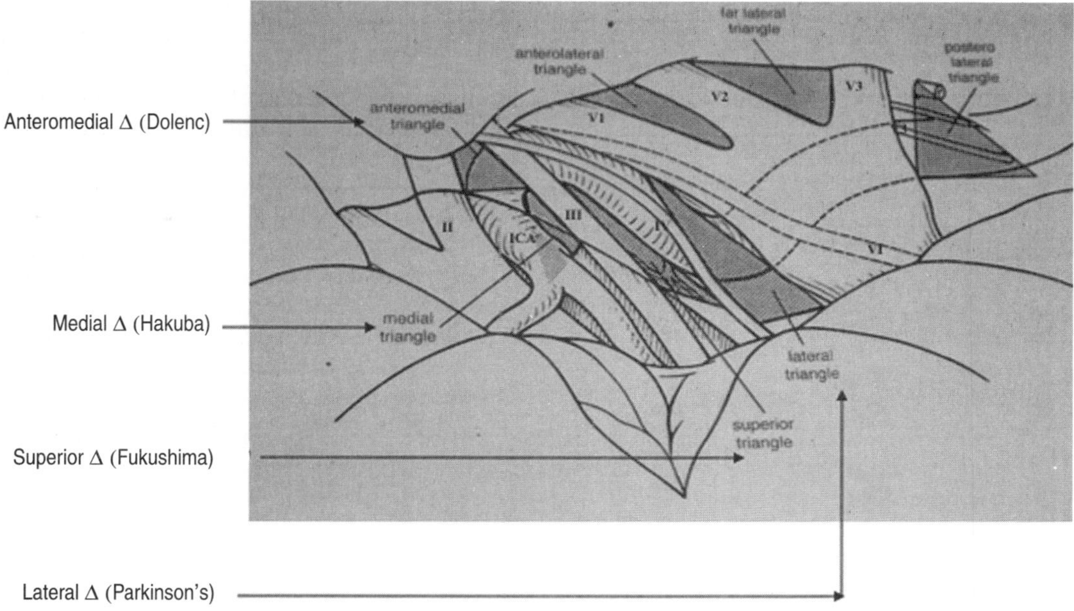

Fig. 1A

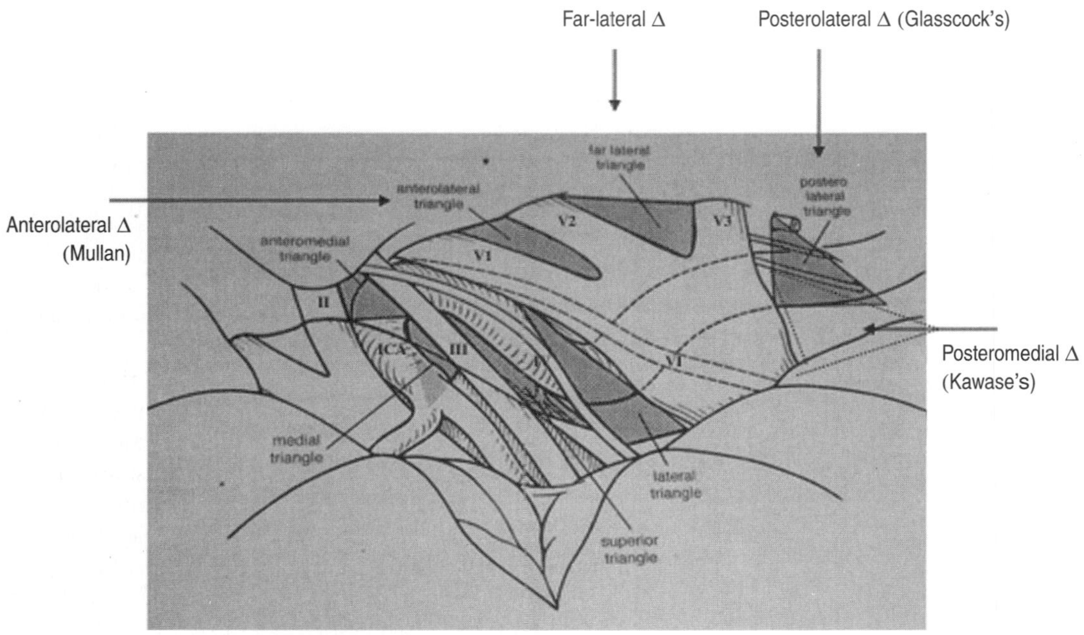

Fig. 1B

Figs 1A and B. Triangles of the cavernous sinus

division distal to the point where the GSPN crosses below it. The posteromedial boundary of the Glasscock's triangle is formed by the GSPN. The petrous carotid artery is situated in the anterior portion of the triangle while the cochlea lies deep to the lateral apex. The posteromedial triangle (Kawase's) is delimited by the GSPN laterally, the proximal mandibular division medially and the petrous ridge posteriorly. The part of the petrous apex within this triangle can be drilled during anterior petrosectomy.

Neural and vascular relationships

The cranial nerves in relation to the CS are from superior to inferior—oculomotor, trochlear, ophthalmic and abducens. The intracavernous ICA is also invested by a sympathetic plexus. The oculomotor nerve enters the CS in the oculomotor triangle, travels through a short cistern

and unites with the inner layer of the lateral wall of the CS only near the posterior tip of the ACP. The trochlear nerve enters the CS at the posterolateral apex of the oculomotor triangle. The oculomotor, trochlear and ophthalmic nerves are embedded within the lateral wall of the CS while the abducens and sympathetic plexus have a pure intracavernous course. The abducens nerve pierces the clival dura and then travels through Dorello's canal to enter the CS where it lies in relation to the lateral aspect of the posterior vertical segment of intracavernous ICA.

The ICA becomes intracavernous superior to the foramen lacerum and lateral to the posterior clinoid process. The intracavernous ICA has five segments (Fig. 2).

1. The posterior vertical
2. The posterior bend
3. The horizontal segment
4. The anterior bend
5. The anterior vertical segment

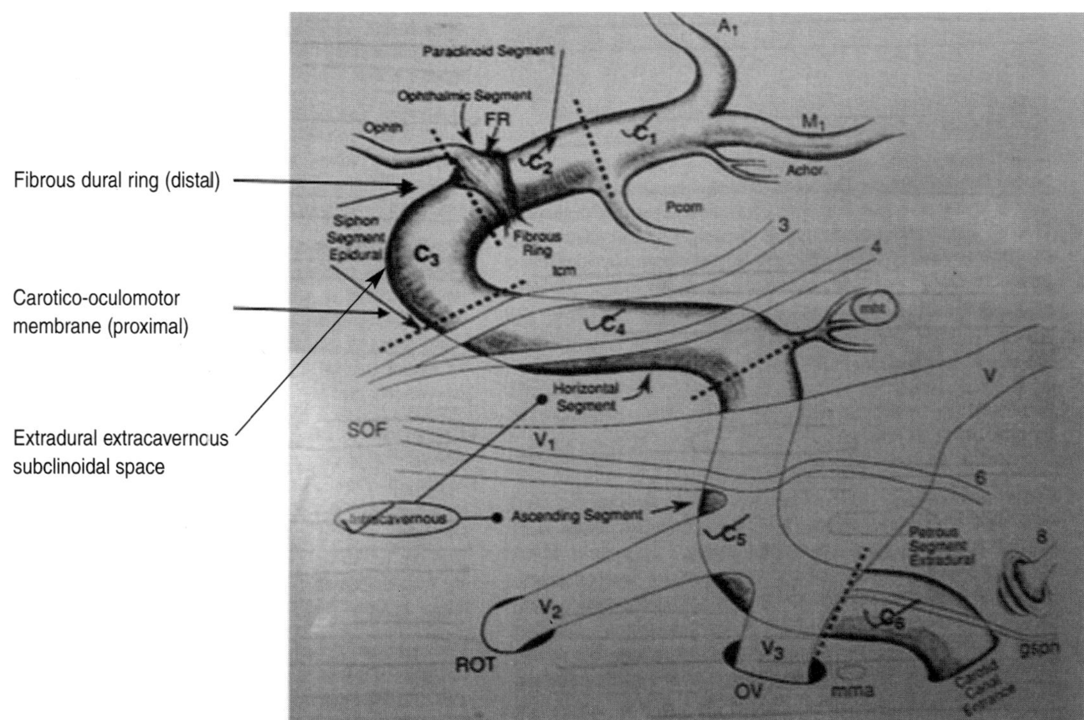

Fig. 2. The segments of the intracranial ICA

The posterior vertical segment begins where the petrous ICA passes below the petro-sphenoid ligament into the CS. The posterior bend is situated lateral to the posterior clinoid process and is sometimes visible as a bulge in the oculomotor trigone. The meningio-hypophyseal trunk originates from the lateral surface of the posterior bend in most cases.[12] Further, the ICA courses along the long axis of the CS forming the horizontal segment, which is also the site of origin of the inferolateral trunk. It then turns upward in the anterior portion of the roof of the CS. The anterior vertical segment corresponds to the clinoidal segment, which is exposed by anterior clinoidectomy.

The venous spaces within the CS are anatomically partitioned into the medial, lateral, postero-superior and antero-inferior compartments, depending on their relationship with the ICA. The CS receives venous drainage from the orbits, posterior fossa, cerebrum and contralateral CS.

Surgical approaches

A number of critical anatomical structures converge in the region of the CS. Hence, a detailed preoperative radiological study incorporating modern techniques such as MRI and MRA are necessary for complete evaluation of abnormalities in this region. Neuronavigational adjuncts such as frameless stereotaxy have excellent applicability to skull base procedures.

In cases where there is an anticipated high risk of carotid artery injury or sacrifice, the patient must undergo provocative angiography and perfusion studies to establish the adequacy of the collateral circulation. Bypass procedures may be indicated in collateral insufficiency.

Sekhar *et al.*[13] have classified CS tumours into five grades depending upon the extent of spread of the tumour and their adherence to the intracavernous ICA (Table 1).

A simpler scheme[13] categorizes CS tumours into confined (size <2.5 cm, predominantly confined to the CS and adjoining regions) and extensive (tumour size >2.5 cm, tumours secondarily invading the CS with the epicentre elsewhere such as a petroclival meningioma with CS extension).

Approaches to the CS are fraught with significant risk of intra-operative carotid artery injury and postoperative cranial nerve palsies. Hence, the decision to surgically explore CS tumours must be made with caution in tumours with extensive CS involvement (grade III, IV, V).

Generally, meningiomas are more difficult to resect than trigeminal schwannomas, pituitary adenomas, epidermoids, cavernous haemangiomas and other benign tumours involving the CS. The latter usually displace the carotid rather than encasing it, which can then be dissected free.

The CS is most conveniently approached through the roof or the lateral wall. Although a variety of surgical approaches have been classically described,[5,12,14] only a few are employed frequently, with the availability of endovascular techniques and radiosurgery. The most relevant approaches today are the cranio-orbito-zygomatic and the middle cranial fossa zygomatic approach.

Table 1. Extent of cavernous sinus and ICA involvement by cavernous sinus tumours

Grade	Cavernous sinus involvement	Cavernous ICA
I	One area only (anterior, posterior, lateral or medial CS)	Not involved
II	More than one area	Displaced, not encased
III	Entire cavernous sinus	Totally encased
IV	Entire cavernous sinus	Encased with narrowing, pseudoaneurysm or occlusion
V	Bilateral cavernous sinuses	Encased

The cranio-orbito-zygomatic approach (Figs 3A, B, C)

The patient is positioned supine with the head fixed in a Mayfield skull clamp. The head is rotated 30° towards the contralateral side and vertex dropped towards the floor so that the malar eminence is the highest point of the head. A fronto-temporal incision is then marked; starting within 1 cm of the tragus at the lower border of the zygoma and gently arching towards the contralateral side across the midline. The posterior limit of the incision may vary according to the extent of temporal exposure required.

After prepping and draping, a sub-galeal flap is elevated with subfascial dissection near the temporalis fat pad to preserve the fronto-temporal branch of the facial nerve.[15–17] The superficial temporal artery stem is carefully preserved to allow for extracranial–intracranial bypass if the need arises. The pericranial flap is elevated separately to provide for latter exteriorization of the frontal sinuses (which are occasionally entered during craniotomy) and also as a dural substitute. A fronto-temporal-orbitozygomatic craniotomy is then performed in 'two-piece' fashion, which has been excellently elucidated by Tanriover *et al.*[18] The two-piece craniotomy permits greater control of the orbital cuts and allows inclusion of a larger portion of the orbital roof in the osteotomy, preventing postoperative enopthalmos.

When proximal control over the ICA is required, it is preferable to obtain it in the neck, which is technically easier than the alternative of petrous carotid exposure in the middle cranial base. Moreover, petrous carotid exposure often requires GSPN sectioning, resulting in dry eye postoperatively.[19]

Superior entry into the CS

After drilling the sphenoid ridge and de-roofing the superior orbital fissure, the orbito-temporal periosteal dural fold is divided and the temporal dura is elevated revealing the base of the ACP.[20] The optic canal is then deroofed and the ACP progressively hollowed out. Care should to be taken during drilling, which must be performed

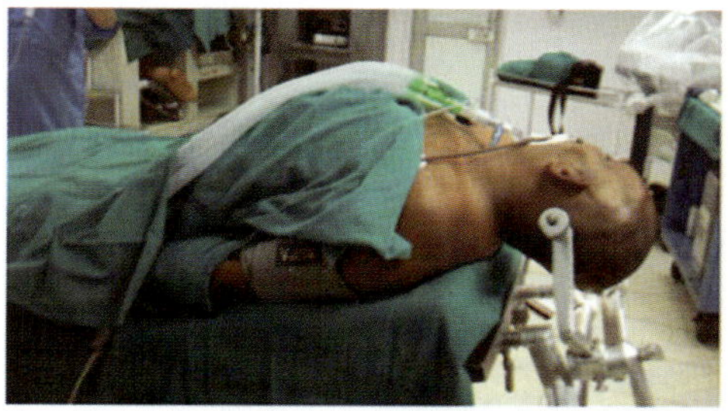

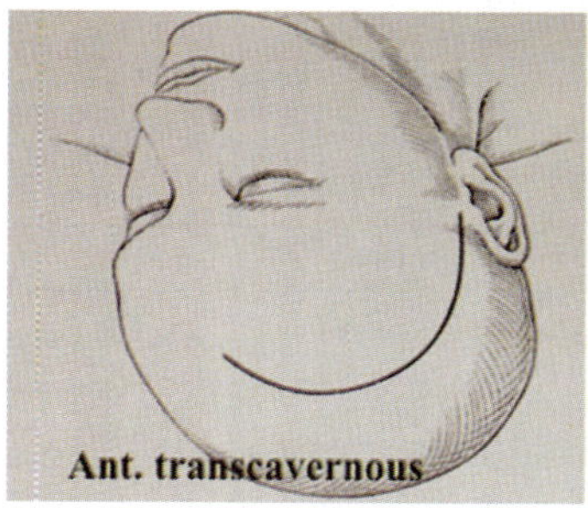

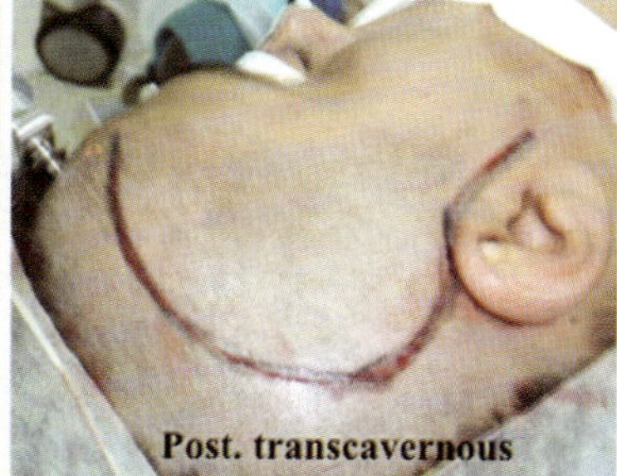

Fig. 3A. Positioning of the patient and incision plan for a superior (anterior)/lateral/posterior cavernous sinus approach

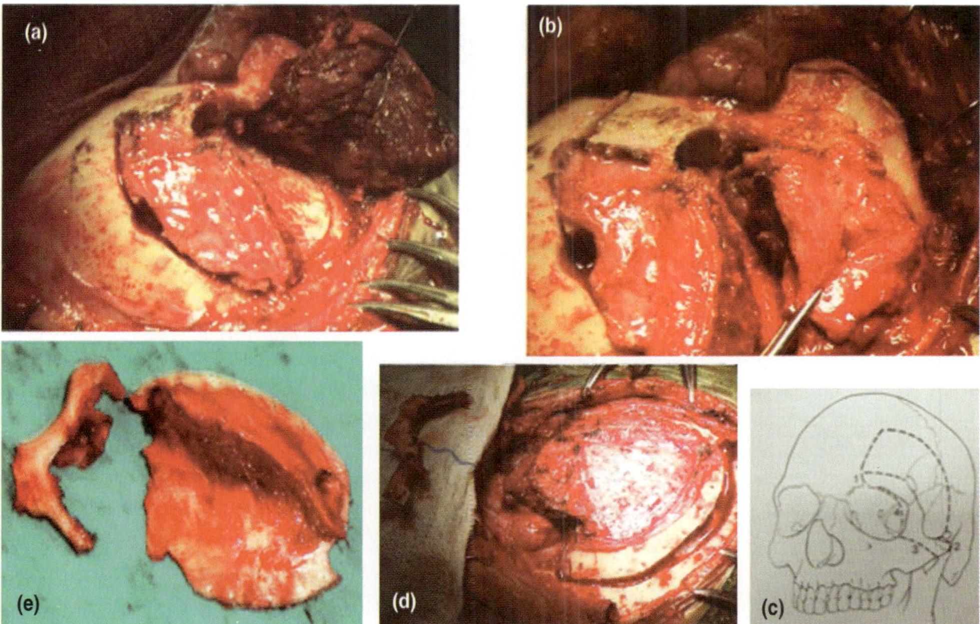

Fig. 3B. Two-piece fronto-temporo-orbitozygomatic craniotomy. **(a)** Fronto-temporal craniotomy; **(b)** orbitozygomatic osteotomy; **(c)** diagrammatic representation of osteotomy cuts; **(d)** osteotomy with osteoplastic craniotomy; **(e)** osteotomy segment and fronto-temporal flap

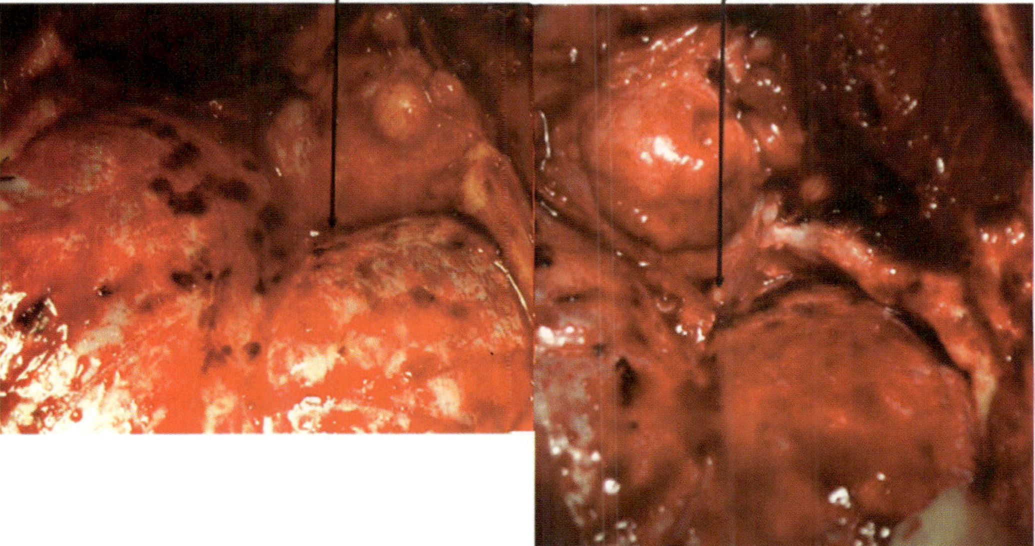

Fig. 3C. Exposure of superior orbital fissure after drilling the sphenoid ridge

with a diamond burr under copious saline irrigation. It must be kept in mind that the COM is intimately related to the tip of the ACP and the ICA is in close contact with the inferior surface of the ACP.[21] For paraclinoid aneurysms with erosion of the ACP evident on preoperative scans, it is preferable to drill the ACP intradurally.

Anterior clinoidectomy exposes the clinoidal space as described earlier. The distal dural ring is then divided circumferentially leaving a cuff around the ICA. A temporary clip may be placed over this mobilized segment of the ICA for proximal control. The optic nerve is then freed by dividing the falciform ligament. Exposure of the posterior half of the roof of the CS requires an intradural approach with a T-shaped dural incision (the vertical arm of the T-directed towards the optic nerve). The dura of the CS roof is then incised along the oculomotor nerve by inserting a 90° angled dissector into the oculomotor cistern and cutting the dura along it.[11] Bleeding from the CS is controlled either with surgicel packing or by injecting fibrin glue.[22] To enhance the exposure for posterior circulation aneurysms, the posterior clinoid process may also be drilled. The approaches through the CS roof provide excellent exposure of lesions located superior and medial to the ICA.

Lateral entry into the CS

The surgical procedure for entering the lateral CS extradurally exploits the loose adherence between the meningeal dura (dura propria) and outer layer of endosteal dura incorporating the cranial nerves. The dura propria can then be easily peeled off from the inner layer. The peeling is begun by incising the outer layer over the V3 region and then proceeding superiorly and anteriorly to progressively expose the V3, V2 and Gasserian ganglion. This can be combined with anterior petrosectomy to access lesions extending into the posterior fossa.

The lateral CS can also be exposed intra-durally, through a dural incision in the Parkinson's triangle, which exposes the posterior bend and the meningohypophyseal trunk.

The middle fossa transzygomatic approach

This approach is utilized in addressing lesions of the lateral CS or when anterior petrosectomy is required to deal with lesions in the posterior fossa. The cranio-orbito-zygomatic approach is more versatile in that it can be used for approaches both through the roof as well as the lateral wall of the CS.

A temporal craniotomy, two-thirds anterior and one-third posterior to the EAM, is performed with removal of the zygomatic process to allow for more inferior reflection of the temporalis muscle. The zygomatic osteotomy can be left attached to the masseter to minimize post-operative masticatory problems. The middle cranial fossa base is then extensively drilled. The middle meningeal artery is coagulated and divided. The dura is then elevated in a posterior-to-anterior direction, sequentially exposing the arcuate eminence, V3 and GSPN; the dura propria is incised over V3 and peeled off to expose the trigeminal ganglion and its divisions. The petrous apex thus exposed is drilled to access the posterior fossa if required as described by Kawase *et al.*[23] During drilling of the petrous apex, care is taken to avoid injuring the ICA, which lies lateral to the GSPN.

Application of CS approaches to various lesions in and around the CS

CS meningiomas (Figs 4, 5)

Meningiomas in this location present with visual disturbance, ocular motility dysfunction or facial numbness. Some of them may be discovered incidentally and may grow very slowly.[24] The CS may also be involved by meningiomas arising in adjoining areas. Thus, clinical observation or surgical resection, and primary or adjunctive

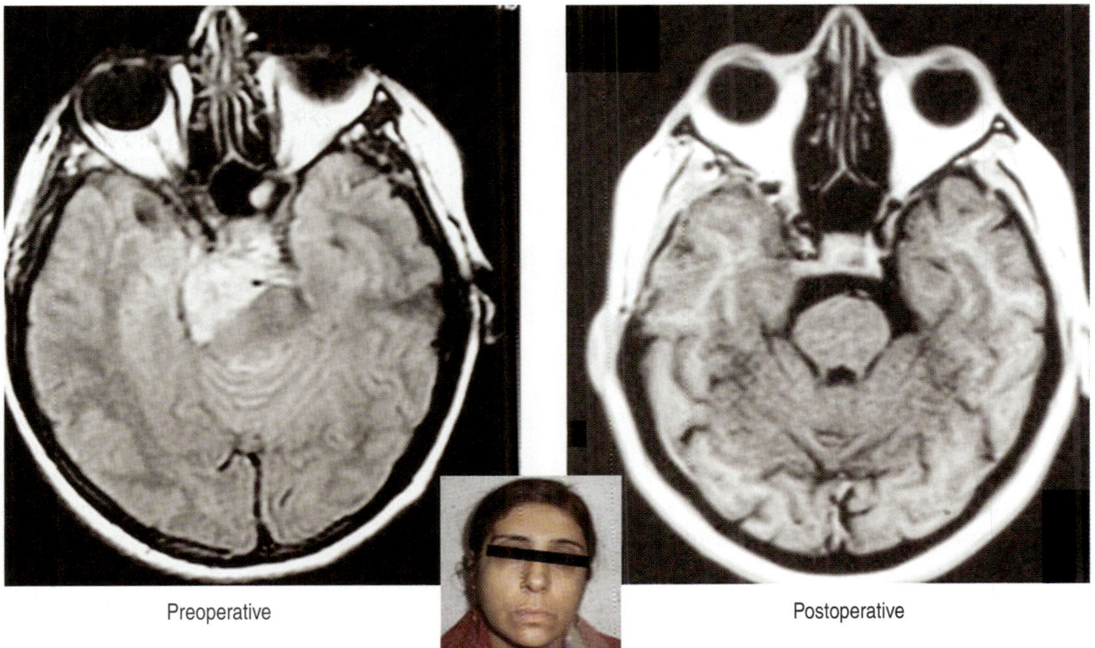

Fig. 4. Petroclival meningioma, example of a posterior fossa lesion which can be addressed through a posterior transcavernous approach

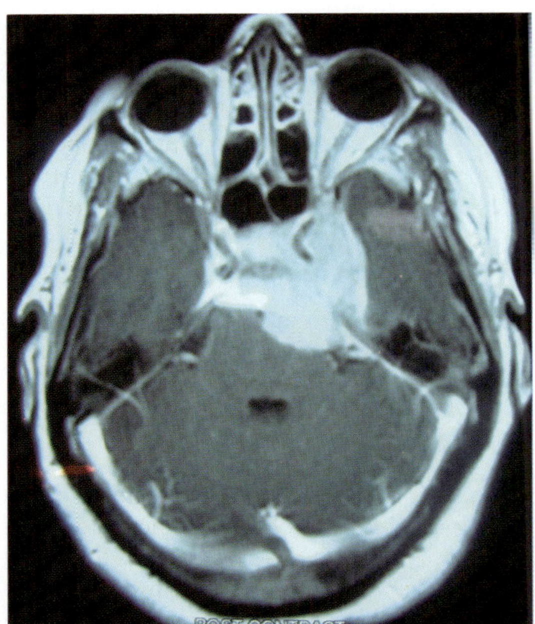

Fig. 5. Sphenocavernous meningioma, requiring exposure of the entire cavernous sinus

stereotactic radiosurgery are valid options for the management of these tumours. However, it is now well recognized that the resection of beningn non-meningeal tumours is easier as compared with meningiomas in the CS.[25] These tumours have a tendency to encase the cavernous ICA and infiltrate the cranial nerves. Complete extirpation of CS meningiomas may require sacrifice of the ICA and cervical–supraclinoid ICA bypass. In a study of 19 patients who underwent ICA sacrifice for resection of CS meningiomas, histological evidence of ICA infiltration was found in 42%.[26] Moreover, morbidity from the cranial nerve palsies resulting from CS exploration is significant.[27,28] The risk of intra-operative ICA injury and postoperative ocular motility dysfunction, major morbidities of CS surgery, correlates with the degree of ICA encasement seen on preoperative imaging.[29] Long-term outcome analysis from various clinical series also indicate that gross total tumour excision could be achieved but only at the cost of high complication rates.[27,28,30] Up to 76%[30] of the tumours could be gross totally excised with ocular motor disability seen in 12%–40% of cases. On the contrary, admirable rates of tumour control and preservation of ocular motor function have been seen with radiosurgery.[31,32] However, surgical exploration of CS meningiomas has the distinct advantage of enabling optic nerve decompression.

On the basis of these observations, we have changed our strategy towards maximum safe debulking of the intracavernous portion of the tumour followed by gamma-knife irradiation.[33,34] The objective of surgical intervention is decompression of the optic nerve and optimization of the residual tumour topography for gamma-knife irradiation, that is, removal of tumour from the proximity of critical structures with poor radiation tolerance; principally, the optic nerve.

These tumours are approached through a cranio-orbito-zygomatic/fronto-temporal craniotomy (depending upon the extent of extracavernous tumour spread). The outer layer of the lateral wall of the CS is peeled off as described and the roof is exposed by a combination of extradural anterior clinoidectomy and intradural exposure. The CS roof is then opened along the course of the oculomotor nerve and the tumour decompressed between the optic nerve and the oculomotor branches. No attempt, however, is made to remove tumour remnants densely adherent to the ICA or the cranial nerves. At least 3 mm of separation between the residual tumour and optic nerve is required for safe gamma-knife irradiation.[35]

Primary gamma-knife irradiation is suitable for small-size tumours without significant encroachment upon the optic nerve.

Pituitary adenomas (Fig. 6)

Pituitary adenomas have the tendency to invade the CS from the medial wall where there is no bony separation between the sella and the CS. Traditionally, intracavernous extension of pituitary adenomas have been considered inoperable and subjected to radiotherapy. However, the latency of the radiation effect is quite long and, in cases of

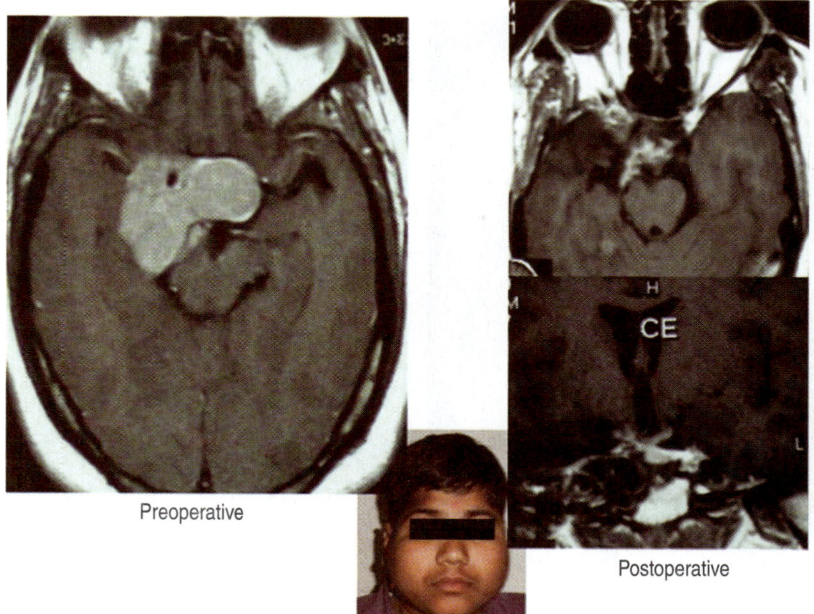

Fig. 6. Multi-compartmental pituitary adenoma surgically treated through a cranio-orbito-zygomatic transcavernous approach

functioning adenomas, the biological effects of hormonal hypersecretion may be disabling or even life-threatening. Dolenc[36] initially described his experience with the transcranial epidural approach to adenomas with parasellar extension. Despite the suitability of radiosurgery for treatment of CS residuals of pituitary adenomas, the CS approaches still remain relevant for functioning pituitary adenomas with CS extension. However, it must be kept in mind that aggressive removal of a pituitary tumour from the CS region is associated with a high risk-to-benefit ratio. Hence, a conservative approach is preferable, which aims for less than 100% tumour removal.

The approach to pituitary tumours with CS invasion is a standard fronto-temporo-orbito-zygomatic approach and anterior clinoidecomy with division of the distal dural ring and mobilization of the ICA. The lateral wall of the CS is then exposed epidurally and transcavernous tumour decompression is carried out through the Parkinson's and antero-medial triangles. Reckless manipulation of infiltrative tumours within the CS may lead to injury to the ICA or cranial nerves. A trans-sphenoidal transcavernous approach through the medial and inferior walls of the CS has also been described, which is postulated to avoid cranial nerve morbidity associated with CS exploration.[37]

Non-meningeal tumours of the CS (Figs 7–10)

As mentioned earlier, non-meningeal benign tumours of the CS such as chordomas, trigeminal schwannomas, epidermoids and haemangiomas tend to displace the CS contents rather than invading them. The surgical resection of these tumours is satisfying, and CS approaches can be applied to them with minimal postoperative morbidity.[25,27] The transzygomatic–transpetrous approach is especially indicated for extradural tumours such as trigeminal schwannomas, which provides a natural corridor for a completely interdural approach minimizing cranial nerve injury.[38–40]

Even tumours with considerable vascularity can be excised safely with the extradural

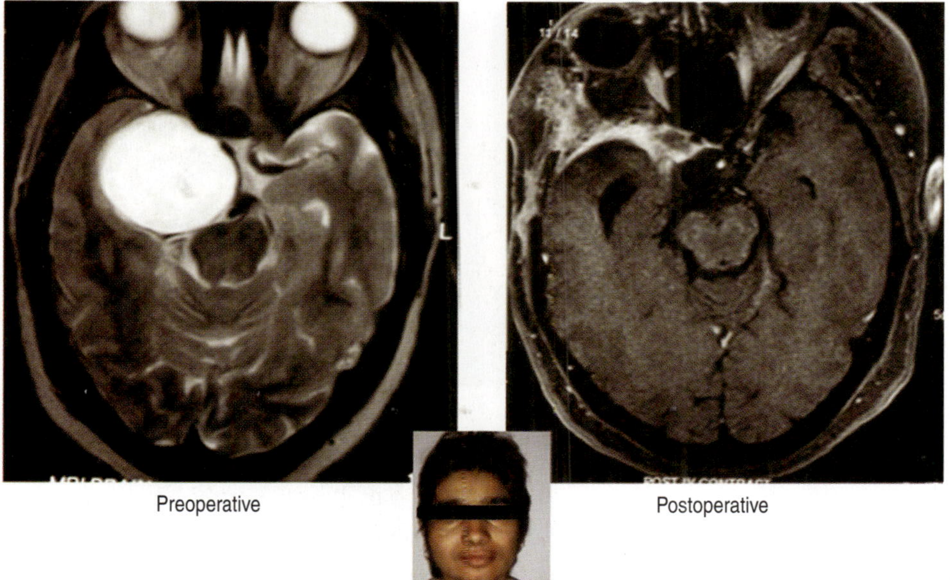

Preoperative   Postoperative

Fig. 7. Cavernous sinus haemangioma surgically treated through the extradural transcavernous approach

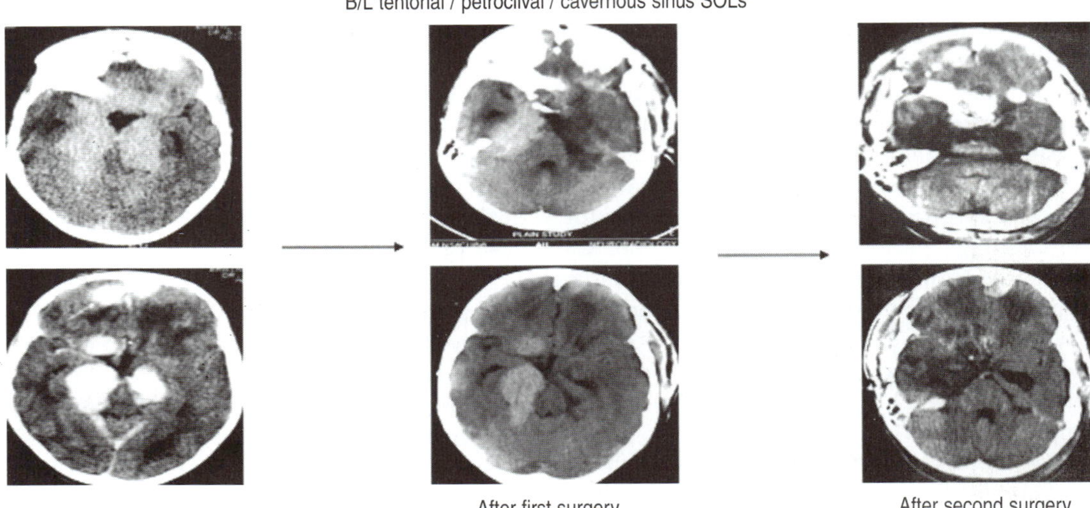

Fig. 8. Rosai–Dorfman d sease (histiocytosis), one of the rare lesions operated by the transcavernous–transpetrous route

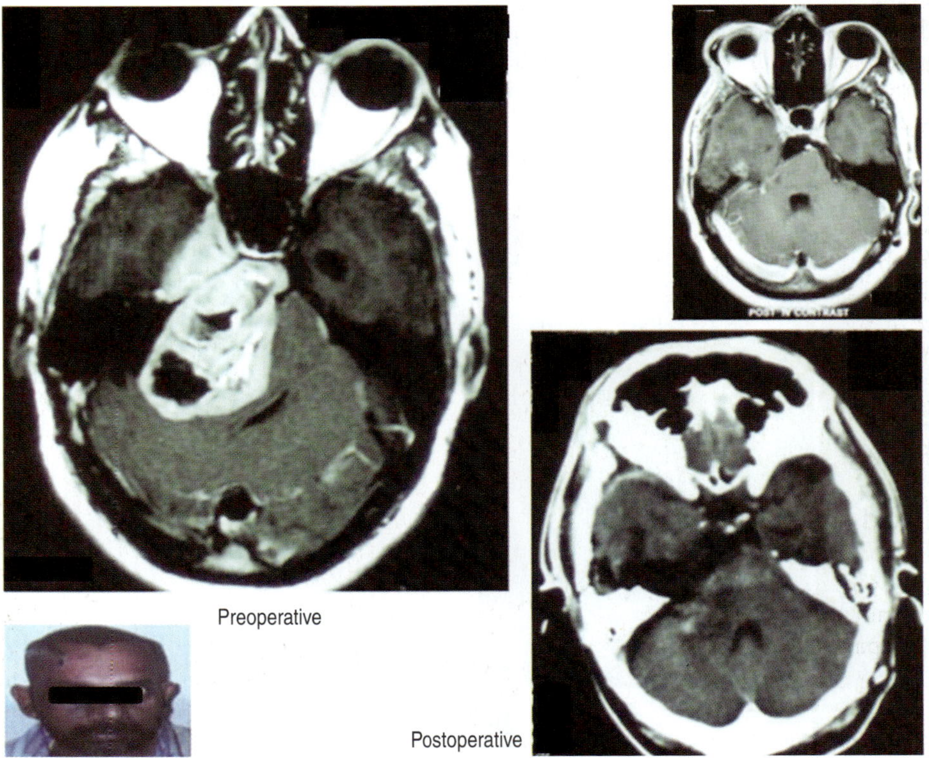

Fig. 9. V nerve schwannoma completely excised through a temporo-zygomatic posterior transcavernous–transpetrous approach

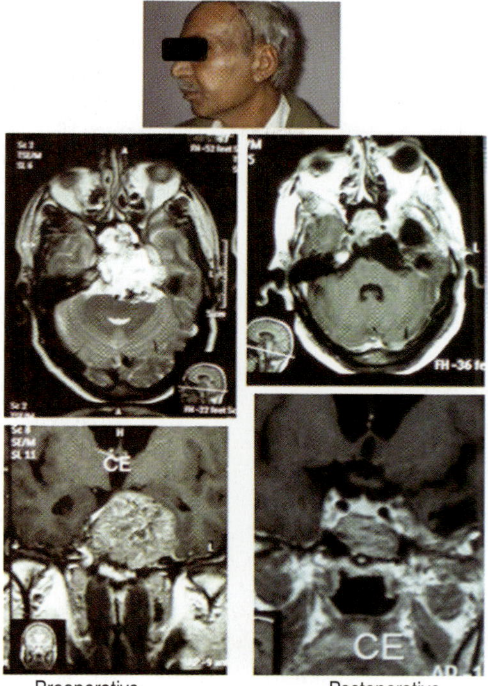

Preoperative   Postoperative

Fig. 10. Sphenocavernous chordoma

approach, which we have highlighted in our own experience with 7 cases of CS haemangiomas.[41] We were able to achieve complete resection of the haemangioma in 6 cases with only a single instance of postoperative VI nerve palsy.

Vascular lesions involving/in proximity of the CS (Figs 11–15)

Paraclinoid aneurysms

Exposure of the clinoidal segment of the extracavernous ICA is routinely required for clipping of paraclinoid aneurysms.[42,43]

Carotid–cavernous fistulas

Carotid–cavernous fistulas (CCFs) are abnormal communications between the carotid arterial system and the venous CS. These fistulas may be divided into spontaneous or traumatic in relation to cause, and direct or indirect (dural) in relation to angiographic findings. Direct CCF (Barrow's type A) is a high-flow communication between the ICA and the CS that occurs after trauma or secondary to a ruptured aneurysm of the cavernous ICA. These patients may present with signs and symptoms such as conjunctival chemosis, proptosis, pulsating exophthalmos, diplopia, ophthalmoplegia, orbital pain and tinnitus. Indirect (dural) CCFs (Barrow's types B, C and D) are low-flow fistulas occurring between the CS, and one or more meningeal branches of the ICA, external carotid artery or both. These dural fistulas usually have low rates of arterial blood flow and may be difficult to diagnose without angiography. These fistulas usually result in less severe symptoms, with insidious onset, mild orbital congestion, proptosis and low or no bruit.

On imaging studies such as CT scan and MRI, CCF may present with an enlarged superior ophthalmic vein, proptosis, thick extraocular muscles and evidence of an enlarged CS with a convexity of the lateral wall. These changes can only make one suspect a fistula. The presence of flow-related enhancement in the CS on MR angiography suggests the diagnosis in the right clinical setting. Digital subtraction angiography (DSA), currently the standard of reference for the diagnosis of dural and direct CCFs, characterizes the blood supply and venous drainage of a CCF. With direct or dural CCFs, the venous drainage may be multidirectional.

Most CCFs are not life-threatening, but the involved eye is at risk. The main indications for treatment include glaucoma, diplopia, intolerable bruit or headache, and severe proptosis causing exposure keratopathy. An indication for urgent treatment is the presence of cortical venous reflux seen on DSA.

Spontaneous closure from thrombosis of the CS is unlikely (especially in direct CCFs). Indirect CCFs may undergo spontaneous closure,

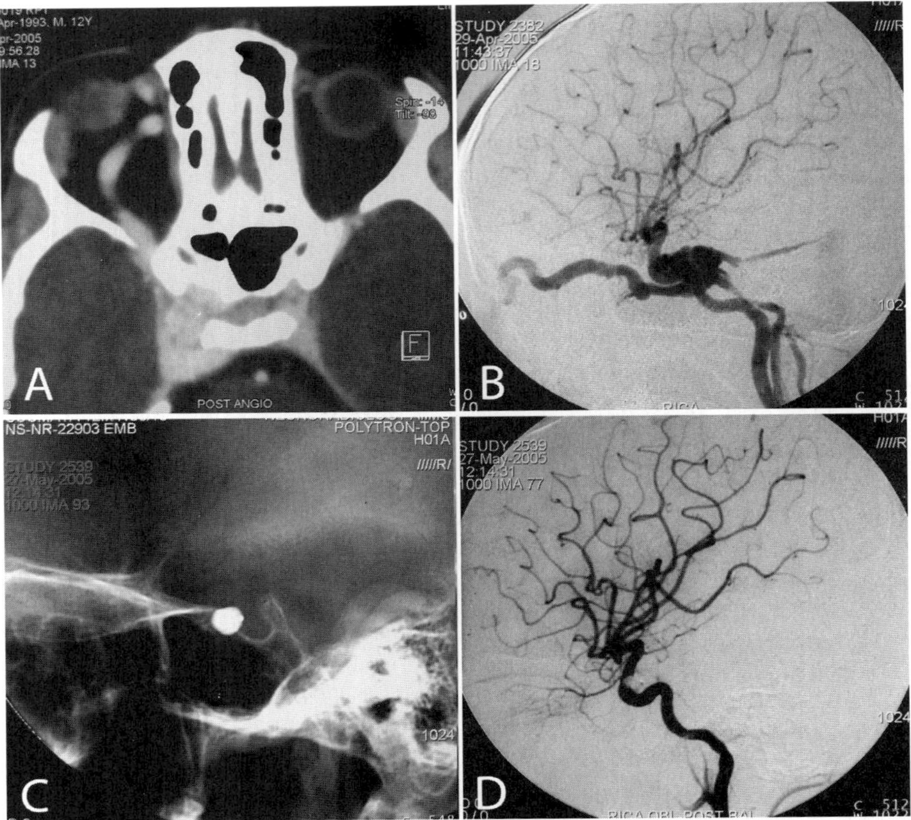

Fig. 11. (A) Contrast CT head showing enlarged cavernous sinus with engorged right superior ophthalmic vein and right eye proptosis;(B) arterial phase DSA exhibiting a direct CCF from C4 carotid segment with engorged superior ophthalmic vein enhancing on contrast, (C and D) post-embolization

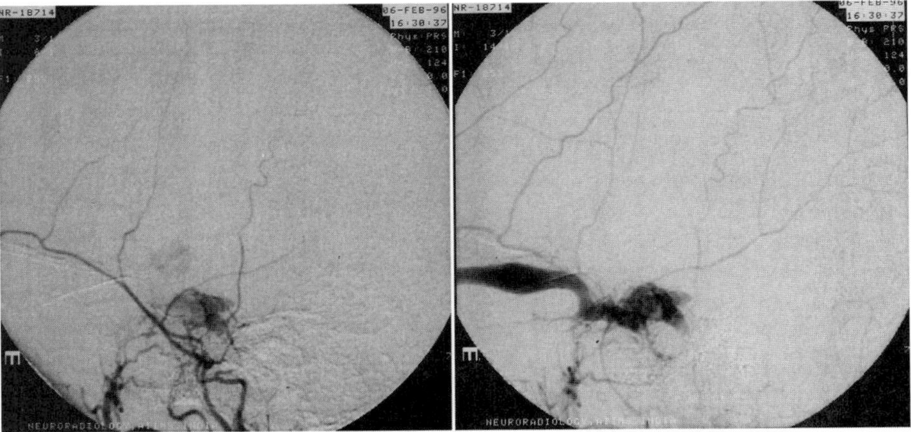

Fig. 12. Indirect CCF fed by the dural branches of the ECA

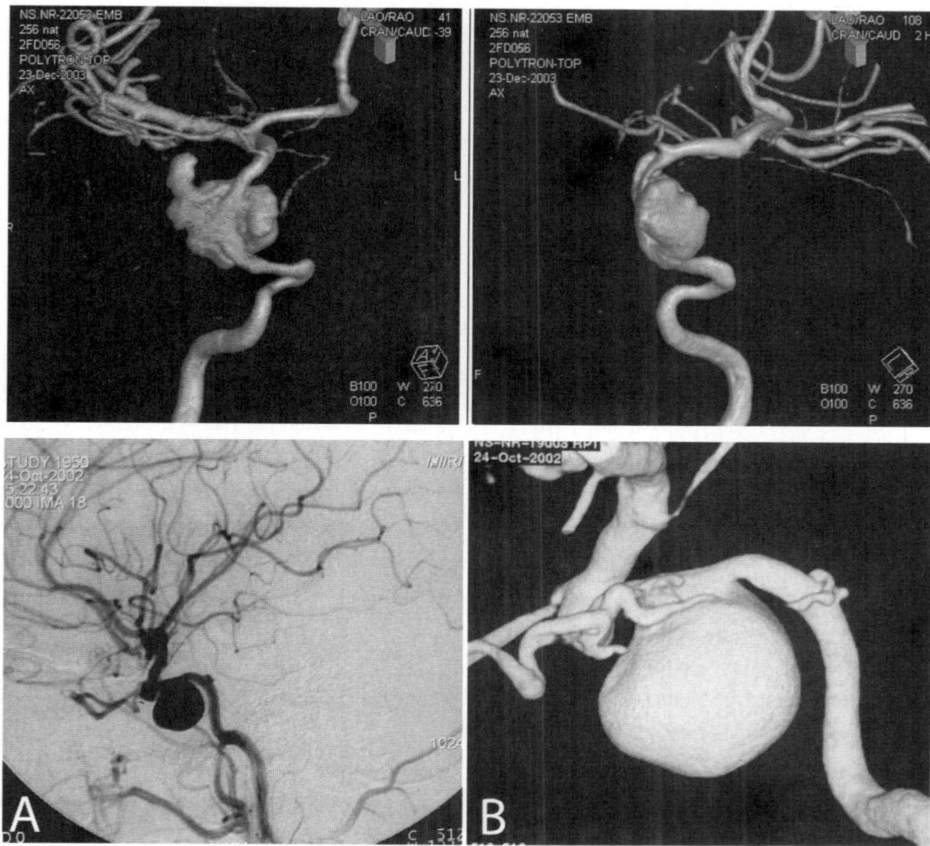

Figs 13 and 14. Cavernous ICA aneurysm

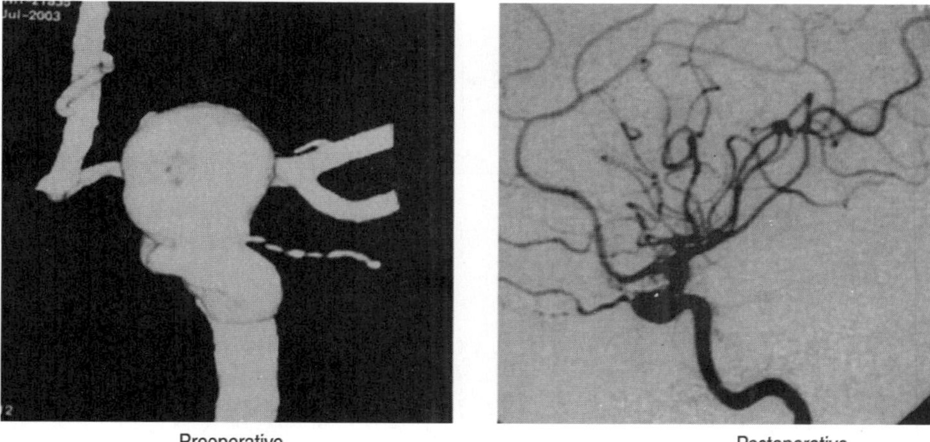

Preoperative

Postoperative

Fig. 15. A giant paraclinoid cavernous ICA aneurysm clipped through a cranio-orbito-zygomatic anterior transcavernous exposure

especially after diagnostic angiography. Carotid compression therapy has also been successful in closure of 17% of direct and 30% of dural CCFs.[44] In the past, various surgical treatments had included ligation of the external and internal carotid arteries; and fistula embolization with particles, glue, detachable balloons and thrombogenic microcoils. Though a transcavernous approach under hypothermic circulatory arrest was described by Parkinson[2] for treatment of CCFs, it was with the pioneering efforts of Dolenc[5] that a direct microsurgical approach to intracavernous vascular lesions became possible without the need for circulatory arrest. However, primary surgical treatment of CCFs is not indicated today with the availability of endovascular techniques.[44] The only surgical indication probably is patients with failed endovascular occlusion of the CCF.

At present, the treatment modality of choice is endovascular intervention. Direct fistulas are best treated with a detachable balloon or coils through an endarterial route. Treatment of cavernous dural arteriovenous fistulas is usually done using a trans-arterial approach with glue or onyx. However, in many complicated cases, treatment using the trans-arterial approach may not be feasible, or are unsuccessful; but dural CCFs can be treated with transvenous embolization via the superior ophthalmic vein.

Cavernous ICA aneurysms

A direct surgical approach to cavernous ICA aneurysms is almost historical. Considering the favourable natural history,[45] treatment is indicated only if they become symptomatic causing considerable cranial nerve deficits, facial pain or extend beyond the dural confines of the CS. Because of the potential morbidity of aggressive surgical approaches, endovascular techniques are preferable wherever treatment is indicated. Parent vessel sacrifice through balloon occlusion/hunterian ligation or aneurysm exclusion through endovascular coiling are the usual therapeutic approaches.

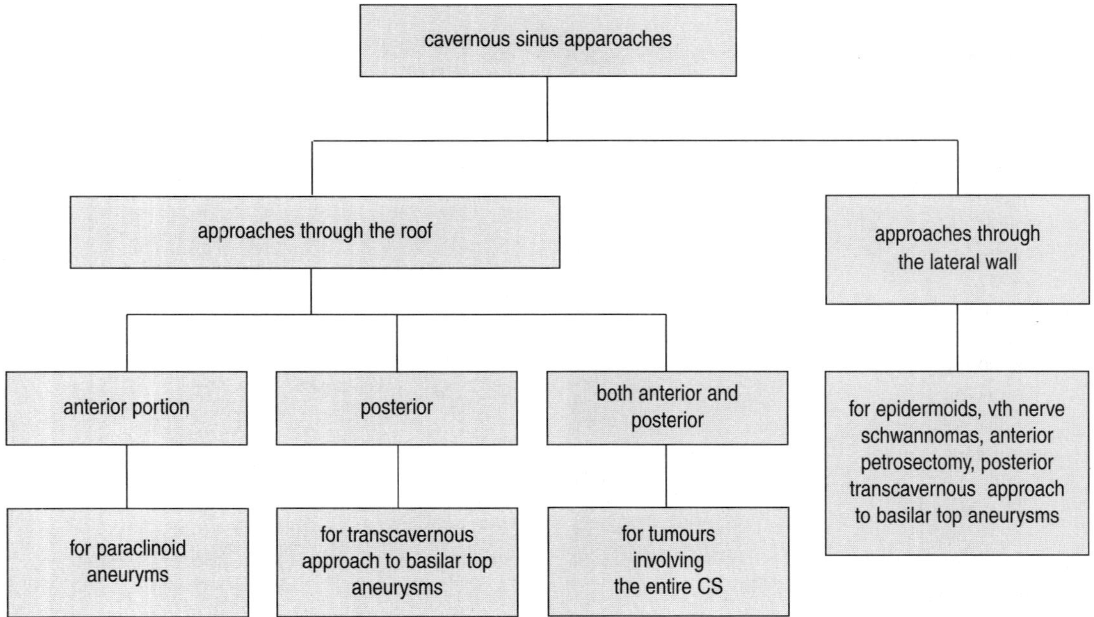

Fig. 16. A simplified scheme representing the application of cavernous sinus approaches

Posterior circulation aneurysms

Transcavernous approaches have wide application in basilar top aneurysms[46] as well as lesions in the upper third of the posterior fossa.[47] Mobilization of the III nerve by incision along the roof of the CS enlarges the operative corridor to the interpeduncular fossa while minimizing III nerve morbidity. Posterior clinoid drilling can further increase access to the posterior fossa.

Conclusion

A detailed knowledge of CS anatomy and various safe microsurgical approaches remains relevant for the neurosurgeon even today.

References

1. Browder J. Treatment of carotid artery–cavernous sinus fistula. Report of a case. *Archs Ophthal, Chicago* 1937;**18**:95–102.

2. Parkinson D. A surgical approach to the cavernous portion of the carotid artery. Anatomical studies and case report. *J Neurosurg* 1965;**23**:474–83.

3. Umansky F, Nathan H. The lateral wall of the cavernous sinus. With special reference to the nerves related to it. *J Neurosurg* 1982;**56**:228–34.

4. Taptas JN. The so-called cavernous sinus: A review of the controversy and its implications for neurosurgeons. *Neurosurgery* 1982;**11**:712–7.

5. Dolenc V. Direct microsurgical repair of intracavernous vascular lesions. *J Neurosurg* 1983;**58**:824–31.

6. Harris FS, Rhoton AL. Anatomy of the cavernous sinus. A microsurgical study. *J Neurosurg* 1976;**45**:169–80.

7. Yasuda A, Campero A, Martins C, *et al.* Microsurgical anatomy and approaches to the cavernous sinus. *Neurosurgery* 2005;**56**:4–27; discus-sion 4.

8. Yasuda A, Campero A, Martins C, *et al.* The medial wall of the cavernous sinus: Microsurgical anatomy. *Neurosurgery* 2004;**55**:179–89; discussion 89–90.

9. Rhoton AL Jr. The cavernous sinus, the cavernous venous plexus, and the carotid collar. *Neurosurgery* 2002;**51**:S1375–S1410.

10. Seoane E, Rhoton AL Jr, de Oliveira E. Microsurgical anatomy of the dural collar (carotid collar) and rings around the clinoid segment of the internal carotid artery. *Neurosurgery* 1998;**42**:869–84; discussion 84–6.

11. Martins C, Yasuda A, Campero A, *et al.* Microsurgical anatomy of the oculomotor cistern. *Neurosurgery* 2006;**58**:ONS-220–7; discussion ONS-7–8.

12. Inoue T, Rhoton AL Jr, Theele D, *et al.* Surgical approaches to the cavernous sinus: A microsurgical study. *Neurosurgery* 1990;**26**:903–32.

13. Raso J, Sekhar LN, Wright DC, *et al.* Anatomy of the cavernous sinus. In: Sekhar LN, Oliveira ED (eds). *Cranial microsurgery: Approaches and techniques.* New York: Theime; 1999:176–81.

14. Rhoton AL Jr, Inoue T. Microsurgical approaches to the cavernous sinus. *Clin Neurosurg* 1991;**37**:391–439.

15. Coscarella E, Vishteh AG, Spetzler RF, *et al.* Subfascial and submuscular methods of temporal muscle dissection and their relationship to the frontal branch of the facial nerve. Technical note. *J Neurosurg* 2000;**92**:877–80.

16. Yasargil MG, Reichman MV, Kubik S. Preservation of the frontotemporal branch of the facial nerve using the interfascial temporalis flap for pterional craniotomy. Technical article. *J Neurosurg* 1987;**67**:463–6.

17. Krayenbuhl N, Isolan GR, Hafez A, *et al.* The relationship of the fronto-temporal branches of the facial nerve to the fascias of the temporal region: A literature review applied to practical anatomical dissection. *Neurosurg Rev* 2007;**30**:8–15.

18. Tanriover N, Ulm AJ, Rhoton AL Jr, *et al.* One-piece versus two-piece orbitozygomatic craniotomy: Quantitative and qualitative considerations. *Neurosurgery* 2006;**58**:ONS-229–37; discussion ONS-37.

19. Fitzpatrick BC, Spetzler RF, Ballard JL, *et al.* Cervical-to-petrous internal carotid artery bypass procedure. Technical note. *J Neurosurg* 1993;**79**:138–41.

20. Froelich SC, Aziz KM, Levine NB, *et al.* Refinement of the extradural anterior clinoidectomy: Surgical anatomy of the orbitotemporal periosteal fold. *Neurosurgery* 2007;**61**:179–85; discussion 85–6.

21. Noguchi A, Balasingam V, Shiokawa Y, *et al.* Extradural anterior clinoidectomy. Technical note. *J Neurosurg* 2005;**102**:945–50.

22. Krayenbuhl N, Hafez A, Hernesniemi JA, *et al.* Taming the cavernous sinus: Technique of hemostasis using fibrin glue. *Neurosurgery* 2007;**61**:E52.

23. Kawase T, Shiobara R, Toya S. Anterior transpetrosal-

transtentorial approach for sphenopetroclival meningiomas: Surgical method and results in 10 patients. *Neurosurgery* 1991;**28**:869–75; discussion 75–6.

24. Kuratsu J, Kochi M, Ushio Y. Incidence and clinical features of asymptomatic meningiomas. *J Neurosurg* 2000;**92**:766–70.

25. Sekhar LN, Pomeranz S, Sen CN. Management of tumours involving the cavernous sinus. *Acta Neurochir Suppl (Wien)* 1991;**53**:101–12.

26. Kotapka MJ, Kalia KK, Martinez AJ, *et al.* Infiltration of the carotid artery by cavernous sinus meningioma. *J Neurosurg* 1994;**81**:252–5.

27. Sekhar LN, Patel S, Cusimano M, *et al.* Surgical treatment of meningiomas involving the cavernous sinus: Evolving ideas based on a ten year experience. *Acta Neurochir Suppl* 1996;**65**:58–62.

28. DeMonte F, Smith HK, al-Mefty O. Outcome of aggressive removal of cavernous sinus meningiomas. *J Neurosurg* 1994;**81**:245–51.

29. Hirsch WL, Sekhar LN, Lanzino G, *et al.* Meningiomas involving the cavernous sinus: Value of imaging for predicting surgical complications. *AJR Am J Roentgenol* 1993;**160**:1083–8.

30. De Jesus O, Sekhar LN, Parikh HK, *et al.* Long-term follow-up of patients with meningiomas involving the cavernous sinus: Recurrence, progression, and quality of life. *Neurosurgery* 1996;**39**:915–19; discussion 19–20.

31. Roche PH, Regis J, Dufour H, *et al.* Gamma knife radiosurgery in the management of cavernous sinus meningiomas. *J Neurosurg* 2000;**93** Suppl 3:68–73.

32. Iwai Y, Yamanaka K, Ishiguro T. Gamma knife radiosurgery for the treatment of cavernous sinus meningiomas. *Neurosurgery* 2003;**52**:517–24; discussion 523–4.

33. Pamir MN, Kilic T, Bayrakli F, *et al.* Changing treatment strategy of cavernous sinus meningiomas: Experience of a single institution. *Surg Neurol* 2005;**64** Suppl 2:S58–S66.

34. Couldwell WT, Kan P, Liu JK, *et al.* Decompression of cavernous sinus meningioma for preservation and improvement of cranial nerve function. Technical note. *J Neurosurg* 2006;**105**:148–52.

35. Nicolato A, Foroni R, Alessandrini F, *et al.* Radiosurgical treatment of cavernous sinus meningiomas: Experience with 122 treated patients. *Neurosurgery* 2002;**51**:1153–9; discussion 1159–61.

36. Dolenc VV. Transcranial epidural approach to pituitary tumors extending beyond the sella. *Neurosurgery* 1997;**41**:542–50; discussion 551–2.

37. Kitano M, Taneda M, Shimono T, *et al.* Extended transsphenoidal approach for surgical management of pituitary adenomas invading the cavernous sinus. *J Neurosurg* 2008;**108**:26–36.

38. Pamir MN, Peker S, Bayrakli F, *et al.* Surgical treatment of trigeminal schwannomas. *Neurosurg Rev* 2007;**30**:329–37; discussion 337.

39. Sharma BS, Ahmad FU, Chandra PS, *et al.* Trigeminal schwannomas: Experience with 68 cases. *J Clin Neurosci* 2008;**15**:738–43.

40. Zhang L, Yang Y, Xu S, *et al.* Trigeminal schwannomas: A report of 42 cases and review of the relevant surgical approaches. *Clin Neurol Neurosurg* 2009;**111**:261–9.

41. Suri A, Ahmad FU, Mahapatra AK. Extradural transcavernous approach to cavernous sinus hemangiomas. *Neurosurgery* 2007;**60**:483–8; discussion 448–9.

42. Heros RC. Anterior paraclinoid aneurysms. *J Neurosurg* 2002;**96**:981–2; discussion 982.

43. Heros RC. Paraclinoid aneurysms. *J Neurosurg* 2002;**96**:647–8.

44. Gemmete JJ, Chaudhary N, Pandey A, *et al.* Treatment of carotid cavernous fistulas. *Curr Treat Options Neurol* 2010;**12**:43–53.

45. Stiebel-Kalish H, Kalish Y, Bar-On RH, *et al.* Presentation, natural history, and management of carotid cavernous aneurysms. *Neurosurgery* 2005;**57**:850–7; discussion 857.

46. Krisht AF, Kadri PA. Surgical clipping of complex basilar apex aneurysms: A strategy for successful outcome using the pretemporal transzygomatic transcavernous approach. *Neurosurgery* 2005;**56**:261–73; discussion 273.

47. Krisht AF. Transcavernous approach to diseases of the anterior upper third of the posterior fossa. *Neurosurg Focus* 2005;**19**:E2.

10

Acoustic neuromas: How I do it

KEKI E. TUREL

No other surgery exemplifies the progress of neurosurgery in the past century better than that of an acoustic neuroma. Neurosurgeons were content with saving the life of the patient with acoustic neuroma in the beginning of the century.[1] The advent of microsurgery in the 1960s, the creation of advanced imaging technology in the 1970s and 1980s, and the addition of intraoperative electrophysiological monitoring almost during the same time has shifted the focus to facial nerve preservation and preservation of serviceable hearing along with gross total tumour removal. The present-day goals of acoustic neuroma surgery are preservation of life, gross total tumour excision, total anatomical preservation of facial nerve, and preservation and even improvement of serviceable hearing, in that order.

Harvey Cushing, with his preoccupation with surgical mortality, had to be content with partial removal of acoustic tumours.[2] However, tumour recurrence led to an overall mortality rate of 56%. Dandy[3,4] succeeded in doing 45 total acoustic tumour removals with a modest mortality rate of 11%. Although facial nerve preservation had begun to be envisioned, it was a rarity. Olivecrona[5] and Nielsen[6] reported facial nerve preservation in a high percentage of cases (65%) with an apparent gross tumour removal. However, a subsequent review of Olivecrona's cases by Horrax and Poppen[7] found half the patients either dead or with subsequent tumour recurrence.[5,6]

The otolaryngologists were the earliest to adopt the surgical microscope in routine practice and demonstrated the advantages of this device with their lower mortality rates and greater numbers of facial nerve preservation using a middle fossa approach.[8,9] However, they were unable to remove large tumours through this approach. When it was attempted, complications such as uncontrollable intraoperative bleeding occurred. The pioneering efforts of William House,[10–12] however, paved the way for renewed optimism in the successful management of acoustic tumours with a low mortality and acceptable morbidity.

Rand and Kurze,[13] Drake,[14–16] and others showed that acoustic tumours could be removed totally, safely, and with preservation of the facial nerve. Rand and Kurze[17] discussed the possibility of anatomical preservation of the cochlear nerve, which they subsequently demonstrated in 1968. Subsequent occasional reports on preservation of cochlear nerve function appeared in the literature, although these were infrequent.

Today's neurosurgeon is able to make an earlier and more precise diagnosis as a result of audiometry, computed tomographic (CT) scan and contrast magnetic resonance imaging (MRI). When combined with modern microsurgical technique, these advances have resulted in the preservation of an increasing number of VII and VIII cranial nerves. The possibility of preservation of useful hearing in some cases of acoustic neuroma (or neurinoma) has important implications regarding the surgical approach.

The translabyrinthine route used by the otolaryngologists to reach the acoustic tumour in the cerebellopontine angle (CPA) must destroy the cochlear organ. It is therefore limited to patients in whom hearing ability has been lost forever. The transtemporal route has the potential of preserving cochlear nerve function but in reality can only be successfully employed to that end if the tumour is <1.5 cm in diameter. Glasscock et al.[18] have reported one case operated by this route with useful postoperative hearing. Fisch[19] preserved cochlear nerve function in 5–12 cases with acoustic tumours, but in retrospect one-quarter of the total cases were not complete removals.

Cochlear nerve preservation has been reported by many authorities in the recent past but there is a lot of ambiguity on the criteria for 'useful hearing'.[20–24] Also there are some who believe that the goal of 'gross total tumour removal' cannot be achieved with cochlear nerve preservation.[25] Gardner and Robertson[26] propose that patients with a speech reception threshold (SRT) of <50 dB and a speech discrimination score (SDS) of >50%, should be considered to have serviceable hearing. Glasscock and Kueton have used the corresponding values of 70 dB and 70%, respectively.[27] However, Nadol et al.[28] uses the criteria of SRT and SDS as 70 dB and 15%. Thus, these studies are not truly comparable.

Sterkers[29] prefers the middle fossa route for intracanalicular tumours and the retrosigmoid approach for large-size acoustic tumours. He operates on all sizes of tumours by either of the two approaches and reported an overall preservation of cochlear nerve function in 33% of the cases of his 94 totally removed tumours.[30]

For the microsurgical removal of acoustic neuroma, we usually use the same unilateral suboccipital approach described by Rand and Kurze[13] in 1965. They felt that it had the following advantages over the middle fossa and translabyrinthine routes: (i) a wide field of

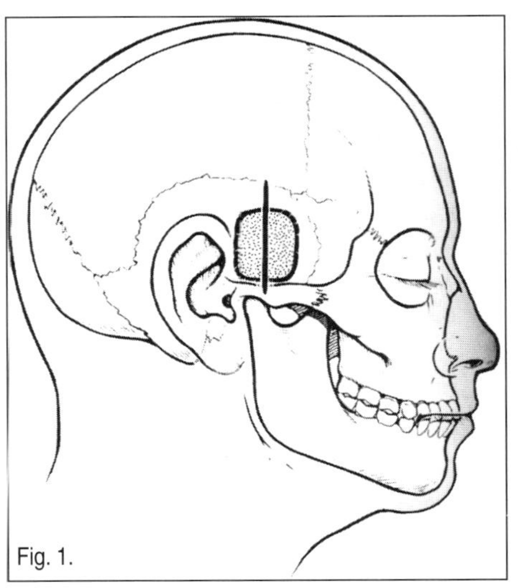

Fig. 1.

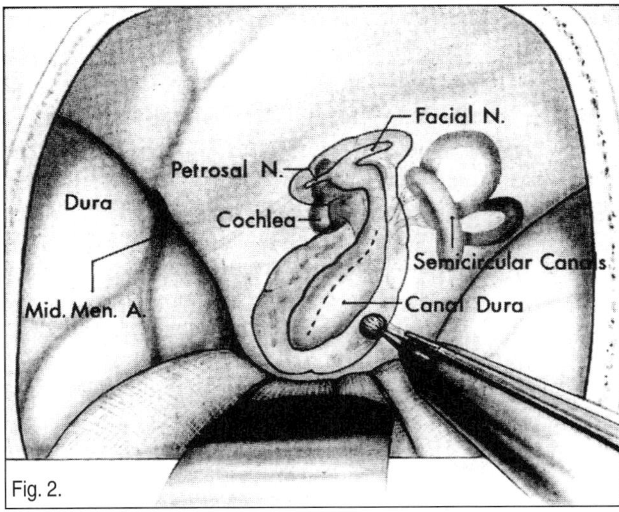

Fig. 2.

Figs 1 and 2. Middle cranial fossa approach to IAC suitable for small tumours (<2 cm)

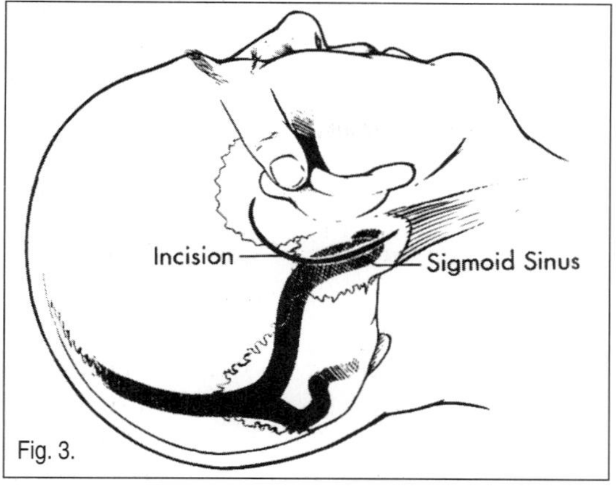

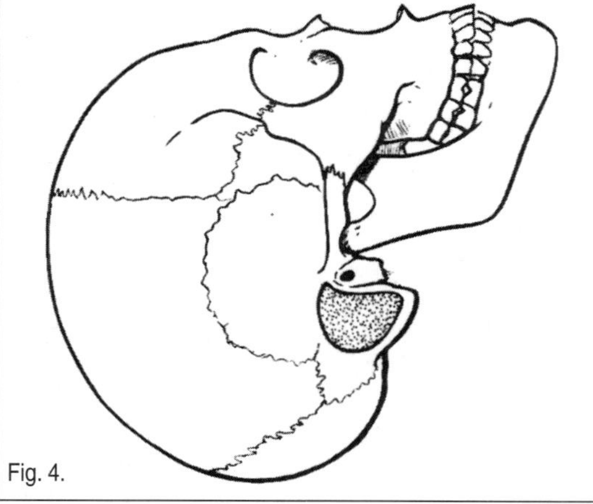

Figs 3 and 4. Translabyrinthine approach to IAC

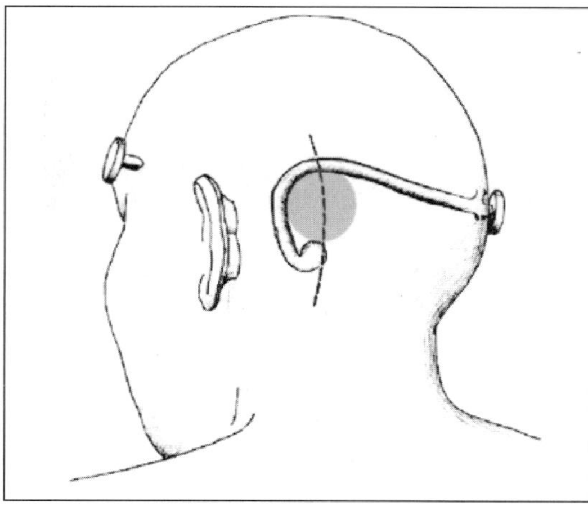

Fig. 5. Suboccipital approach

action; (ii) direct visualization of the anterior inferior cerebellar artery (AICA) and other brain stem vessels; (iii) dissection of all surfaces of the acoustic tumour always under direct vision; (iv) identification of the facial nerve in the lateral angle of the internal auditory canal (IAC); and (v) ready access to the facial nerve when either anastomosis or graft reconstruction is necessary.

More than 95% of acoustic neuromas[23] arise from vestibular fascicles, hence the term 'vestibular schwannoma' would be most appropriate. However, the term acoustic neuroma continues to be used because of its historic importance and popularity. Samii *et al.*,[21] in their series of 1000 acoustic neuromas, have observed that 1.1% of the CPA tumours arose from cochlear nerve. In our series presented below, we had one patient of a schwannoma arising from the facial nerve which did not enter the canal.

Patients and Methods

In the past 25 years (1985–2010), 1002 cases of CPA tumours were surgically treated by one surgeon (the senior author, KET), thus eliminating the 'operator bias' for statistical purposes. An overwhelming majority of these were acoustic neuromas (890), while meningiomas and epidermoids constituted the remaining few.

Break-up of 1002 CPA tumours

Acoustic neuromas	890	(88%)
Meningiomas	64	(7%)
Epidermoids	30	(3%)
Haemangioblastomas	4	
Tuberculoma	6	
Secondaries	6	
Neurenteric cyst	2	
Total	**1002**	

The above series also includes:

- 8 cases of acoustic neuroma who had undergone gamma knife radiosurgery earlier on with no symptomatic relief over a couple of years

- 6 cases of residual acoustic neuromas (operated elsewhere)
- 16 cases of Bil. acoustic neuromas with NF-2
- 2 cases of trigeminal neuralgia accompanying but not caused by acoustic neuroma on ipsilateral side
- 36 cases of purely intracanalicular acoustic neuroma.

Preoperative work-up

All patients of CPA tumours in our series underwent:

- Contrast MRI
- CT scan (with bone windows)
- Audiometry
- Brainstem auditory evoked response (BAER)

Contrast MRI

Contrast-enhanced MRI is the most sensitive imaging modality for assessment of CPA and IAC lesions. This is because of its excellent soft tissue delineation, multiplanar imaging capability and absence of streak artifacts from bone as with CT scan. Acoustic schwannomas are iso- to hypo-intense on T_1-weighted images with respect to adjacent brain. Occasionally, the tumour is brighter on T_1-weighted images, if there has been haemorrhage into the tumour or the tumour contains a proteinaceous fluid.

On T_2-weighted image, their appearance is more variable, with larger tumours tending to be more heterogeneous in morphology and signal intensity. Acoustic schwannomas are composed of Antoni A and Antoni B histological patterns in variable proportions. The former has a compact texture resulting in areas of homogeneous signal on T_2-weighted images. The Antoni B tissue contains a loose myxoid matrix with degenerative changes, resulting in heterogeneous hyper-intensity on T_2-weighted images. Mild-to-

moderate degrees of oedema may be seen in the adjoining brain. The principal differential diagnosis here is a meningioma. Table 1 gives the differentiating features between the two. Small pure intracanalicular tumours as well as early recurrences are best picked up by a contrast MRI.

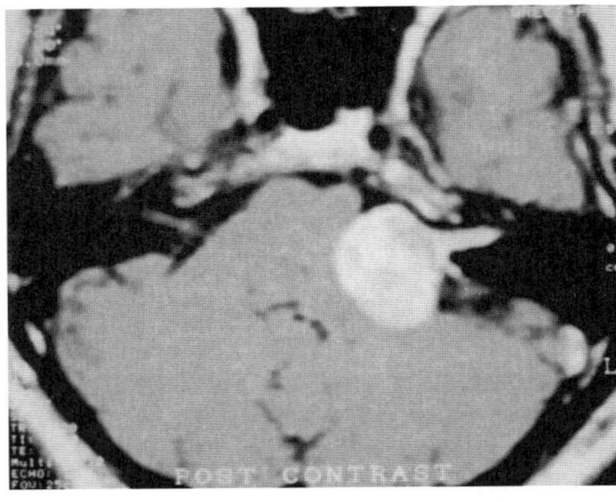

Fig. 6. Schwannoma

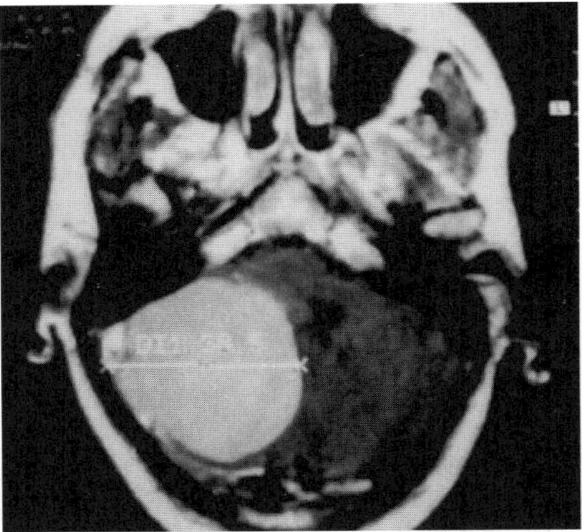

Fig. 7. Meningioma

CT scan

The principal disadvantage of CT in evaluating posterior fossa lesions is the presence of streak artifacts. However, it still retains its place in evaluating the canalicular portion of acoustic neuromas. It shows the exact length of IAC as

Table 1. The differentiating features

	Schwannoma	Meningioma
CT scan		
Widening and/or erosion of porus	Present	Absent (usually)
Intratumoral calcification	Absent	Present
Hyperostosis of petrous bone	None	May be seen
MRI		
Centering over IAC	Well centered	Eccentric with regard to IAC
Extension into IAC	Always	Very rare
Dural base	None	Broad-based
Angle with the petrous bone	Acute	Obtuse
Dural tail	Absent	Present
Heterogeneity and cystic change	Often	Rare
Angiography		
Blush	Uncommon	Common
Large feeding vessels	Uncommon	Common

well as the degree of its widening. This information is helpful in guiding the surgeon on how far laterally to drill the IAC. Two important landmarks demonstrated by CT scan are the location of semicircular canals and placement of jugular bulb, which if huge will forewarn the wary surgeon to be careful whilst drilling the inferocaudal part of IAC.

Audiometry

A complete audiometric evaluation involves pure tone audiometry, speech discrimination scoring, testing the acoustic reflex and measurement of reflex decay. However, we routinely perform only the first two parameters mentioned above. Pure tone audiometry will demonstrate high frequency sensory neural hearing loss or total deafness in the involved ear. But, hearing loss is not proportionate to the size of the tumour. Speech discrimination score refers to difficulty in understanding the speech and is quantified by measuring patient's response to a list of familiar words. A poor speech discrimination that is out of proportion to the pure tone loss is the audiological hallmark of acoustic neuroma.

A simple bedside test of hearing, which we have found useful in our practice, is to check the patient's ability to use the telephone, on the affected side.

Brainstem auditory evoked response (BAER)

This technique measures the electrical potential from mastoid and vertex electrodes in first 15 ms following an acoustic stimulus. In a normal patient, it is possible to delineate 7 waves of which wave 'V' is the largest and most reproducible. In CPA tumours when the cochlear nerve is stretched by the tumour, these waves are delayed. The interwave period between wave I and V may be used to detect a retrocochlear lesion. The technique most commonly used to detect acoustic tumours is to compare wave forms from the suspected ear with the contralateral side. An

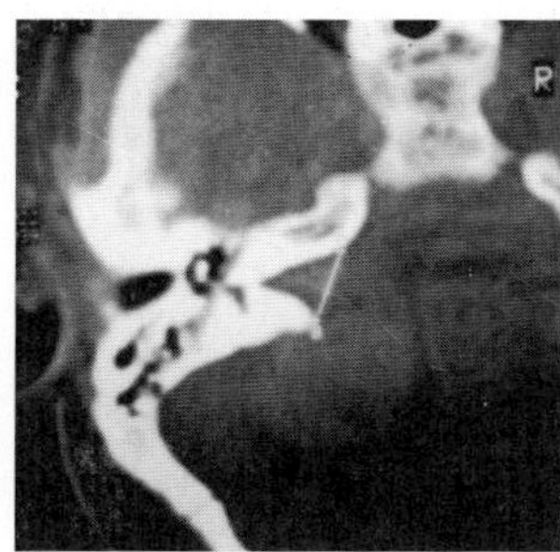

Fig. 8.

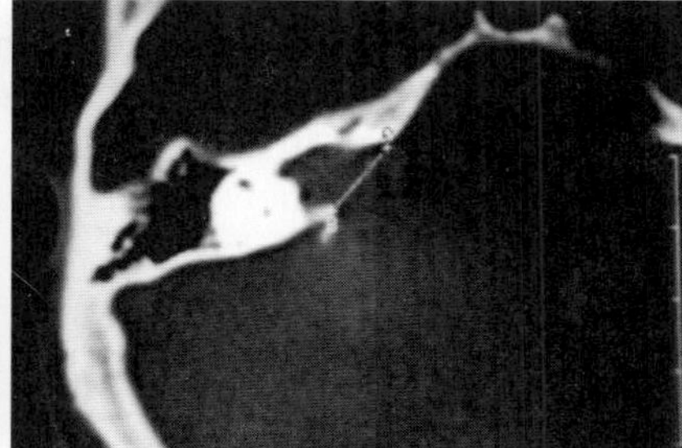

Fig. 9.

Figs 8 and 9. Various degrees of erosion of porus and IAC

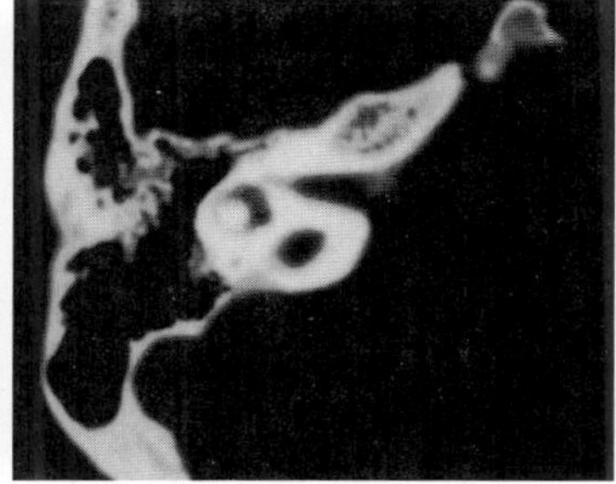

Fig. 10. Situation of semicircular canal and jugular bulb

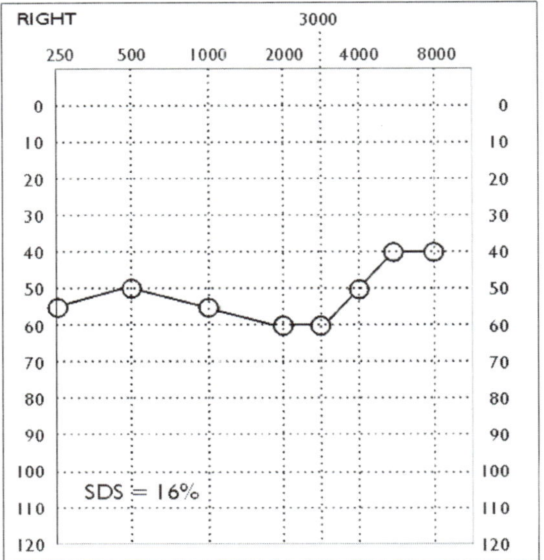

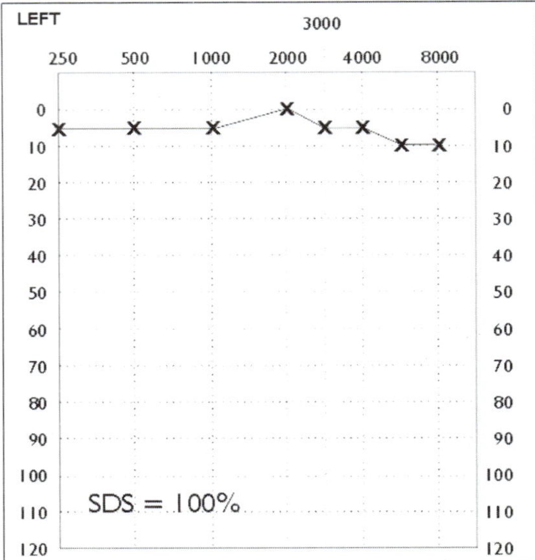

Fig. 11. Typical audiometric findings in an acoustic neuroma right ear

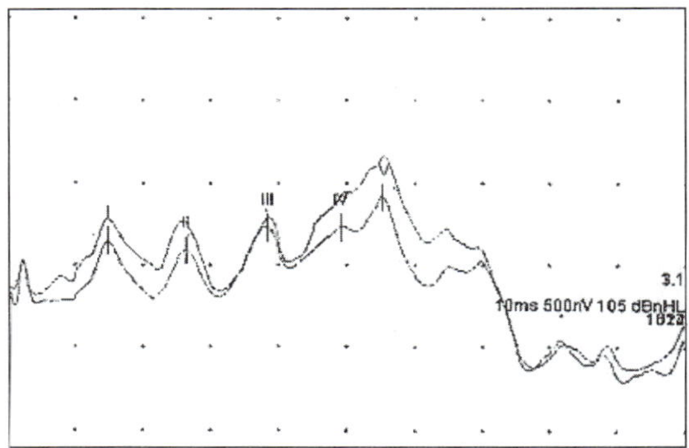

Fig. 12. A normal BAER

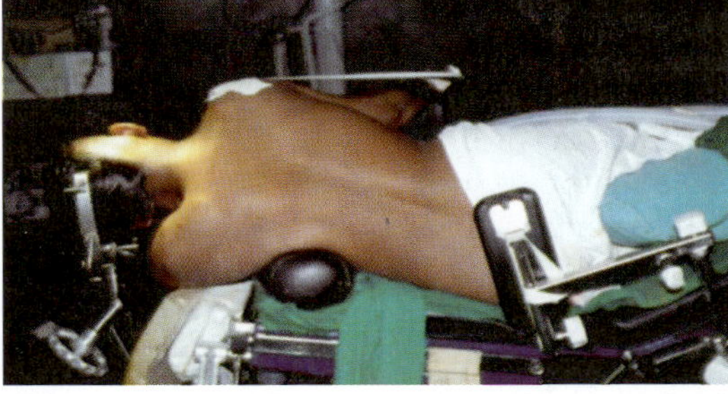

Fig. 13. A normal BAER

inter-aural latency difference between waves I and V of more than 0.2 ms is most sensitive as well as a specific test for acoustic neuroma.

Operative management

Position

Following administration of general anaesthesia, patient is placed in a lateral 'park-bench' position, with a roll kept under the lower axilla. The shoulders and hips are strapped to the table to allow table manipulation in all planes. Gentle traction is applied to the ipsilateral shoulder by pulling it caudally and anteriorly, to move the shoulder out of the surgeon's way. The head is now fixed on a 3-pin Mayfield clamp or a 4-pin Sugita head holder, and is flexed, tilted down 5° to 10°, so as to bring mastoid tip to the top of the operative field.

Exposure

Skin incision is a lazy 'S' shaped and is a thumb's breadth behind the mastoid. It is about 10 cm long, its upper limit extending just beyond where

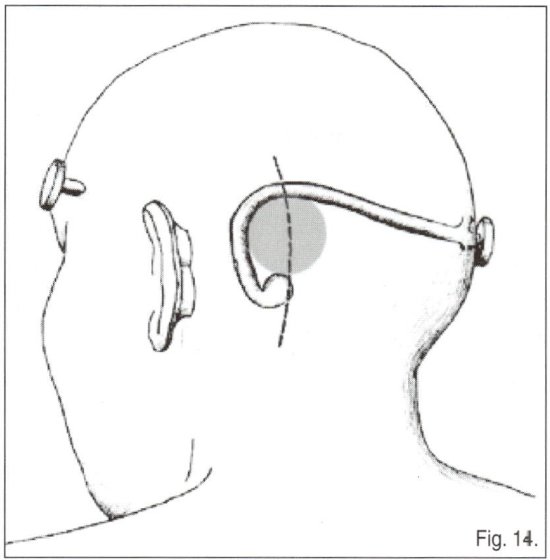

Fig. 14.

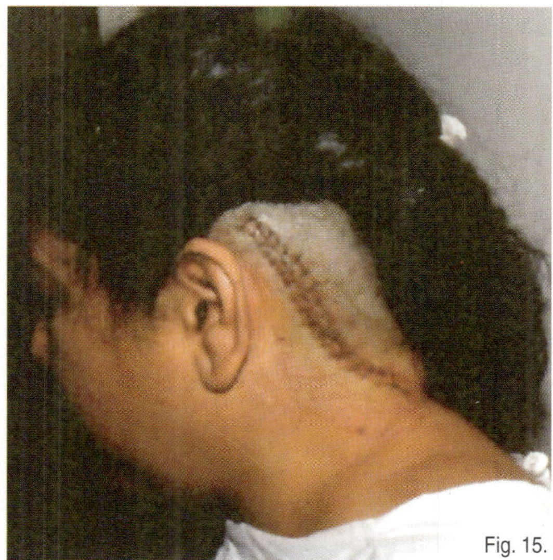

Fig. 15.

Figs 14 and 15. Skin incision and craniectomy

the transverse sinus is expected to lie (which means roughly reaching the top of the pinna). Its lower limit extends as low as is necessary to gain the lower limit of occiput. Subsequent muscle layers are cut progressively higher to make the plane of the wound somewhat oblique downwards. A small strip of uncoagulated muscle used to be excised for later use to cover the IAC, though now we use subcutaneous fat to fill of the canal after tumour removal as a safe guard against CSF rhinorrhoea.

The nearly circular craniectomy is 2.5–3 cm in diameter. We open the foramen magnum in all cases to open the cisterna magna, unless the tumour is very small. It is directed laterally to the border of the sigmoid sinus. Superiorly, it extends to the transverse sinus. This bone opening is irrespective of the size of acoustic tumour, and, in fact for a very small tumour a slight medial extension of this craniectomy may be even more convenient. The secret of a good exposure is in being as lateral as possible (flush with the borders of the transverse and sigmoid and sinuses) in order to have the shortest and most direct access to the IAC. The dural incision is Y shaped, runs obliquely from the transverse sigmoid junction towards cisterna magna, and

the lateral triangle further divided into two by a perpendicular cut.

The surgical microscope is draped in a sterile transparent cover and brought into the operating field. A 250 or 300 mm objective is used. The microscope is equipped with cameras (still and video) and an observer tube. In addition to the microscope, other microsurgical aids are: (i) an armrest to support the surgeon's arms and prevent fatigue; (ii) long microinstruments (sharp angulated dissectors of varying breadth, bayonet tumour-holding forceps, plain and bayonet microdissectors, bayonet scissor, dura knife); (iii) a suction-irrigator; (iv) bipolar cautery with long forceps; (v) nerve stimulator; (vi) air drill with diamond burrs ranging from 1 to 5 mm; and (vii) self-retaining Leyla retractors. Finally, the operating table should be capable of being remotely controlled in all positions to enable the surgeon to view the tumour and surrounding structures from a variety of positions.

The cerebellum is retracted by a single, broad-bladed, self-retaining retractor. The CSF from the basal cisterns is allowed to flow out. This facilitates relaxation of the brain and lessens the force of retraction. The extracanalicular tumour is visualized. Since the vast majority of our CPA tumours are acoustic neuromas, we shall first consider operative strategy of this tumour in this presentation.

Opening of the IAC

It is mandatory to open the IAC. The dura over the petrous bone is incised in a semicircular flap, with the centre of its base over the porus acusticus. The dural flap is stripped off the bone. The dura continues into the canal, and the raised semicircular dural flap is snipped at the porus. The roof of IAC is now drilled. A high-speed steel burr and diamond drill placed on a light, angulated handset is used. Some surgeons place cotton patties under the spatula and over the lower cranial nerves as an added protection against any accident, such as injury inflicted by a slippage of the drill. We condemn the use of cotton patties during drilling as it can get caught in the drill and rotate ferociously, blurring the surgeon's vision and even unnerving him and causing complications. We begin with a 4–5 mm steel burr and then switch over to a diamond burr one approaches the last bit of the root of the canal.

A large size of burr is used at the beginning and, as one approaches the contents of the IAC, the burr size is reduced. While the drill works, the suction-irrigator is kept close to it to cool the bone. Heating of the bone damages the nerves within and should never be permitted. The drilling is oriented in the direction of the roof of the canal rather than its floor. With the thickness of the bone being drilled away, the last thin shell of bone is cracked out in bits with a sharp and finely angulated dissector. While drilling, it is most important to know the superolateral disposition of the semicircular canals and the inferoposterior relationship of the jubular bulb. A high-resolution CT scan provides the location of these structures with respect to the IAC. The exact length and widening of the IAC are also obtained by such a scan so that the surgeon

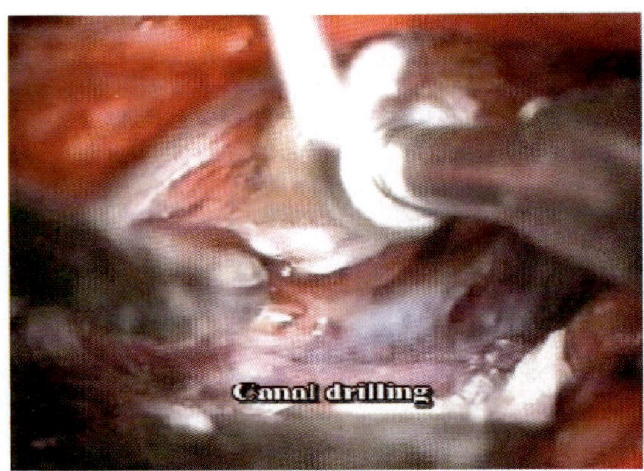

Fig. 16. Canal drilling

knows how far laterally he can drill. The lateral extent of opening of the canal is guided during operation by the bulging presence of the tumour within the dura inside the IAC. The tumour extends to a variable degree within the canal. However, it rarely reaches right up to the fundus. Hence, a full lateral opening is not routinely or randomly made. If the tumour bulge seems to persist far laterally, it may be advisable to stop somewhat short of the fundus and to resume drilling only after exposing and evacuating the tumour from the canal. Further drilling may then be performed with a very fine 1 mm burr from within the IAC. Finally, drilling along the floor of the canal must be performed cautiously and with the recognition of the possibility that the jugular bulb may be placed quite high, although this is an uncommon occurrence.

Surgical anatomy of CPA

Before continuing with further operative strategy it would not be out of place to recall a few points on the surgical anatomy of the region. The VII and VIII cranial nerves arise from the pons proximal to the olive. The VII nerve arises about one half centimetre caudal to the emergence of the trigeminal nerve and slightly rostral and anterior to the origin of the VIII. It slopes gently downwards and dorsally to lie in front of the VIII nerve in the porus acusticus. Its course spans 12–

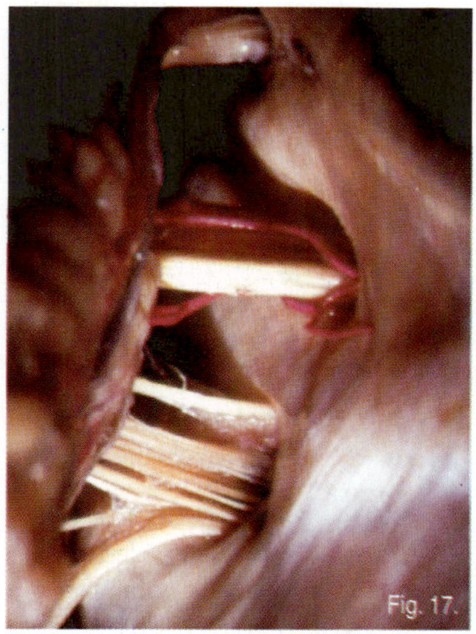

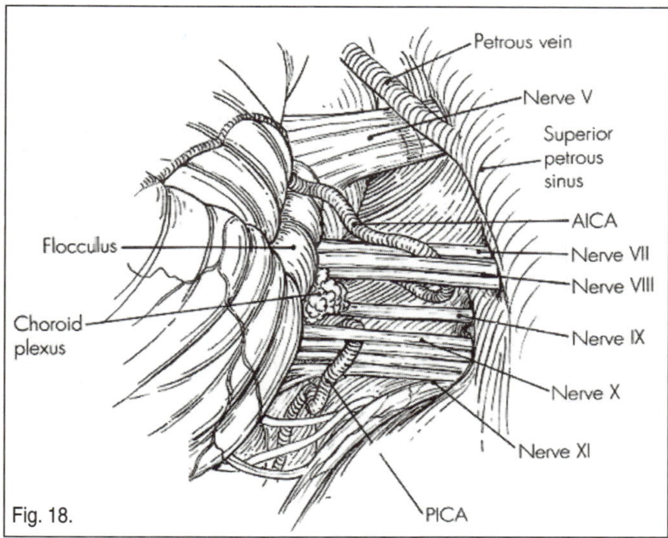

Figs 17 and 18. Anatomy of CPA angle

14 mm in the CPA and 8–10 mm in the IAC. If the cross-section of the IAC is to be divided into four quadrants, the facial nerve lies in the superior and anterior quadrant. The cochlear nerve lies below the facial nerve, while the superior and inferior vestibular divisions lie in the appropriate posterior (dorsal) quadrants. The central part of the facial nerve, for 2–3 mm, has no Schwann sheath, but acquires it, thereafter, during its course through the CPA, appearing to make it look more white and strong. The VIII nerve assumes the Schwann cell covering not in the CPA but only after entering the canal. Anatomical damage or discontinuity occurs easily and the nerves must be handled extremely gently. Both nerves have a covering of arachnoid within which arterioles follow the nerve. The AICA has enormous variations, but in at least two-thirds of normal CPAs its loop lies just in front of the porus or well within the canal.

Most acoustic neuromas arise from the Schwann cell sheath of one or more of the vestibular nerve fascicles. In only 5%–7% of them it arises from the cochlear (in very rare instances a neurinoma in the CPA could arise from the VII or V cranial nerves). The facts that emerge with acoustic neuroma now are:

- The neoplasm almost always originates in the IAC.
- Its growth may cause widening of the canal if the bone is relatively less dense. Unyielding bone may cause the tumour to compress the sensitive cochlear nerve and its vascularity more easily and to such an extent as to cause profound, rapid, or even sudden hearing loss. Such tumours carry poor prognosis with regard to recovery of hearing and at operation are also more difficult to dissect from the cochlear nerve.
- Since most tumours arise from vestibular nerves, the VII nerve is pushed from an anterosuperior to an anteroinferior position. However, within the IAC the position of facial nerve remains unaltered. The cochlear nerve is displaced from that position to a more caudal or caudodorsal location.
- As the tumour grows out of the canal it pushes the anterior inferior cerebellar artery (AICA) progressively medially.
- The tumour tends to grow symmetrically, with the porus generally remaining in the middle of the tumour with the tumour likened to a mushroom.
- The V nerve lies only 5 mm away from the VII,

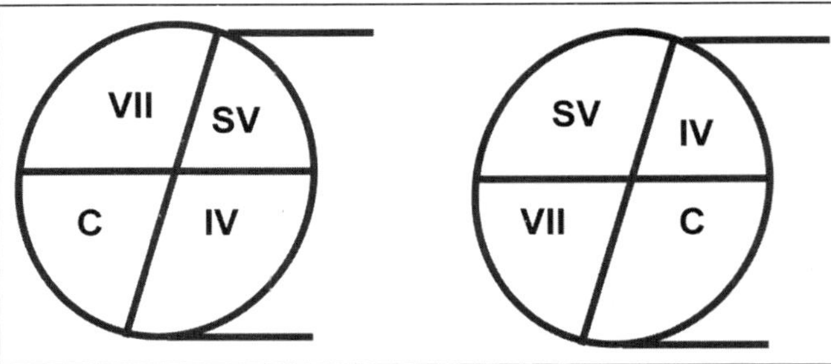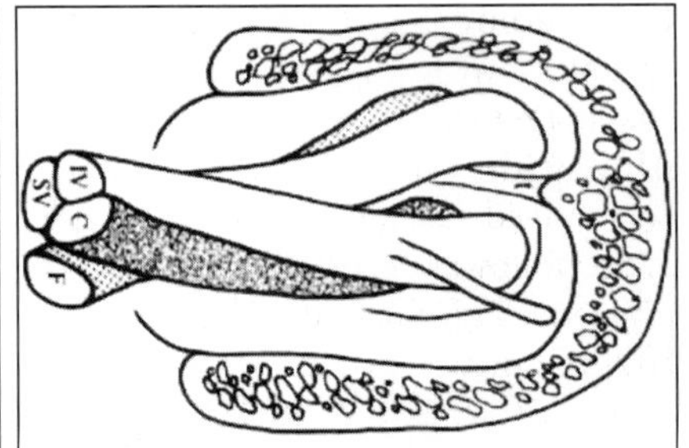

Fig. 19. Displacement of facial nerve in acoustic neuroma

and despite its thickness, its disturbance, in case of an expansive growth, is next to follow.

- The overlying petrous vein may also get stretched.
- The caudal cranial nerves are less frequently compressed, and even when stretching occurs, their symptomatic involvement is uncommon.
- The pons is the most medial structure and is reached when the extracanalicular tumour growth exceeds 1.5 cm.
- A long-standing compression in such tumours may result in stretching and compression of tiny blood vessels bridging between tumour and the brain stem. Handling of the pons during tumour separation or traction of such connecting blood vessels could rupture them farther away in the substance of the pons, and could even result in brain stem damage.
- The structures around are generally only displaced and compressed. Adhesion of the tumour to them is not the rule, except in the case of the facial and cochlear nerves with which the tumorous vestibular nerves are in very intimate and chronic contact. Rarely, though, there may also be adhesions to the brain stem.

Surgical removal of acoustic tumours

The basic principles of surgical technique are common to all sizes of tumour, including: (i) opening of the IAC is mandatory; (ii) enter tumour through posterior part of the capsule and systematically debulk it, thus making a large tumour small and a small tumour smaller; (iii) achieve progressive shrinkage of tumour capsule from the neighbouring compressed but non-adherent nerves; and (iv) approach the parts of tumour capsule most densely adherent with neural tissue at the very end.

Tumour size is a decisive factor in the operative strategy of acoustic tumours.

Small tumours which remain within the IAC or just protrude out of the porus do not alter the anatomy of the medial CPA. The cerebello-pontine cistern is opened in order to visualize and identify the structures. Having obtained this orientation, one should cover it with fibrin sponges. The nerves and the tumour in the canal are enclosed by the dura, which is slit horizontally across. The tumour bulges out, as it usually arises from the vestibular nerves, which face the surgeon. The tumour capsule is coagulated with bipolar current and is opened, and its core is debulked with microdissectors and tumour forceps. This reduces its volume and tension on the neighbouring structures. Once the tumour bulk is reduced, the surrounding nerves become relaxed. The tumour capsule is grasped in forceps and dissected away from the adjacent nerves using a microdissector which is designed to present its rounded smooth surface to the nerve, using its internal surface bearing a sharp edge for tumour dissection. One therefore avoids handling the nerve as much as possible. The fascicles from which the tumour arises can be identified and transected in their healthy portion.

Slightly larger tumours, although still under 3 cm in size, occupy the CPA and cause a medial shift of the AICA. The VII and VIII nerves are of course intimately related, but the remainder of the anatomy is unchanged. The AICA feeds the tumour with small branches which are coagulated and cut as they enter the tumour. The AICA is thus freed from its tumour attachment and moved to safety. Further operative management follows the same pattern as for smaller tumours. Tumours larger than 3 cm form almost 60% of our series of acoustic tumours.

The VII nerve is usually not visible at the outset, being translocated anteriorly by the tumour, which obscures the surgeon's view. Large tumours may push all structures away beyond the view obtained through the microscope. Reduction of the size of the tumour in the CPA is therefore the immediate goal. An opening is made in the posterior part of the capsule using microscissors. Tumour substance is then evacuated. CUSA may be helpful in debulking with less effort but one has to be aware of not going through the capsule on the far side.

One must constantly be aware of the possibility of encountering the vestibular, cochlear, and facial nerves. The dissector, which seems to excavate the tumour, should, in reality, be aiming to dissect the involved nerves. The tumour excision, in relative terms, should be a secondary issue. The dissector should be worked systematically and equally in all directions, from the centre outwards. As the core is removed, the capsule starts to collapse towards the centre. In doing so, it spontaneously falls away from the nerves it had been stretching. The capsule is also excised piecemeal. With shrinkage of the tumour, the nerves which were compressed and stretched begin to appear quite slack. They can be identified separate from the tumour more easily at the two extremes. Rather than discuss whether to remove tumour from lateral to medial, or vice versa, we would emphasize a symmetric internal decompression which, 'deflates' the tumour. Once it is sufficiently small, the space created in the CPA permits the tumour to be moved in all directions. The tumour capsule is therefore constantly manipulated with an attempt at freeing it from the nerves on all sides. In doing so, the operator gradually converges to the most

densely adherent point. Generally, such adherence of the tumour with the facial nerve is most prominent at a couple of millimetres proximal to the porus. This point is never approached at an early stage of the operation and ideally the last point to be reached.

Occasionally, during the process of separation of the seventh nerve from the tumour, fine fascicles of the nerve may be entangled within the capsule and may resist dissection. They are best transected to avoid further traction and damage to the rest of the facial nerve on some occasions.

With large tumours the nerve may be so thinned as to look like a veil of arachnoid. Anticipation and nerve stimulation will help to identify and save it. Even such very thinned out nerves can still be capable of function but need great perseverance at preservation.

The tumour may also be adherent to the brain stem. Until the CPA is almost completely evacuated of the space-occupying tumour, there is not enough freedom of movement nor the ability to appreciate the location of the most densely adherent points. Ideally one would focus its activity on these points only at the very end.

During tumour dissection vestibular fascicles may be seen entering the tumour. These fascicles are transected in their non-tumorous segment. The cochlear nerve, which is usually pushed under the tumour, may be identified there, and the tumour capsule may be separated away from it. It is best to dissect the tumour away from the nerve, and not vice versa, as handling the nerve could disturb its function. The strategy of removal of the intracanalicular portion has already been discussed. The point to be stressed, however, is that small and soft though the tumour may be, it should always be dissected and cut, and not 'rolled over'. There may be times when the intracanalicular portion extends right up to the fundus. If the canal opening has not been sufficiently lateral, it can now be done from within outwards, using a 1 mm burr. It is a good practice to remove all the tumours under direct vision. At the same time, lateral drilling must be performed carefully so as not to damage the vestibule.

Blood vessels supplying the tumour are usually branches of the AICA. They are coagulated very close to the tumour surface, using the bipolar cautery, and are then transected. When the tumour lies close to or is attached to the brain stem, blood vessels may directly bridge between the two. Traction on these vessels may sometimes lead to intrapontine haemorrhages which can have grave consequences. Hence, the above strategy should be rigidly followed in this area. Occasionally, the connection of the tumour with the VIII nerve is dense and difficult to dissect. In such a situation, it is preferable to transect the nerve in its healthy portion rather than cause the nerve to pull on and possibly damage the brain stem. Nuclear lesions by such traction mechanisms may explain nerve palsies despite their apparent anatomical continuity after total tumour removal. BAEPs signal VIII nerve disturbance and are a useful tool at surgery.

Large tumours often stretch and flatten the facial nerve. As a rule, its physiological status must be checked after the tumour is removed. The nerve is stimulated at the medial end near the brainstem, and facial contraction is observed by the anaesthetist under the covering drapes. A positive contraction is a sure sign of intact facial function.

If the facial nerve is damaged at operation, there are three possible situations:

1. the proximal and distal stumps are both available
2. only the proximal stump is available; or
3. the proximal stump is not available.

When proximal and distal stumps are both available and there is no gap between the nerve ends, a direct end-to-end anastomosis is performed. A nerve gap within the CPA can be bridged by a graft obtained from the sural nerve.

If only the proximal stump is available and it is at least 3–5 mm long, the procedure of choice is an intracranial–intratemporal facial nerve grafting. If the proximal stump is not available, we must resort to peripheral anastomotic procedures preferably faciohypoglossal. It is also necessary to ensure that the hypoglossal nerve is intact. When using the latter, it is possible to dissect just one fascicle, the ansa, so that the tongue function is not compromised. The phrenic nerve has also been utilized but is not as popular because the number of axons is less and the patient has to learn to coordinate voluntary breathing in order to have the face contract.

Bilateral acoustic neuromas

Bilateral acoustic neuromas comprise about 2.5% of all cases of acoustic neuroma (24 cases in our series). They differ from the conventional unilateral tumour in several ways. These tumours may represent a part of generalized von Recklinghausen disease (VRD). Interestingly enough, most patients are detected rather late in their course. Preservation of the VII and VIII cranial nerves in this situation is of even greater importance due to bilateral involvement, and to make matters worse, these tumours are even more difficult to operate. Unlike unilateral neuromas which arise from one side of a nerve sheath, displacing other nerves around it, the neurofibromas of VRD is a result of an unencapsulated proliferation of Schwann cells, fibrous connective tissue, and neural tissue (axons). They are lobulated and tend to grow between and around nerve fascicles. Moreover, their multifocal origin over the length of the same nerve or nerves makes their total removal

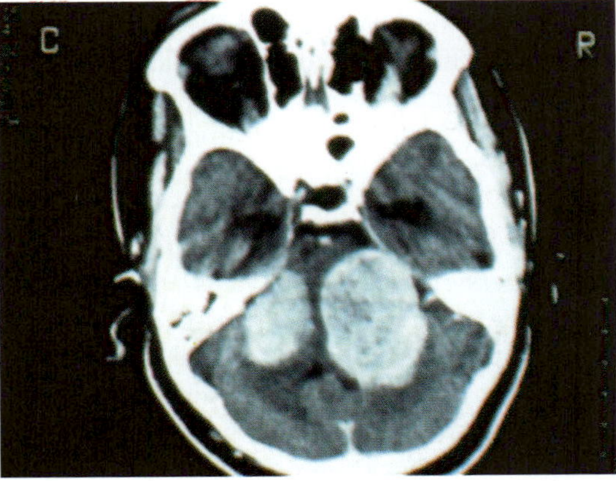

Fig. 20. Bilateral acoustic neuromas

formidable. The consequent morbidity tends to be higher than which accompanies unilateral neuronomas. Most of our patients came with large tumours, and only 4 patients had tumours measuring <3 cm in diameter.

Of 16 patients with bilateral tumours, 3 had already been operated on one side at another clinic and had lost their hearing on that side. The tumours on their remaining unoperated side, as well as bilateral tumours of the remaining 10 patients, were all totally excised. Hearing was preserved bilaterally in 4 of these patients and unilaterally in 2 patients.

The strategy of operation does not differ significantly. However, the question that often confronts us in patients with bilateral acoustic neurinomas is which side should be operated first.

Two factors come into consideration: (i) hearing ability and (ii) tumour size. They may be interrelated or independent. One may have a smaller tumour with profound hearing loss, or the reverse, a larger tumour with relatively better hearing.

Patients with functional hearing still have a chance of its preservation, and since that is the goal of surgery, one should prefer to operate on that tumour first. On the other hand, the operative morbidity of larger tumours is decid higher than that of smaller ones. The process of decision-making necessarily must consider both of these factors.

Results

Of the 1002 CPA tumours, 890 were acoustic neuromas, 64 were meningiomas, and 30 were epidermoids. The remaining 18 were a heterogeneous group of rare tumours.

Facial nerve function

Facial Nerve function was assessed on three occasions after surgical excision of acoustic neuroma.

1. Immediate postoperatively
2. At the time of discharge
3. After 6–12 months of surgery.

Facial nerve function at each time was quantified using the House–Brackmann facial nerve grading system (Table 2).[31]

Of the 890 acoustic neuromas, 12 patients had come with facial palsy and residual tumour following attempted surgical excision elsewhere. These patients were excluded while evaluating our operative results. Of the remaining 878, 284 (32%) had various degrees of facial paresis (Table 3) preoperatively.

Evaluation of facial function at the end of 6 months vis-à-vis size of the tumour has been given in Table 4.

It was observed that facial function deteriorated by one or two grades postoperatively, i.e. a facial paresis of grade II went down to grade III or IV over the next 5 days. However, it gradually recovered to grade II again over the next 6 weeks. The cause of this phenomenon is yet unexplained. Similar observations have been made by Lalwani *et al.*[32]

There were 8 patients in this series whose facial nerves were found extremely attenuated

Table 2. The House–Brackmann facial nerve grading system

Grade	Descriptions	% facial function
I	Normal	100
II	Slight weakness	80
III	Obvious but not disfiguring	60
IV	Obvious and disfiguring	40
V	Barely perceptible movements	20
VI	Total paralysis	0

Table 3. Preoperative facial paresis (284 / 878 cases)

Size	Cases	Grade II or III	Grade III or IV
Intracanalicular	18	16	2
<3 cm	64	56	8
> 3 cm	202	158	44
Total	284	230	54

Table 4. Size-related facial function in 878* acoustic neuromas

Size	Cases	Postoperative		
		Grade I/II+	Grade III or IV+	Grade V+
Intracanalicular	36 (4%)	30 (83%)	6 (17%)	–
< 3 cm	336 (38%)	170 (53%)	150 (44%)	12 (3%)
> 3 cm #	506 (58%)	180 (35%)	246 (46%)	84 (19%)
Total	878	380	402	96

* 12 patients who came with residual tumours with facial palsy following surgery performed elsewhere were excluded from the study

+ Figures quoted refer to assessment of facial function done at the end of 6 months.

Refers to the size of extracanalicular tumour only

and were looking like the tumour arachnoid. They would have been surely severed otherwise but for the facial nerve stimulation and experience-based judgement of the surgeon. These patients regained adequate facial function after a prolonged period of 8–12 months. The anatomical continuity of facial nerve was lost in 16 patients. In all of these 16 cases the ends were identified and sutured primarily. In 6 of these patients a delayed facio-hypoglossal anastomosis was done, after a waiting period of 1 year at the end of which facial EMG did not show any sign of regeneration of nerve.

Cochlear nerve preservation

The following audiometric parameters define the term serviceable hearing, some hearing and total deafness (Table 5).[23,24]

In the present study, we have followed the same guiding principles. All the 890 patients of acoustic neuroma underwent audiometry and BAER preoperatively and again one week after the operation. Out of them, 280 patients (31.5%) turned out to be totally deaf, of the remaining 610 (68.5%), 378 (42.4%) had serviceable hearing, while 232 (26.1%) had some hearing (Table 6).

The 610 patients who had either serviceable or some hearing preoperatively were catagorized into three groups, those with tumours >3 cm or <3 cm and intracanalicular tumours (Table 7). The results of hearing preservation in each of these groups are as follows.

Although functional preservation of hearing was possible only in 33% of 610 patients, anatomical preservation of cochlear nerve was possible in 48% of these patients. One patient who was totally 'deaf' with an intracanalicular tumour of 11 mm size regained a serviceable hearing postoperatively. Audiograms and BAEPs of this patient are depicted in Table 8.

Extent of tumour removal

In all the 890 patients total excision of tumour was given priority over preservation of VII or VIII nerve. There were 16 patients with residual tumours detected on postoperative MRI (done

Table 5. Audiometric parameters

	Serviceable hearing	Some hearing	Deaf
Pure tone average* (loss)	<50 dB	50–80 dB	>80 dB
Speech discrimination score	>50%	50%–20%	<20%

* is an average of scores obtained at 500 Hz, 1500 Hz, 2000 Hz and 4000 Hz.

Table 6

Hearing	Number	Percentage (%)
Serviceable	378	42.4
Some	232	26.1
Deaf	280	31.5
Total	890	

Table 7

	Pre-operatively	Post-operatively	Percentage (%)
Intracanalicular	16	12	75
< 3 cm	324	142	43
> 3 cm	250	48	19
Total	610	202	33

Table 8. Preservation of VIII nerve in acoustic neuromas (hearing preserved)

	Cases	Pre-operatively	Post-operatively
Acoustic neuromas	890	610	202

after 3 months of surgery). None of these needed resurgery. All these patients were kept under observation by performing regular MRI scans every year.

Spontaneous regression of a small residual tumour was seen in one of our patients, in whom a small bit of tumour was left behind near the canal. This was done because near the end of the surgery cerebellar swelling occurred obscuring the field. Surprisingly, on a follow up MRI done 3 months later, the tumour had vanished.

Complications (excluding VII/VIII nerve non-preservation)

Considering its intricate anatomy, surgery in the CPA is certainly fraught with life-threatening consequences. Advances in microsurgical technique have made many of these procedures less risky. The list of complications includes:

- *CSF leak* (rhinorrhoea or from the wound): 36 cases (3.5%) was the commonest complication encountered. Twenty patients had retrograde rhinorrhoea (through a patent eustacian tube) while 8 leaks occurred from the wound. In the latter category, resuturing of the wound and lumbar drainage stopped the leak in all 16 cases. Of the 20 with CSF rhinorrhoea, only 4

patients needed re-exploration of the wound and waxing of the mastoid air cells. Rest of them settled with complete bed-rest, lumbar drainage and acetazolamide. Four patients developed a delayed CSF rhinorrhoea appearing 4 and 6 years after surgery. These patients too were treated conservatively.

- *Bacterial meningitis:* Occurred in 16 of whom 6 had CSF rhinorrhoea. Severe headache coupled with vomiting and photophobia were the usual heralding features. The organisms responsible were mostly grain negative bacilli (enterococci, pseudomonas, *E. coli*). In two patients *Staphylococcus aureus* was isolated. Early institution of intravenous antibiotics and lumbar puncture and drainage helped in all patients, but intravenous antibiotics had to be continued for 2 weeks.

- *Lower cranial nerve paresis:* Lower cranial nerve paresis was observed in 16 patients, 3 of whom preoperatively had palatal weakness and an absent gag reflex. All these patients needed tracheostomy and tube-feeding (percutaneous endoscopic gastrostomy or nasogastric tube) for prolonged periods (3–6 weeks).

- *Hydrocephalus/VP shunt:* Communicating hydrocephalus occurred in 76 patients; 32 of them had hydrocephalus preoperatively too which failed to regress postoperatively. Hydrocephalic symptoms included gait apraxia, incontinence pseudomeningocoele at the operative site and a boggy. Twenty-four of these patients were treated for either aseptic or bacterial meningitis previously. Sixteen of these were treated with lumbo-peritoneal shunt while others were treated with a VP shunt.

- *Exposure keratitis/tarsorraphy:* Combined V and VII nerve paresis causing severe exposure keratitis occurred in 12 cases who needed tarsorraphy.

- *Others:* Empyema thoracis was detected postoperatively in one of our patients. However, he recovered with timely drainage (2 litres at first tap) by an intercostal tube.

- Mortality rate in this series of 890 acoustic neuromas was zero (0%).

Table 9. Complications in the current series of 445 acoustic neuromas

	Cases	Percentage
CSF leak	36	3.5
Bacterial meningitis	16	1.8
Aseptic meningitis	18	1.9
Hydrocephalus/VP shunt	76	7.3
Exposure keratitis	12	1.2
Mortality	0	0

Summary and conclusion

Microsurgical techniques have made a significant contribution in the advancement of surgery. Since then, the field of neurosurgery has made great and rapid strides. Neurosurgeons now venture through the deep and delicate regions of the brain, where they dared not venture only a few years ago. In particular, the morbidity and mortality of surgery in CPA has seen a progressive decrease.

This presentation deals with 890 acoustic neuromas. Preoperative investigation has been aimed at arriving at a diagnosis which is as exact as possible to plan the operative strategy. All patients ranging in age from 8 to 82 years have been operated upon, in either a sitting position (the initial 23% of cases) or in a lateral park bench position through a unilateral suboccipital craniectomy.

The basic surgical technique, irrespective of the tumour, is to decompress it from within to relieve its tension and pressure on surrounding nerves, vessels, and the brain stem. The structures which are only compressed are spontaneously relieved of compression. This helps define their full anatomical course. Having been identified, they are protected from damage. The most adherent points between the acoustic tumour and nerves are recognized and handled last under direct vision when there is sufficient space to allow manipulation of the tumour. In the occasional event of facial nerve being interrupted, primary end-to-end repair or repair using sural nerve cable grafts are attempted during the same procedure if both ends are available. On other occasions, we have resorted to delayed facial neurotization using facio-hypoglossal or occasionally facio-phrenic anastomosis producing acceptable results. The cochlear nerve lacks a Schwann cell cover in the CPA and is more prone to being affected, either by tumour processes or surgical manipulation. Preservation of cochlear nerve is the ultimate hallmark of acoustic neuroma surgery.

Of the 890 acoustic neuroma tumours 58% were larger than 6 cm in size. Two important factors with regard to predicting the preservation of VII and VIII cranial nerves are tumour size (<6 cm) and preoperative hearing status (serviceable, 'some' or totally deaf). Facial nerve preservation anatomically, after total tumour removal was achieved in 91% cases. With regard to hearing preservation, anatomical preservation of cochlear nerve was possible in 48% of cases who had preoperative hearing while functional preservation was possible in 33% of patients with preoperatively preserved hearing. It is important to note that

Table 10. Results of VII/VIII nerve preservation in other series

	Total cases	VII nerve (%)	VIII nerve Anatomical (%)	Functional (%)
Samii et al.[33]	1000	93.0	68	39
Post et al.[24]	123	96.4	53	39
Cerullo et al.[22]	102	86.0	64	18
Gormley et al.[23]	179	92.0	69	48
Present series	**890**	**91.0**	**48**	**33**

tumour removal in all but 16 of these patients was complete.

Complications due to surgery including the dreaded complication of brain stem damage or lower cranial nerve injury have been mild, infrequent and reversible (except VII and VIII nerve morbidity which has been extensively discussed above). One should appreciate the fact that mortality in this series of 890 consecutive patients of acoustic neuromas was 0%.

References

1. Balance CA, Duel B. The operative treatment of facial palsy by the introduction of nerve grafts into the fallopian canal and by the other intratemporal methods. *Arch Otolaryngol* 1932;**15**:1.
2. Cushing H. Tumors of the nervus acusticus and the syndrome of the cerebellopontine angle. Philadelphia, London: W.B. Saunders; 1917.
3. Dandy WE. An operation for the total removal of cerebellopontine (acoustic) tumors. *Surg Gynecol Obstet* 1925;**41**:129–48.
4. Dandy WE. Results of removal of acoustic tumors by the unilateral approach. *Arch Surg* 1941;**42**:1026–33.
5. Olivecrona H. Acoustic tumors. *J Neurol Neurosurg Psychiatry* 1940;**3**:141–6.
6. Nielsen A. Acoustic tumors. *Ann Surg* 1942;**115**:849–63.
7. Horrax G, Poppen JL. The end results of complete versus intracapsular removal of acoustic tumors. *Ann Surg* 1949;**130**:567–75.
8. House WF. Middle cranial fossa approach to the petrous pyramid. *Arch Otolaryngol* 1963;**78**:460–9.
9. Kurze T, Doyle JB. Extradural intracranial (middle fossa) approach to the internal auditory canal. *J Neurosurg* 1962;**19**:1033–77.
10. House WF. Monograph I. Transtemporal bone microsurgical removal of acoustic neurinomas. *Arch Otolaryngol* 1964;**80**:597–756.
11. House WF. Monograph II. Acoustic neurinoma. *Arch Otolaryngol* 1968;**88**:575–715.
12. House WF, Hitselberger WW. Preservation of the facial nerve in acoustic tumour surgery. *Arch Otolaryngol* 1968;**88**:655–8.
13. Rand R, Kurze T. Microneurosurgical resection of acoustic tumors by a transmeatal posterior fossa approach. *Bull Los Angeles Neurol Soc* 1965;**30**:17–20.
14. Drake CG. Acoustic neuroma: Repair of facial nerve with autogenous graft. *J Neurosurg* 1960;**17**:836–42.
15. Drake CG. Intracranial facial nerve reconstruction. *Arch Otolaryngol* 1963;**78**:456–60.
16. Drake CG. Total removal of large acoustic neuromas. *J Neurosurg* 1967;**26**:554–61.
17. Rand R Kurze T. Preservation of vestibular, cochlear and facial nerves during microsurgical removal of acoustic tumors: Report of two cases. *J Neurosurg* 1968;**28**:158–61.
18. Glasscock ME, Hays JW, Murphy JP. Complications in acoustic neuroma surgery. *Ann Otol* 1975;**84**:530–40.
19. Fisch U. Otochirurgische Behandlung des Acusticus-neurinomas. In: Plester D, Wende S, Nakayama N (eds). *Kleinhirnbrick-enwinkeltumoren*. Berlin: Springer Verlag; 1978:196–14.
20. Samii M, Matthies C. Management of 1000 vestibular schwannomas: Surgical management and results. *Neurosurgery* 1997;**40**:11–23.
21. Samii M, Matthies C, Titigaba M. Intracanalicular acoustic neuroma. *Neurosurgery* 1991;**29**:181–99.
22. Cerullo LJ, Grutsch J, Heifermann K. *Surg Neurol* 1993;**39**:485–93.
23. Gormley WB, Sekhar L, Wright D. *Neurosurgery* 1997;**41**:50–61
24. Post KD, Eiseaberg M, Catalano P. Hearing preservation in vestibular schwannoma surgery: What factors influence the outcome? *J Neurosurgery* 1995;**83**:191–6.
25. Tos M, Thomsen J, Harmsen A. Is preservation of hearing acoustic neuroma worthwhile? *Acta Otolaryngol (Stockh)* 1988;**452**:57–68.
26. Gardner G, Robertson JH. Hearing preservation in unilateral acoustic neuroma surgery. *Ann Otol Rhinol Laryngol* 1998;**97**:55–66.
27. Glasscock ME, Kueton JF. A systemic approach to surgical management of acoustic neuromas. *J Neurosurg* 1993;**78**:864–70.
28. Nadol JB, Chinog CM, Ojemann RG. Preservation of hearing and facial function in resection of acoutic neuroma. *Laryngoscope* 1992;**102**:1153–8.
29. Sterkers JM. Retrosigmoid approach for preservation of hearing in early aoustic neuroma surgery. In: Samii M, Jannetta PJ (eds). *The cranial nerves.* Berlin: Springer-Verlag; 1981:579–85.
30. Sterkers JM. Facial nerve preservation in acoustic neuroma surgery. In: Samii M, Jannetta PJ (eds). *The cranial nerves.* Berlin: Springer-Verlag; 1981:451–5.
31. House J, Brackman DE. Facial nerve grading system. *Otolaryngol Head Neck Surg* 1985:**93**:146–7.

32. Lalwani AK, Butt FY, Jackler RK, *et al. Am J Otol* 1995;**16**:758–64.

33. Samii M, Turel KE, Peakeak G. Management of 7th and 8th nerve involvement by cerebello pontine angle tumors. *Clin Neurosurgery* 1985;**32**:242–72.

Suggested reading

34. Di Tullio MV, Jr Malkasian D, Rand RW. A critical comparison of neurosurgical and otolaryngological approaches to acoustic neuromas. *J Neurosurg* 1978; **48**:1–12.

35. Dott NM. Facial paralysis: Restitution by extra-petrous nerve graft. *Proc Roy Soc Med* 1958;**51**:900–2.

36. Dott NM. Facial nerve reconstruction by graft bypassing the petrous bone. *Arch Otolaryngol* 1963; **78**:426–8.

37. Draf W, Samii M. Intracranial-intratemporal anastomosis of the facial nerve after cerebellopontine angle tumour surgery. In: Graham MD, House WF (eds). *Disorders of the facial nerve.* New York: Raven Press; 1982:441–9.

38. Jacobson JH. Microsurgical technique in the repair of the traumatized extremity. *Clin Orthop* 1963;**29**:132.

39. McCarty CS. Acoustic neuroma and the suboccipital approach. *Mayo Clin Proc* 1975;**50**:15–16.

40. Rhoton AL. Microsurgical removal of acoustic neuromas. *Surg Neurol* 1976;**6**:211–19.

41. Sachs E. Translabyrinthine microsurgery for acoustic neuromas. *J Neurosurg* 1965;**22**:399–401.

42. Samii M. Neurochirurgische Gesichtspunkte bei der Behandlung der Akustikusneurinome mit besonderer Berucksichtigung des N. facialis. *Laryng Rhinol* 1979; **59**:97–106.

43. Samii M. Nerves of the head and neck. In: Omer GE (Jr), Spinner M (eds). *Management of peripheral nerve problems.* Philadelphia: W.B. Saunders; 1980:507–47.

44. Samii M. Facial nerve grafting in acoustic neurinoma. *Clin Plastic Surg* 1984;**11**:221–5.

45. Smith MFW, Ray NM, Cox DJ. Suboccipital microsurgical removal of acoustic neurinomas of all sizes. *Ann Otol* 1973;**82**:407–14.

46. Malis LI. Nuances in acoustic neuroma surgery. *Neurosurgery* 2001;**49**:337–41.

47. Yasargil MG. Mikrochirurgie der Kleinhirnbrucken-winkel-Tumoren. In: Plester D, Wende S, Nakayama N (eds). *Kleinhirn-bruckenwirkelntumoren.* Berlin: Springer-Verlag; 1978:215–57.

48. Fischer G, Fischer C, Remond J. Hearing preservation in acoustic neurinoma surgery. *J Neurosurg* 1992;**76**: 910–17.

11

Translabyrinthine approach for vestibular schwannoma

SURESH SANKHLA, NARAYAN JAYASHANKAR, K.P. MORWANI

ABSTRACT

Objectives: In this chapter, we describe the microsurgical technique of the translabyrinthine approach and evaluate the access offered by this approach for removal of vestibular schwannomas. We also review the results of this surgical approach in 35 patients with large vestibular tumours.

Materials and methods: A retrospective evaluation was made of the clinical data from 35 patients who had undergone translabyrinthine surgery at our institution for removal of large vestibular schwannomas with extrameatal diameters of ≥3 cm, between January 2004 and December 2008.

Results: Thirty-four patients (97.1%) had a complete tumour removal, which was confirmed by imaging studies. Anatomical facial nerve preservation was achieved in 31 patients (88.6%). Four patients (11.4%), in whom the facial nerve was interrupted during surgery, were treated with immediate surgical nerve repair techniques, including an end-to-end anastomosis in 3 patients and nerve grafting in 1 patient. At 1-year follow up, 28 patients (80%) had good facial function (grades I and II, House–Brackmann [H–B] grading). Postoperative complications were minimal and included cerebrospinal fluid (CSF) leak in 1 patient (2.9%) and a slow recovery in gait in another (2.9%). Paresis persisted postoperatively in 1 patient with preoperative cranial nerves IX and X paresis.

Conclusions: The translabyrinthine approach is a safe surgical procedure in patients with large acoustic neuroma who do not have useful hearing on the affected side. Complete tumour removal with a very low morbidity in our series suggests that the enlarged translabyrinthine approach offers excellent control of the neurovascular structures in the cerebellopontine angle (CPA). It also offers the advantage of management of the interrupted facial nerve during the primary procedure itself, as the proximal and distal segments are in the operative field.

The surgical management of vestibular schwannoma (acoustic neuroma) has evolved significantly over the past few decades. In recent years, advances in neuroimaging and neuro-anaesthesia, introduction of intra-operative neurophysiological monitoring, and the development of microsurgical techniques have transformed what was a highly difficult operation into one associated with low morbidity and mortality.[1–6] The improvement in surgical results has, indeed, changed from the earlier goal of saving life in the treatment of acoustic neuroma to the current objectives of total tumour removal without major morbidity, preservation of the facial function and service-able hearing, and a good quality of life.

Three basic surgical approaches are used currently for the removal of acoustic neuromas. The middle fossa exposure allows complete exposure of the internal auditory canal (IAC) and thus facilitates total removal of intra-canalicular tumours with an excellent chance for preserving hearing.[7] The retromastoid (sub-occipital) approach requires cerebellar retraction but can be used to treat all sizes of tumours.[8,9] The major limitation of this approach is the obstruction produced by the posterior semi-circular canal which prevents viewing of the lateral end of the IAC and thereby interferes with complete tumour removal. An additional risk of injury to the distal cranial nerves exists because of their location in the surgical access route. The translabyrinthine exposure inevitably destroys residual hearing, if any.[10,11] However, the possibility of a complete tumour dissection from the facial nerve in the IAC, with a reduced incidence of tumour recurrence, and excellent success in anatomical preservation of the facial nerve, coupled with the ready ability to perform a direct end-to-end facial nerve anastomosis or grafting, when necessary, are all appealing features of the translabyrinthine technique.[10,12–14]

We describe the surgical technique used at our institute (Dr Balabhai Nanavati Hospital, Mumbai) during the past 5 years of the trans-labyrinthine approach in the surgical management of 35 patients with acoustic neuroma. The technical details of the procedure and surgical outcomes in these patients were evaluated, and comparisons were made by reviewing the literature.

Materials and methods

Clinical records of 35 patients with large acoustic neuroma who had been treated surgically at our institute in a 5-year period from January 2004 to December 2008 were reviewed retrospectively. All these patients had unserviceable hearing (speech reception threshold of <50 dB and/or speech discrimination score of <50%); they were operated upon using an enlarged translabyrin-thine approach. Data were collected to evaluate the extent of tumour removal, surgical compli-cations, and postoperative results in the immediate postoperative period and at a minimum follow up of 1 year.

The tumour removal was classified as total or subtotal, according to the surgeon's impression and the findings of a postoperative contrast magnetic resonance imaging (MRI) scan. The tumour removal was considered subtotal even if only a tiny sleeve of tumour capsule was left over the brainstem or the facial nerve. Cranial nerve functions (V, VII, VIII, IX–XI) were documented in the following periods: preoperative, imme-diate postoperative and at 1-year follow up. H–B grading scale was used to evaluate facial nerve function.

Surgical technique

All operations were performed by a team of experienced neuro- and neuro-otological surgeons. The surgical technique of the trans-labyrinthine approach used was essentially the same as described by House but with certain modifications.[10,11]

After induction of general anaesthesia, the patient is placed in a supine position with the head rotated away, towards the opposite side. The abdomen or ipsilateral thigh is prepared for harvesting fascia lata and fat graft at the time of wound closure. A C-shaped temporal and retro-auricular incision is made, beginning 1 cm superior to the helix and extending posteriorly ~4–5 cm behind the postaural groove (Fig. 1). This incision allows adequate exposure of the temporal squama, mastoid process and the adjacent retrosigmoid region. A sharp T-shaped

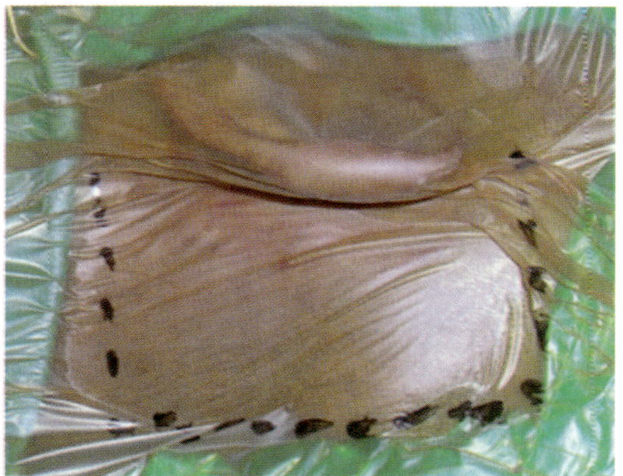

Fig. 1. Patient position and skin incision during surgery for left acoustic neuroma

musculoperiosteal incision with subperiosteal dissection is used to expose the mastoid process and the adjacent bone (Fig. 2). The horizontal limb of this musculoperiosteal incision is ~1 cm inferior to the corresponding skin incision level, and the vertical limb of the T-shaped incision is midway between the postaural groove and the corresponding retromastoid limb of skin incision. This prevents overlap of the skin and the musculoperiosteal incisions and allows a water-tight approximation of the soft tissue layer

at the time of the wound closure.

A mastoidectomy is first performed, followed by removal of the cortical bone over the sigmoid sinus, superior petrosal sinus, and the dura of the pre- and retro-sigmoid regions and middle cranial fossa. The drilling of bone is continued to skeletonize the mastoid segment of the facial nerve (Figs 3a and b). The bone is skeletonized from the area of the jugular bulb. In the case of a high jugular bulb, it is necessary to expose the bulb completely in order to achieve adequate exposure inferiorly. The bone anterior to the high jugular bulb is first drilled away until the entire inferior lip of the IAC has been removed. To avoid injury to cranial nerve IX, care is taken not to proceed anterior and inferior to the cochlear aqueduct. This is followed by removal of bone posteriorly, in the area of the sigmoid sulcus. The bulb can now be decompressed completely by simply pushing it inferiorly; it is kept in place by using bone wax. If properly decompressed, a high jugular bulb is not particularly restrictive in the translabyrinthine approach.

A labyrinthectomy is then performed during which the lateral aspect of the IAC is completely uncovered (Fig. 4). Complete bone removal

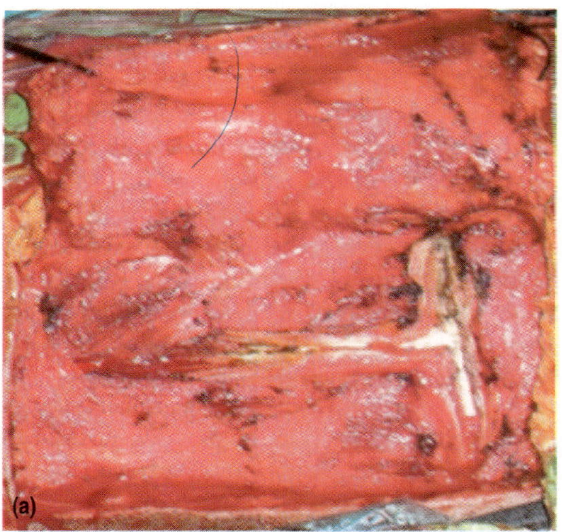

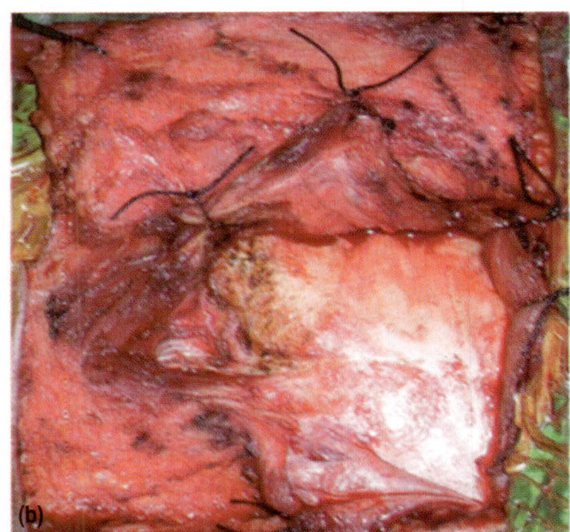

Fig. 2. Intraoperative photographs showing a sharp T-shaped musculoperiosteal incision (a) and a subperiosteal dissection to expose the mastoid region (b)

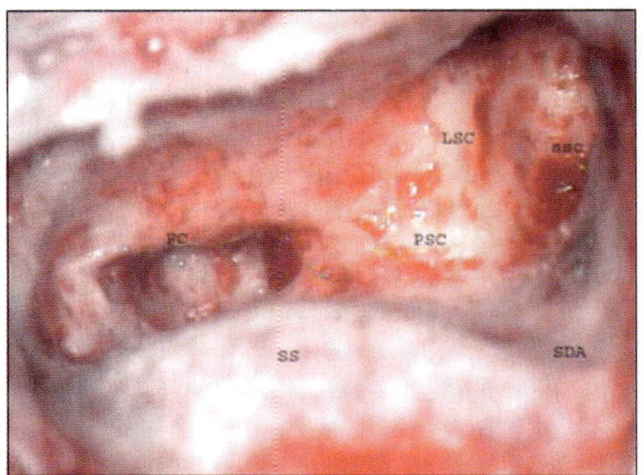

Fig. 3a. Microphotograph showing left cortical mastoidectomy

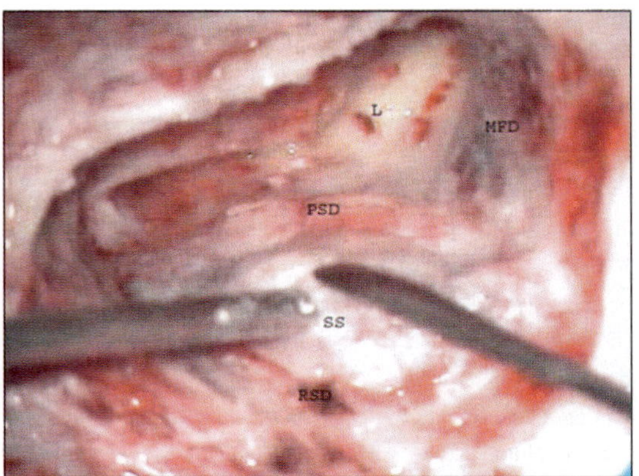

Fig. 3b. Microphotograph showing skeletonization of the left presigmoid, retrosigmoid and middle fossa dura

FC=fallopian canal; LSC=lateral semicircular canal; PSC=posterior semicircular canal; SSC=superior semicircular canal; SDA=sinodural angle; SS=sigmoid sinus; L=labyrinth; MFD=middle fossa dura; PSD=presigmoid dura; RSD=retrosigmoid dura; SS=sigmoid sinus

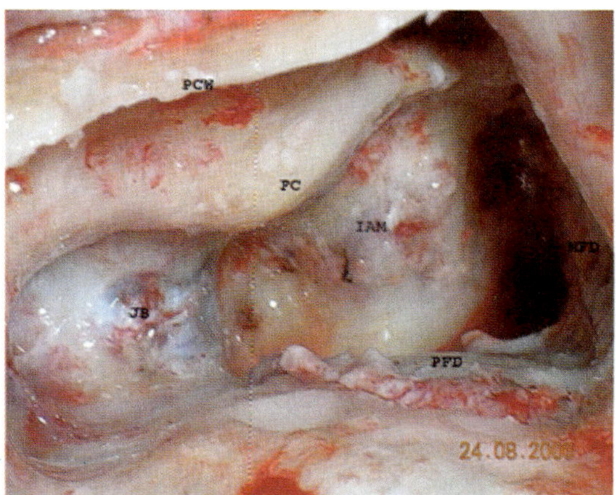

Fig. 4. Microphotograph showing left-sided labyrinthectomy with exposure of the internal auditory meatus

FC=fallopian canal; IAM=internal auditory meatus; JB=jugular bulb; MFD=middle fossa dura; PCW=posterior canal wall; PFD=posterior fossa dura

from the areas between the superior wall of the IAC and the dura of the middle cranial fossa, and between the inferior wall of the IAC and the jugular bulb is essential to obtain proper exposure. It cannot be overemphasized that the key to this approach is having the necessary wide exposure obtained by removing bone superiorly and posteriorly. We prefer to unroof the bony IAC as much as possible, usually between 270°

(enlarged translabyrinthine approach) to 300° (transapical extension type I) (Figs 5a and b). After the Bill's bar has been identified in the fundus, further dissection proceeds from the superior ampullary nerve towards the superior vestibular nerve, thereby creating a plane of cleavage between the superior vestibular nerve and facial nerve (Fig. 6). It is at this point that the facial nerve is farthest away from the superior vestibular nerve. This anatomical orientation helps in early identification, and thus preservation, of the facial nerve at the lateral end of the IAC. The superior or inferior vestibular nerve and the tumour can then be dissected safely from the posteriorly placed facial and cochlear nerves until the medial end of the IAC.

We prefer a standard dural incision, as shown in Fig. 7. However, when a larger exposure is required, the dural incision can be extended along the tentorium by dividing the superior petrosal sinus. Care should be taken at this stage to avoid injury to the trochlear nerve and the vein of Labbe. The need for cerebellar retraction is obviated by releasing the CSF after dural opening, which results in immediate brain relaxation. This approach provides a wide exposure of the lateral skull base from the anterior aspect of the brainstem and the trigeminal roots superiorly to

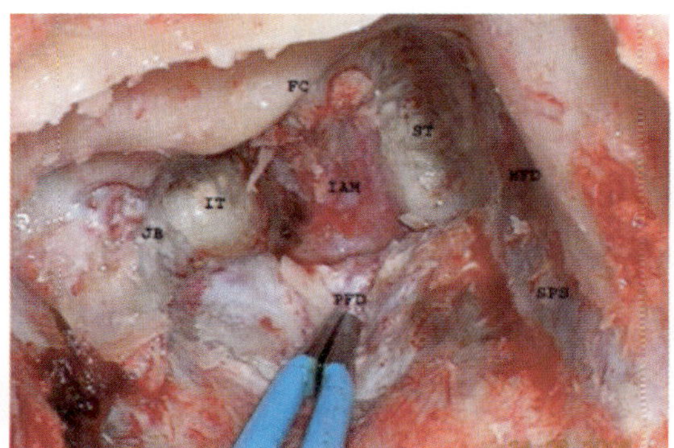

Fig. 5a. Intraoperative microphotograph showing 270° exposure of the internal auditory canal (enlarge translabyrinthine approach)

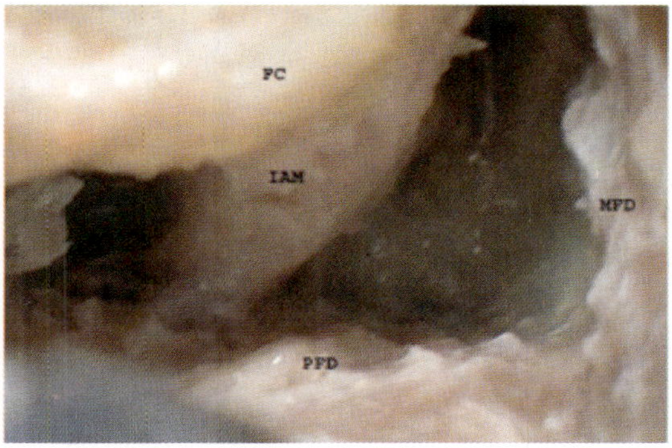

Fig. 5b. Cadaveric photograph showing 300° exposure of the internal auditory canal (transapical extension type I approach)

FC=fallopian canal; IAM=internal auditory meatus; IT=inferior trough; JB=jugular bulb; MFD=middle fossa dura; PFD=posterior fossa dura; SPS=superior petrosal sinus; ST=superior trough

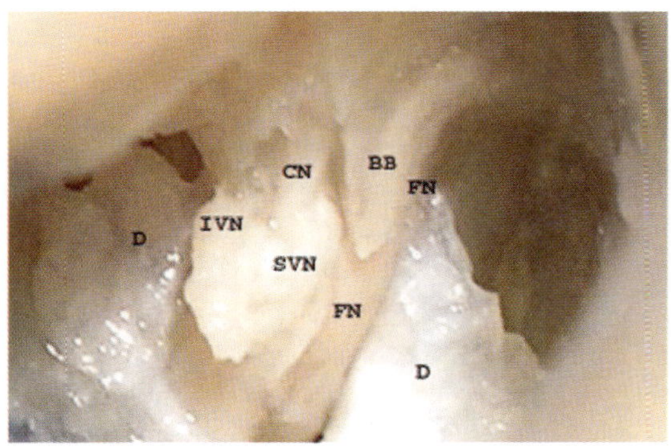

Fig. 6. Cadaveric dissection showing contents of the internal auditory canal (IAC)

BB=Bill s bar; CN=cochlear nerve; D=dura; FN=facial nerve; IVN=inferior vestibular nerve; SVN=superior vestibular nerve

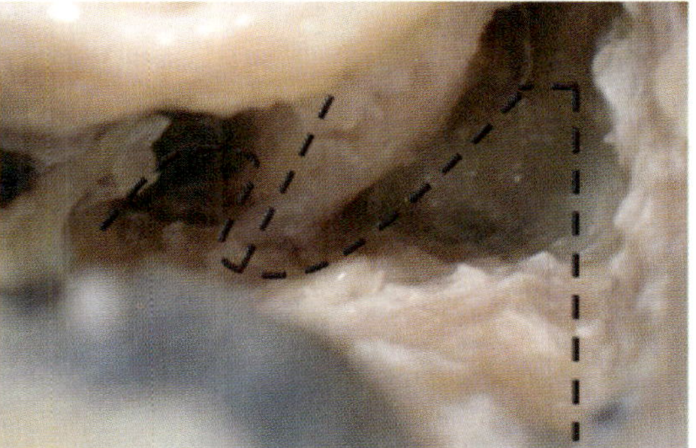

Fig. 7. Intraoperative photograph showing dural incision with a dotted line

the lower cranial nerves inferiorly (Figs 8a and b). Effective decompression of the jugular bulb inferiorly, as mentioned above, helps in an unhindered access to the area of the lower cranial nerves. Exposure of the tumour after opening the dura is shown in Fig. 9.

The tumour capsule is then incised and intra-capsular tumour decompression is performed using the regular microsurgical techniques (Fig. 10). Cerebellar retraction is not needed and the use of bipolar coagulation is reduced to a minimum during tumour decompression to ensure maximal safety of the brainstem and the

vascular supply to the nerve. A continuous irrigation with warm saline during tumour resection helps in maintaining a clear operative field. As soon as the tumour mass is largely debulked, the redundant tumour capsule can be easily mobilized without a significant risk of increasing tension on the already compressed neural structures. A plane of cleavage is identified between the capsule and the arachnoid sheath, which usually separates and protects the neurovascular structures. We prefer a bimanual technique of dissection at this stage. The residual tumour capsule is dissected out by gripping it with the tumour-holding forceps with one hand and gently sliding the overlying arachnoid sheath

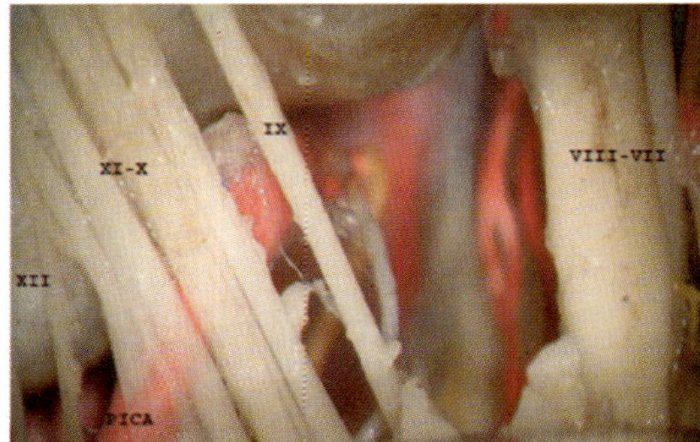

Fig. 8a. Cadaveric photograph showing the left VII–VIII cranial nerves complex and the lower cranial nerves (IX, X, XI, and XII) at the inferior part of the translabyrinthine exposure

PICA=posterior inferior cerebellar artery; SCA= superior cerebellar artery; T= tentorium.

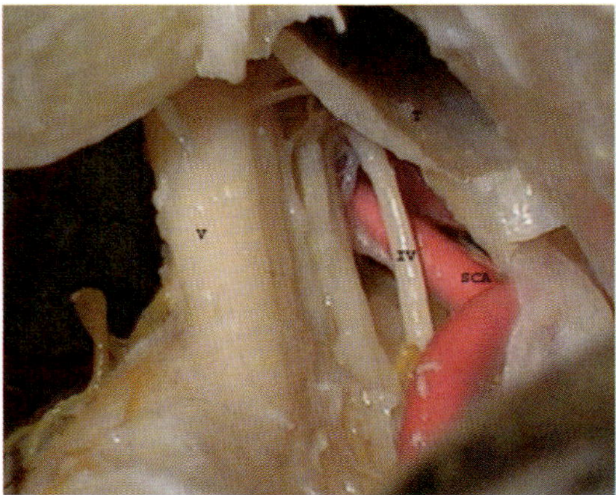

Fig. 8b. Cadaveric photograph showing cranial nerves IV and V at the superior part of the translabyrinthine exposure

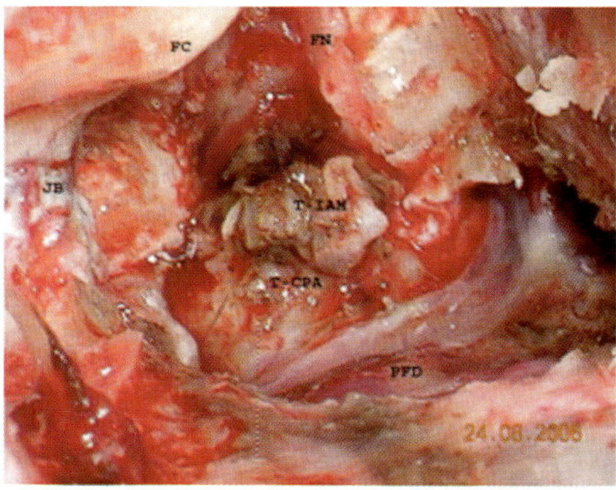

Fig. 9. Microphotograph showing complete exposure of the tumour in the CP angle

FC=fallopian canal; FN=facial nerve; JB=jugular bulb; PFD=posterior fossa dura; T-CPA=tumour in cerebello-pontine angle; T-IAM=tumour in internal auditory meatus

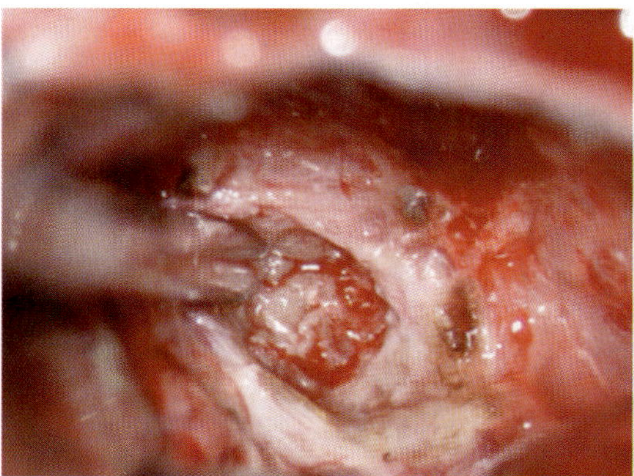

Fig. 10. Intraoperative microphotograph showing intracapsular decompression of a large left-sided acoustic neuroma

away using a blunt dissector or a non-traumatic suction cannula with the other hand (Fig. 11). Intermittently, a sharp arachnoid dissection is used to separate delicate neurovascular structures.

The facial nerve is kept under direct vision at all times during the entire process of tumour removal. The mastoid portions of the nerve are identified in the early stage of the procedure. The labyrinthine part is localized at the meatus and is followed further medially in the CPA along the tumour capsule. When identification of the facial nerve is difficult in the CPA, an attempt is made to identify the medial part of the nerve as it emerges from the brainstem (root exit zone) (Fig. 12). The utmost care should be taken to preserve the arachnoid coverings and vascularity of the facial nerve along its entire course, and that of the trigeminal and the lower cranial nerves. Finally, a meticulous haemostasis should be obtained, preferably by using a jugular venous compression technique.

Our technique of closure is fairly standard and essentially includes the basic steps of prevention

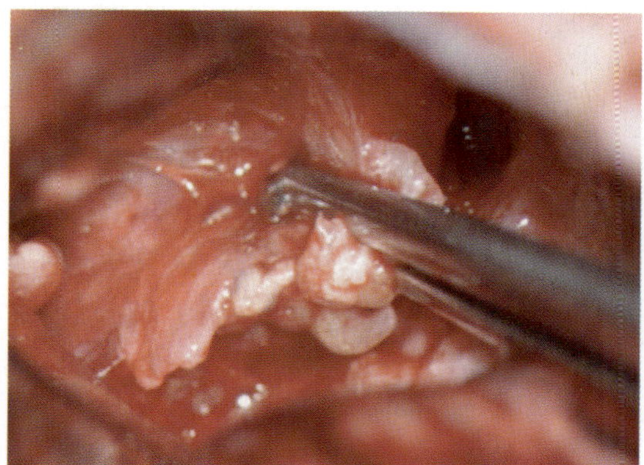

Fig. 11. Intraoperative microphotograph showing the microdissection technique using the tumour capsule—arachnoid interface

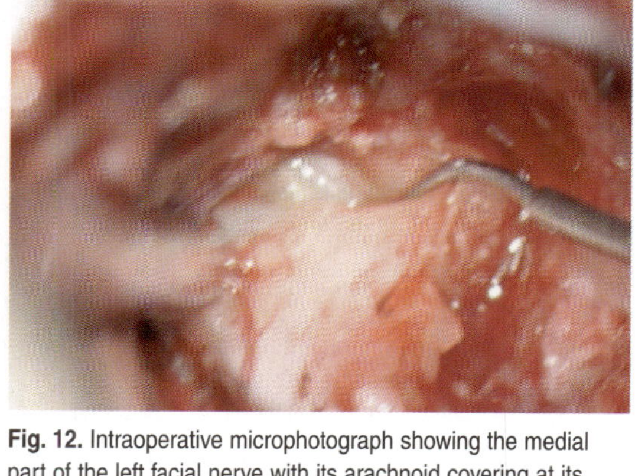

Fig. 12. Intraoperative microphotograph showing the medial part of the left facial nerve with its arachnoid covering at its root-exit zone

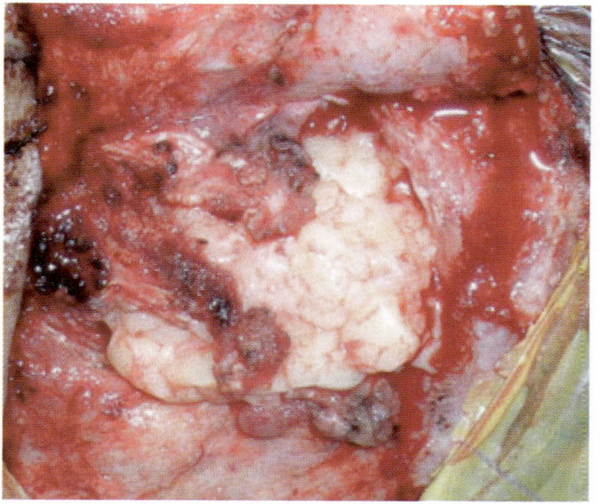

Fig. 13a. Intraoperative photograph showing wound closure with long strips of autologous fat

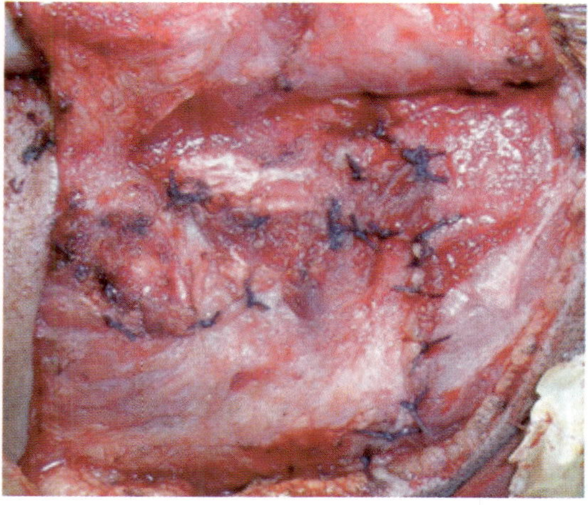

Fig. 13b. Intraoperative photograph showing water-tight closure of the musculoperiosteal layer

of CSF leak. This includes exenteration of air cells, blockage of any remnant cells with bone wax and obliteration of antrum with fat, bone dust and bone wax. Large strips of fat are placed from the mastoid until the CPA to achieve air-tight closure. Musculoperiosteal, subcutaneous and skin layers are sutured separately and meticulously to prevent CSF leak (Figs 13a and b). We frequently use fibrin glue during wound closure; a continuous lumbar CSF drainage is used for 3–5 days only when a postoperative CSF leak is encountered.

Results

Of the 35 cases studied, 20 (57%) were men and 15 (43%) were women, with ages ranging from 17 to 65 years. Tumour removal was complete (Fig. 14) in 34 (97.1%) patients and incomplete in 1 (2.9%) patient, in whom a small residual tumour capsule was left alone because of its adherence to the brainstem. Table 1 summarizes the results of the facial nerve functions. Preoperatively, 4 of 35 patients (11.4%) had H–B

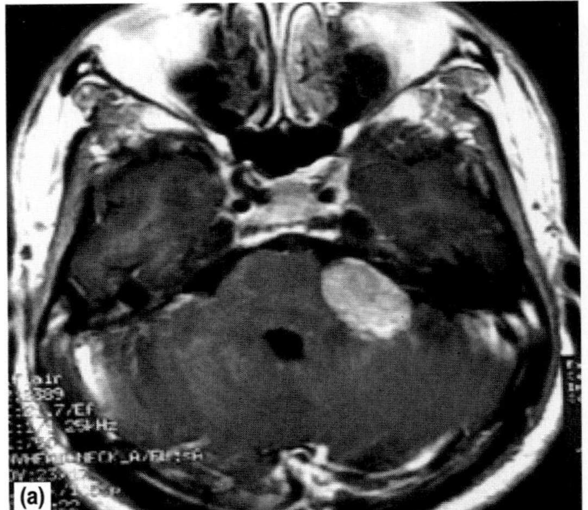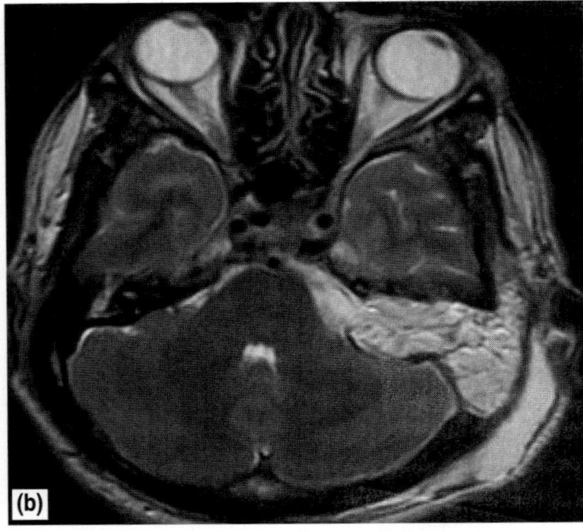

Fig. 14. Contrast MRI scan of a 47-year-old man with headache, vertigo and diminished left-sided hearing, showing a large acoustic neuroma in the left CP angle (a) and complete tumour resection postoperatively (b)

Table 1. Facial nerve preservation results (tumours of >3 cm in extrameatal diameter; n=35)

House–Brackmann grading	Preoperative no. of patients (%)	Immediate postoperative no. of patients (%)	1-year follow up no. of patients (%)
Grade I	31 (88.6)	15 (42.9)	24 (68.6)
Grade II	4 (11.4)	8 (22.9)	4 (11.4)
Grade III	0	6 (17.1)	6 (17.1)
Grade IV	0	2 (5.7)	0
Grade V	0	0	0
Grade VI	0	4 (11.4)	1 (2.9)#

Patient underwent VII–XII anastomosis much later after failure of anastomosis at primary surgery

grade II facial function. This was primarily because of the large size of the tumours (>4.5 cm). It may be noted that our anatomical preservation of the facial nerve was not good in our early cases, but has been improving progressively with experience. Inadvertent interruption of the facial nerve was encountered in 4 patients (11.4%). End-to-end apposition with fibrin glue was performed in 3 patients and interposition nerve grafting was done in 1. At 1-year follow up, 3 patients recovered to grade III, whereas one patient did not show any improvement. This patient, who developed grade

VI palsy and had a failed interposition nerve graft, was subjected to facial hypoglossal anastomosis subsequently. Nearly 80% of all patients recovered to functionally acceptable results between grades I and II at 1-year follow up (Fig. 15).

None of the patients in this study had developed any life-threatening intracranial complications, such as postoperative haematomas, brain oedema, cerebral infarction, meningitis or hydrocephalus. All postoperative complications were minor and treatable. Postoperative CSF leak from the wound was encountered in 1 patient

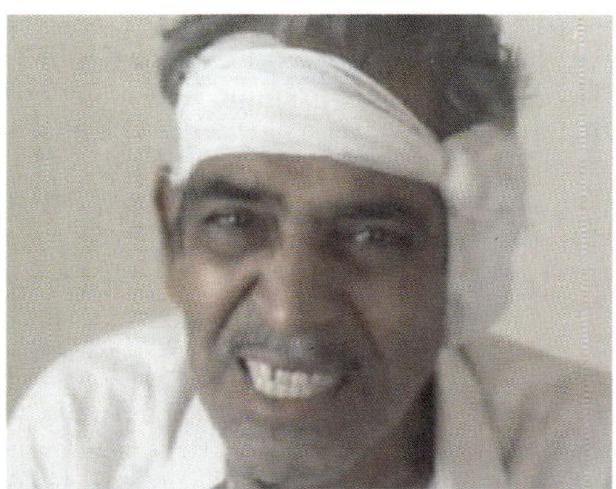

Fig. 15a. Postoperative photograph of a 60-year-old-man who underwent surgery for total resection of his left acoustic neuroma, showing H–B grade I facial function on the left side

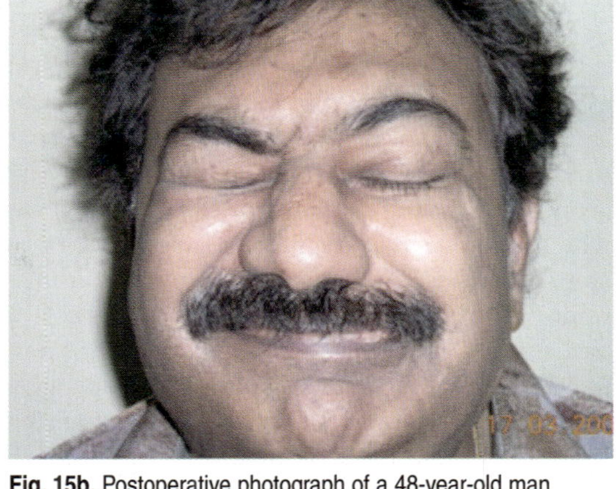

Fig. 15b. Postoperative photograph of a 48-year-old man showing H–B grade II facial paresis on the right side after removal of a right acoustic neuroma

(2.9%); conservative treatment using a lumbar drain was successful. Another patient (2.9%), who had preoperative cranial nerves IX and X pareses, did not improve after surgery and required swallowing therapy for a longer period.

Postoperative gross cerebellar ataxia was not observed in any of these patients. Although, the majority (97.1%) of patients resumed normal gait, albeit a slow walk, by postoperative day 6, one patient (2.9%) required >2 weeks to be able to walk without support; bipolar coagulation of one of the superficial arterial branches to the cerebellum during tumour removal was probably responsible for this delayed recovery in gait.

Discussion

The translabyrinthine technique was first introduced by House in 1964 for microsurgical removal of acoustic neuroma.[10,11] His approach was based on the principles of removing bone rather than retracting the brain in order to achieve wide surgical exposure at the base of skull. In his report of 41 operations, tumour excision was complete in >90% of cases with 0% mortality, and all patients experienced some return of facial function. He concluded that this approach provides a more direct route to the CPA, and has the advantage of achieving facial nerve exposure on either side of the tumour.

The translabyrinthine approach was earlier criticized by many surgeons for its narrow and limited surgical exposure, and was therefore not favoured for resection of medium or large-sized acoustic neuromas. However, recent advances in the surgical techniques facilitating wide temporal bone dissection, and the improved illumination and magnification offered by the operating microscope, have gradually changed the general perception. With introduction of several modifications to the original technique over the years, the translabyrinthine approach has now become one of the most commonly used surgical approaches for acoustic neuromas and other CPA tumours.[1,3,5,14–22,24,25]

In 1980, King and Morrison reported the results of surgical treatment of 150 acoustic neuromas using a modified technique known as the combined translabyrinthine–transtentorial approach, in which a wide surgical exposure was obtained by combining the translabyrinthine approach with the middle fossa exposure without exposing the brain.[23] They believed that their rates of tumour removal, morbidity, and mortality were comparable to the best reported rates using the posterior fossa approach.

While describing a similar technical modification in which the translabyrinthine approach is extended by adding the subtemporal route to gain a wider view, Sluyter *et al.* concluded that this approach is a safe route for removing acoustic neuromas with a diameter of ≥2 cm for which the translabyrinthine approach was considered less appropriate.[21] Complete tumour removal in their study was achieved in 110 patients (91.7%), with facial nerve preservation in 97 patients (80.8%). The main postoperative complications were CSF leakage (13.3%) requiring surgical revision in 2.5%, meningitis (9.2%), CSF rhinorrhoea (6.7%) requiring surgical revision in 2.5%, and epileptic seizures (3.3%) requiring medication. No deaths occurred that were directly related to the surgery in this series; the long-term follow-up examination of the facial nerve revealed recovery of function to the level of H–B grade I or II in 56.2% of the patients.[21]

Gormley and colleagues published another modification in this approach by combining transpetrosal and retrosigmoid exposures for the tumours that extend superiorly well into the tentorial notch.[3] Complete tumour resection in their study was accomplished in 99% of the patients and the facial outcome of grade I or II was achieved in 71%. These authors and others claimed that a combination of various angles of access afforded by this approach allows good visualization of the entire tumour and related anatomy.[3,22]

The modification in the translabyrinthine approach described here is based on the technique published by Sanna and co-workers and is slightly different to those reported by others.[3,21–25] Our technique of enlarged translabyrinthine, transapical extension type I approach includes dural exposure of the middle fossa, pre-sigmoid and retrosigmoid regions, and involves drilling of bone around the IAC by 270°–300°, as opposed to 180° in the classic translabyrinthine approach. The extra bone removal allows a free lateral to medial dissection for exposure of the CPA and offers excellent

visualization of the surgical field from the trigeminal nerve superiorly to the lower cranial nerves inferiorly, and from the CPA posteriorly to the prepontine cistern anteriorly, without any cerebellar retraction. The anterior surface of the brainstem and the tumour–brainstem interface can be visualized clearly without any cerebellar retraction. This manoeuvre has been found to be extremely useful in dealing with the large acoustic neuromas. Using this technique, we have been able to resect tumours of >4 cm in size. Our rate of complete tumour resection is comparable to those of others.[5,18,21] However, facial nerve preservation in our series was evidently marginally less than other series.[5,9,18,21,25] Likewise, the technique-related complication rate in our series also appears to be more or less similar to that described in the literature.[1,5,9,21,22]

Besides providing a wide surgical exposure without brain retraction, the other main advantage of the translabyrinthine approach is the early identification of the facial nerve, which is possible because of the presence of constant bony landmarks in that region. Control of the facial nerve in the early part of the dissection helps in the preservation of its anatomical and functional integrity during tumour removal. There are several reports in the literature demonstrating excellent facial nerve function using this approach.[1,3,5,14–22,24,25] In addition, the translabyrinthine approach also provides adequate exposure and accessibility to perform facial nerve repair, direct end-to-end or with-nerve grafting, if necessary.

Compared with the suboccipital or retro-sigmoid craniotomy, this approach offers a shorter distance between the surface and the neoplasm, demands a relatively simpler position of the patient, and is comfortable for the surgeon. The risk of injury to the lower cranial nerves is significantly lower compared with the posterior approaches. The incidence of complications, such as postoperative haematomas in the trans-labyrinthine approach, is not significantly different from the retrosigmoid approach.[26] However, it should be noted that if a haematoma develops postoperatively, it may be simpler to drain it via a translabyrinthine route compared with the retrosigmoid route in which a swollen cerebellum may be encountered. The major disadvantage of this method is that the removal of labyrinthine structures causes deafness in the affected ear. However, preservation of serviceable hearing is rarely feasible using any approach in tumours of >2.5 cm extrameatal diameter.[27]

Conclusion

The translabyrinthine approach is a safe route for removing acoustic neuromas in cases in which the hearing is unserviceable. With recent refinements in the technique, it is now possible to remove large and giant-sized acoustic neuromas with minimal morbidity. The enlarged translabyrinthine technique offers a very good approach for removal of large tumours and those with extension anterior to the internal acoustic meatus, which were previously thought to be unapproachable via the classic translabyrinthine approach. Because the key goals when dealing with removal of large acoustic neuromas are total tumour removal and facial nerve preservation, the translabyrinthine exposure, when properly performed, has an important advantage among the available approaches and may be considered as an alternative to the retrosigmoid approach.

References

1. Briggs RJS, Luxford WM, Atkins JS Jr, *et al.* Translabyrinthine removal of large acoustic neuromas. *Neurosurgery* 1994;**34**:785–92.
2. Darrouzet V, Guerin J, Aouad N, *et al.* The widened retrolabyrinthine approach: A new conception acoustic neuroma surgery. *J Neurosurg* 1997;**86**: 812–21.
3. Gormley NB, Sekhar LN, Wright DC, *et al.* Acoustic neuromas: Results of current surgical management. *Neurosurgery* 1997;**41**:50–60.
4. Kaylie DM, Gilbert E, Horgan MA, *et al.* Acoustic neuroma surgery outcomes. *Otol Otoneurol* 2001;**22**: 686–9.
5. Lanman TH, Brackmann DE, Hitselberger WE, *et al.* Report of 190 consecutive cases of large acoustic tumors removed via the translabyrinthine approach. *J Neurosurg* 1999;**90**:617–23.
6. Ojemann RG. Management of acoustic neuromas (vestibular schwannomas): Honored guest presentation. *Clin Neurosurg* 1991;**40**:498–535.
7. Gantz BJ, Parnes LS, Harker LA, *et al.* Middle cranial fossa acoustic neuroma excision: Results and complications. *Ann Otol Rhinol Laryngol* 1986;**95**: 454–9.
8. Harner SG, Beatty CW, Ebersold MJ. Retrosigmoid removal of acoustic neuroma: Experience 1978–1988. *Otolaryngol Head Neck Surg* 1990;**103**:40–5.
9. Samii M, Matthies C. Management of 1000 vestibular schwannomas (acoustic neuromas): Surgical management and results with an emphasis on complications and how to avoid them. *Neurosurgery* 1997;**40**:11–23.
10. House WF. Transtemporal bone microsurgical removal of acoustic neuromas. Evolution of transtemporal bone removal of acoustic tumors. *Arch Otolaryngol* 1964;**80**:731–42.
11. House WF. Translabyrinthine approach. In: House WF, Luetje CM (eds). *Acoustic tumors. Management.* Baltimore: University Park Press; 1979;**2**:43–87.
12. Hardy DG, MacFarlane R, Bagulay D, *et al.* Surgery for acoustic neurinoma: An analysis of 100 translabyrinthine operations. *J Neurosurg* 1989;**71**: 799–804.
13. Whittaker CK, Luetje CM. Vestibular schwannomas. *J Neurosurg* 1992;**76**:897–900.
14. Chen TC, Giannotta SL, Brackmann DE. Acoustic neuromas. Translabyrinthine approach. In: Apuzzo MLJ (ed). *Brain surgery. Complication avoidance and management.* New York: Churchill Livingstone 1993; **2**:1772–1800.
15. Brackmann DE, Green JD. Translabyrinthine approach for acoustic tumor removal. *Otolaryngol Clin North Am* 1992;**25**:311–29.
16. Giannotta SL. Translabyrinthine approach for removal of medium and large tumors of the cerebellopontine angle. *Clin Neurosurg* 1992;**38**: 589–602.
17. Hitselberger WE. Translabyrinthine approach to acoustic tumors. *Am J Otol* 1993;**14**:7–8.
18. Mamikoglu B, Wiet RJ, Esquivel CR. Translabyrinthine approach for the management of large and giant vestibular schwannomas. *Otol Neurotol* 2002;**23**:224–7.
19. Naguib MB, Saleh E, Cokkeser Y, *et al.* The enlarged translabyrinthine approach for removal of large

vestibular schwannomas. *J Laryngol Otol* 1994;**108:** 545–50.

20. Tos M, Thomsen J. The translabyrinthine approach for the removal of large acoustic neuromas. *Arch Otorhinolaryngol* 1989;**246:**292–6.

21. Sluyter S, Graamans K, Tulleken CAF, *et al.* Analysis of the results obtained in 120 patients with large acoustic neuromas surgically treated via the translabyrinthine-transtentorial approach. *J Neurosurg* 2001;**94:**61–6.

22. Anderson DE, Loenetti J, Wind JJ. Resection of large vestibular schwannomas: Facial nerve preservation in the context of surgical approach and patient-assessed outcome. *J Neurosurg* 2005;**102:**643–9.

23. King TT, Morrison AW. Translabyrinthine and transtentorial removal of acoustic nerve tumors. Results in 150 cases. *J Neurosurg* 1980;**52:**210–16.

24. Sanna M, Agarwal M, Mancini F, *et al.* Transapical extension in difficult cerebellopontine angle tumors. *Ann Otol Rhinol Laryngol* 2004;**113:**676–82.

25. Sanna M, Russo A, Taibah A, *et al.* Enlarged translabyrinthine approach for the management of large and giant acoustic neuromas: A report of 175 consecutive cases. *Ann Otol Rhinol Laryngol* 2004; **113:**319–28.

26. Sade B, Mohr G, Dufour JJ. Vascular complications of vestibular schwannoma surgery: A comparison of the suboccipital retrosigmoid and translabyrinthine approaches. *J Neurosurg* 2006;**105:**200–4.

27. Khrais T, Sanna M. Hearing preservation surgery in vestibular schwannoma. *J Laryngol Otol* 2006;**120:** 366–70.

12

Medium-size acoustic schwannomas: Preferred approach—the retrosigmoid

V.K. JAIN, SAMIR K. KALRA

Acoustic schwannomas are situated within the narrow confines of the cerebellopontine angle (CPA). Though benign, these tumours are located in critical locations intimately close to the cranial nerves, cerebellum and the brainstem. They were once considered the most difficult brain tumours to remove without producing additional neurological deficits. Sir Charles Ballance first successfully resected an acoustic schwannoma in 1894 and Dandy performed the first total excision of this tumour in 1925, when the aim of surgery was only prolongation of life. In the current era, with the advent of modern surgical techniques, the goal has shifted to preservation of cranial nerve function.

Schwannomas constitute about 8% of all intracranial tumours that present clinically.[1,2] The majority of acoustic schwannomas are sporadic and unilateral.[3,4] They present commonly in the fourth to sixth decades.[5–7] Bilateral tumours are hereditary and constitute <5% of all schwannomas.[8]

The past 10 years have seen remarkable advances in the diagnosis and management of these tumours. They are diagnosed at an early stage whereby management becomes much easier and rewarding both for the patient and easier and rewarding both for the patient and doctor, since smaller the tumour the better the results.

Pathological anatomy

Acoustic schwannomas arise most commonly from the vestibular nerves.[9] The origin of the tumour is from the junctional (Obersteiner–Redlich) zone where the central and peripheral myelin meet each other. This zone is situated at the auditory meatus or within the internal auditory canal in most instances. The tumour grows initially within the canal and, thereafter, extrudes into the CPA. Inside the internal auditory canal, the tumour may compress the cochlear component of the nerve or the labyrinthine artery, causing hearing loss.[10] Growth of the tumour into the CPA results in anterior displacement of the facial and cochlear nerves. As the anterior inferior cerebellar artery (AICA) most often passes below the VII and VIII nerves, it is displaced inferiorly. In large lesions, the AICA may be seen lying in close relation to the IX and X cranial nerves. The superior cerebellar artery is displaced rostrally and the posterior inferior cerebellar artery (PICA) caudally. The veins surrounding the tumour form bridging veins which empty into the superior petrosal sinus. While small tumours can be removed without sacrifice of these veins, in large tumours it may be necessary to sacrifice one, if not more, or even the superior petrosal vein to reach the superior pole of the tumour.

Once the tumour emerges from the canal, it pushes the lateral layer of the arachnoid inwards till it comes into contact with the more important vessels and nerves of the CPA. This arachnoid plane is an important aid to dissection.

Grading of acoustic schwannoma

Ojemann *et al.*[11] classified tumours as:

- Small tumours that extend <2 cm into the cerebellopontine cistern and generally cause symptoms of only the VIII nerve.
- Medium-sized tumours which extend 2–3 cm into the cerebellopontine cistern, cause trigeminal symptoms and reach up to the brainstem.
- Large tumours which extend for >3 cm into the cistern and produce signs of brainstem compression and of raised intracranial pressure.

All patients should have the following for decision-making.

Pure tone audiogram (PTA): May be useful as the first step screening test. Air conduction assesses the entire system, bone conduction assesses from the cochlea and proximally. PTA assesses the functionality of hearing (to help in treatment decision-making) and acts as a baseline for future comparison. The single numerical score is an average of the thresholds for frequencies across the audio spectrum.

Speech discrimination: Maintained in conductive hearing loss, moderately impaired in cochlear hearing loss, poorest with retrocochlear lesions. A score of 4% suggests a retrocochlear lesion, as does a score that is worse than would be predicted based on PTA testing.

If audiogram and speech discrimination score do not qualify in the same class, use the lower class.

A generous definition of functional hearing requires thresholds at least <50 dB or speech discrimination >50%

Useful hearing is unlikely to be preserved if (i) preoperative speech discrimination is <75% or preoperative threshold loss is >25 dB.

Treatment options

1. *Expectant management:* follow symptoms, hearing (audiometrics) and tumour growth on serial imaging (CT or MRI 6 monthly for 2 years, then annually if stable). Intervention is performed for progression. The growth patterns observed are:
—*little or no growth:* usually those contained within the IAC
—*slow growth:* 2 mm/year
—*rapid growth:* 10 mm/year.
Sudden profound hearing loss from surgery seems to have a far greater psychological and social impact than the same loss that has occurred slowly from tumour growth. The best way to preserve hearing is not to remove the tumour but this requires conscientious follow-up with repeat scans and even then there is an incidence of spontaneous severe sensorineural hearing loss with these tumours.
2. *Radiation therapy* (alone, or in conjunction

Table 1. Gardner and Robertson modified hearing classification

Class	Description	Pure tone audiogram (dB)	Speech discrimination (%)
I	Good-excellent	0–30	70–100
II	Serviceable	31–50	50–59
III	Non-serviceable	51–90	5–49
IV	Poor	91–max	1–4
V	None	Not testable	0

with surgery)
—External beam radiation therapy (EBRT)
—Stereotatic radiosurgery
3. *Surgery:* approaches include the following
—*Retrosigmoid (or suboccipital):* may be able to spare hearing
—*Translabyrinthine (and its several variations):* sacrifices hearing, may be slightly better for sparing the VII nerve
—*Extradural subtemporal, (middle fossa approach):* only for small intracanalicular tumours

Selection of treatment option

In addition to the usual factors influencing the decision process with brain tumours, e.g. the patient's general medical condition, age (some use age >65 years as a cut-off for surgery, but there is not universal agreement on this), etc., other factors that must be weighed include: chances of hearing preservation in those with serviceable hearing and chances of preserving VII and V nerve function (all of which are related to tumour size), demonstrated tumour growth on serial imaging, the presence of NF2, local control rates of the various treatment modalities and long-term side-effects of treatment.

Surgical approaches

Total excision of tumour is usually the goal of surgery. The only indications for planned subtotal resection is a large tumour on the side of the ear with good hearing or those patients who require debulking with little chance of recurrence because of limited life expectancy, especially if the facial nerve is densely adherent to the tumour.[12,13] Microsurgical resection of acoustic schwannomas can be accomplished via three operative approaches: the translabyrinthine approach, middle fossa approach, and retrosigmoid sub-occipital approach.

1. *Translabyrinthine:* useful for tumours with primarily intracanalicular component with little CPA extension. Often preferred by neuro-otologists.
2. *Retrosigmoid:* This approach is often preferred by neurosurgeons.[14] This usually offers the best opportunity for preservation of hearing (when possible) with a possibility of preserving facial nerve as well. The disadvantages are higher morbidity than that by the translabyrinthine approach and it is difficult to remove small tumours from the lateral recess of the IAC without entering the vestibule producing inner ear dysfunction. The facial nerve usually presents on the blind (anterior) side of tumour and is encountered late.
3. *Extradural subtemporal (middle fossa approach):* This is limited to the removal of small, laterally located intracanalicular tumours. The approach has poor access to posterior fossa, and has higher risk of VII nerve palsy (injury at geniculate ganglion). It however provides good chances for preservation of hearing.

Table 2. Advantages and disadvantages of the translabyrinthine approach

Disadvantages	Advantages
• Sacrifices hearing (acceptable when hearing is already non-functional or unlikely to be spared by other approaches)	• Early identification of the facial nerve may result in higher preservation rate
• Limited exposure (limits maximal tumour size that can be approached)	• Less risk to cerebellum and lower cranial nerves
• May take longer than suboccipital approach	• Patients do not get as ill from blood in cisterna magna (essentially an extracranial approach)
• Possibly higher rate of postoperative CSF leak	

Selection of surgical approach

The choice of surgical approach is influenced by the size and position of the tumour, the surgeon's preference and experience, and the likelihood of preserving hearing on the affected side.

Retrosigmoid versus translabyrinthine approach for medium size tumours

1. Most neurosurgeons prefer to use the retrosigmoid approach whereas the translabyrinthine approach is used more by neuro-otologists.
2. The translabyrinthine approach cannot be used in the presence of otitis media.
3. The translabyrinthine approach cannot be used if the aim of surgery is to preserve hearing.
4. The chances of developing CSF leak are much higher in the translabyrinthine approach.
5. With the translabyrinthine approach, the visualization of critical vessels as well as the brainstem is late.
6. The chances of sacrifice of the superior petrosal vein are much higher in the trans-labyrinthine approach.

Therefore, it looks more plausible to choose the retrosigmoid approach for medium-size acoustic schwannomas.

The future

The advances in imaging technology have made the detection of small tumours much easier, and this in itself has posed problems as to what to do with the relatively asymptomatic growths in young people. To be able to reliably predict the rate of growth of an individual tumour would be a great advantage, and work is in progress to identify specific tumour markers that may be helpful. These could be obtained endoscopically through small posterior cranial fossa burr holes.

It may be that precision radiotherapy will then be able to prevent the further growth of these small tumours and surgery will be relegated to treat those tumours that have escaped early detection or fail to respond to radiotherapy. At present, however, one great benefit would be the ability to reliably preserve residual hearing during surgery.

Intraoperative monitoring of the electrical function of the cochlea and auditory brainstem is possible (although difficult) and is practised by some groups. Whether widespread acceptance of this technique occurs will depend on the usefulness of the residual hearing after such surgery, and there is much debate as to what constitutes useful residual hearing, but in those few people with absent or poor hearing in the other ear such techniques may become mandatory. The development of brainstem auditory implants, whereby electrodes are placed on the brainstem cochlear nuclei (which conveniently lie on the surface of the brainstem), might mean that hearing can be preserved even though the cochlear nerve is damaged.

References

1. Ramamurthi B. Intracranial tumors in India. Incidence and variations. *Intern Surgery* 1973;**58**:542.
2. Tandon PN. Intracranial neurofibromas. In: Ramamurthi B, Tandon PN (eds). *Textbook of neurosurgery*. Delhi: National Book Trust (India); 1980:946.
3. Pool JL, Pava AA, Greenfield EC. *Acoustic nerve tumors: Early diagnosis and treatment.* Charles C. Thomas; 1970:183.
4. Robinson K, Rudge P. The differential diagnosis of cerebellopontine angle lesions. *J Neurol Sci* 1983;**60**:1.
5. Harner SG, Ebersold MJ. Management of acoustic neuromas. *J Neurosurg* 1985;**63**:175.
6. Ramamurthi B, Balasubramaniam V, Kalyanaraman S. Acoustic neurinomas. *Neurol (India)* 1970;**18**:176.
7. Sambasivam M, Mathai KV Chandy J. Surgical experience with eighty cases of acoustic neurinomas. *Neurol (India)* 1966;**14**:125.
8. Eldridge R, Parry D. Summary: Vestibular schwannoma (acoustic neuroma) consensus

development conference. *Neurosurgery* 1992;**30**:962.

9. Samii M, Turel KE, Penkert G. Management of VII and VIII nerve involvement by cerebellopontine angle tumors. *Clin Neurosurg* 1985;**32**:242.

10. Sataloff RT, Davies B, Myers DL. Acoustic neuroma presenting as a sudden deafness. *Am J Otol* 1985;**6**:349.

11. Ojemann RG, Levine RA, Monogomery WM, *et al.* Use of intraoperative auditory evoked potentials to preserve hearing in unilateral acoustic neuroma removal. *J Neurosurg* 1984;**61**:938.

12. Lownie SP, Drake CG. Radical intracapsular removal of acoustic neurinomas. Long-term follow-up review of 11 cases. *J neurosurg* 1991;**74**:422–5.

13. Wazen J, Silverstein H, Norrell H, *et al.* Preoperative and postoperative growth rates in acoustic neuromas documented with CT scanning. *Otolaryngol Head Neck Surg* 1985;**93**:151–5.

14. Rhoton AL Jr. The cerebellopontine angle and posterior fossa cranial nerves by the retrosigmoid approach. *Neurosurgery* 2000;**47** (3 Suppl): S93–S129.

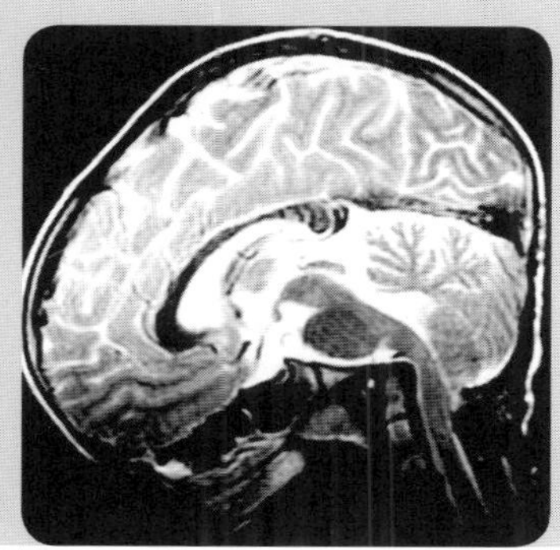

Neuroendoscopy

13

Endoscopic transoral excision of odontoid process in irreducible atlanto-axial dislocation

YAD RAM YADAV, RAVIKIRAN SHENOY, GAURAV MUKERJI, SNEHAL SHEREKAR, VIJAY PARIHAR

ABSTRACT

Introduction: The surgical approaches available for irreducible atlanto-axial dislocation (AAD) or basilar invasion are the transoral microscopic resection, endoscopic transnasal excision and endoscopic transoral excision of the odontoid process. Palatal splitting or prolonged retraction is required in the microsurgical technique whereas palatal splitting can be avoided by the minimally invasive technique of endoscopic transoral excision of the odontoid, which has been found to be effective and safe. We report our preliminary experience of performing endoscopic odontoidectomy.

Materials and methods: This is a prospective study of 22 patients treated during the 3-year period from July 2006 to June 2009. A detailed history was taken and a thorough physical and neurological examination was made to record preoperative status. The patients had a preoperative X-ray of the cervical region, and computed tomography (CT) and magnetic resonance imaging (MRI) scans. Postoperative evaluation in all patients included CT scans, recording postoperative complications and neurological status at 1, 6 and 12 months, respectively.

Results: During the study period, 22 patients between 15 and 56 years of age (mean 42 years) underwent this procedure. There were 18 male and 4 female patients. Duration of symptoms at presentation ranged from 6 to 18 months (mean 14 months). All patients had quadriparesis. Three patients also had cranial nerve X paresis. Fourteen patients had AAD, 7 had basilar invasion, and 1 had tubercular invasion. Palatal splitting was not required in any of the patients. All patients improved after surgery and no deaths occurred. One patient had a cerebrospinal fluid (CSF) leak, which stopped after external lumbar drainage.

Conclusion: Endoscopic transoral odontoidectomy is a direct, minimally invasive technique that is safe and effective. Angled scope improved exposure of the clivus, and palatal splitting is not required even in basilar invasion.

Introduction

Pathology, such as AAD and basilar invagination, affecting the cranio-vertebral junction can result in compression of the cervical spinal cord, brainstem or the vertebro-basilar vessels, which if left untreated can be fatal. Surgical treatment of these disorders is indicated in the presence of intractable neck and head pain, vertebral artery compromise, neurological deficits with instability or evidence of cord compression on MRI scans. The goal of surgery is to decompress the neural tissue and stabilize the involved joints. Following the successful treatment of atlanto-axial instability by Mixter and Osgood in 1910, other techniques, such as the Gallie technique and the Brooks and Jenkins methods, have been used to stabilize the atlanto-axial joint.[1] Achieving adequate anterior decompression of an irreducible atlanto-axial joint is difficult with such techniques. Anterior access to the cranio-vertebral junction is commonly achieved through the transoral–transpharangeal approach. The most frequent surgical approach used for irreducible AAD or basilar invasion is the transoral microscopic resection.[2] Recently, endonasal and transoral endoscopic approaches to the cranio-vertebral junction have been described.[3–7] A minimally invasive microendo-scopic anterior approach has recently been reported to be safe and reliable for treating irreducible AAD.[8] We report our initial experience in performing endoscopic transoral odontoidectomy in a series of 22 patients.

Materials and Methods

Ours was a prospective study of patients treated during a 3-year period from July 2006 to June 2009. Detailed history was taken and a thorough physical examination, including preoperative neurological status, was recorded. The neurological deficits were documented and patients were graded using the Ranawat classification.[9] Preoperatively, all patients had an X-ray of the cervical spine lateral view (in neutral, flexion and extension), anterior–posterior and transoral view for the odontoid process. Other investigations, including CT and MRI scan, were performed in all cases. A CT scan was carried out post-operatively in all patients. All postoperative complications were recorded. Postoperative neurological status was recorded at intervals of 1, 6 and 12 months, respectively. Follow up ranged from 12 to 48 months (mean 26 months).

Clinical features

AAD can result from associated bony abnormalities caused by abnormal development or ossification of the odontoid, or after a fracture. It can also be found in conditions associated with transverse ligament laxity, as in Down syndrome. Inflammation of the ligament can weaken the joint and predispose to subluxation. Patients with AAD can present with a cock-robin deformity or torticollis in rotatory dislocation, occipital pain or vertigo. They can also present with features of myelopathy, such as hyper-reflexia, clonus, and extensor plantar reflexes. The brainstem symptoms can occur with either basilar invaginations or with occlusion of the vertebral artery. Various clinical gradings of patients are described, such as Di Lorenzo grading, Frankel grading system, the Ranawat grading scale and the Japanese Orthopaedic Association scores.[10–12]

Diagnosis

AAD is defined as an atlantodens interval (ADI; i.e. distance between the odontoid process and the posterior border of the anterior arch of the atlas) of >3 mm in adults and of >5 mm in children, as measured on plain radiography. Chamberlain line (palato-occipital line) joins the posterior tip of the hard palate to the posterior rim of the foramen magnum. Normally, the tip of the dens lies 3.6 mm below this line. Up to

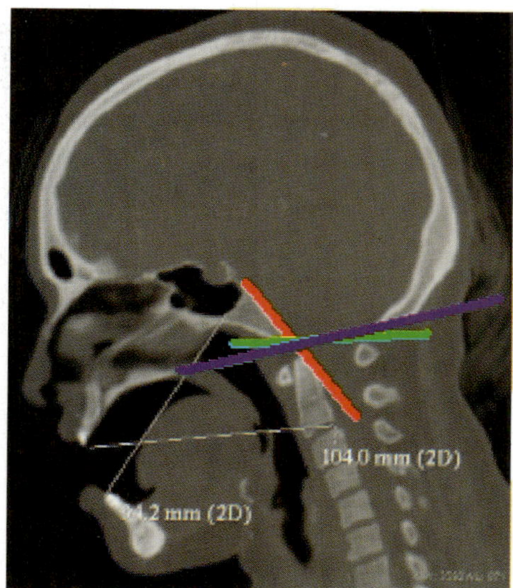

Fig. 1. Various lines used in radiological diagnosis of cranio-vertebral anomaly

one-third of the dens may be above this line (Fig. 1). McRae line (foramen magnum line) joins the anterior and posterior edges of the foramen magnum. The average sagittal diameter of the foramen magnum is 35 mm; the tip of the dens must be below this line. Neurological deficit is usually present if the effective sagittal space for the cervicomedullary junction is <20 mm in a child >8 years of age. McGregor line (basal line) joins the hard palate to the lowest point of the occipital bone. The tip of the dens should not be >5 mm above this line. Wackenheim line (clivus canal line) extends along the clivus and extrapolated into the cervical spinal canal. The odontoid process should be ventral or tangential to it. The odontoid process transects this line in basilar invagination, AAD and anterior occipito-atlantal dislocation. Irreducible AAD is diagnosed when the dislocation does not reduce even after a period of applying traction.

Operative technique

The transoral approach primarily provides midline exposure of the inferior one-third of the clivus, the anterior cranio-vertebral junction, and the C1–C2 complex.[2] Its main advantage is that it provides a direct extradural approach. The lateral limits of this exposure are defined by the mandible and the tonsillar pillars. The superior and inferior limits are usually the lower clivus and the middle to lower C2 vertebral body, respectively, although this will vary with each individual. Basilar invagination allows exposure further down the spinal column. Restricted jaw opening, such as that found in patients with rheumatoid arthritis, may reduce the extent of exposure, especially inferiorly.

A careful review of radiographic images, including MRI and fine-cut 3D-reconstructed CT scans of the cranio-vertebral junction are required before selecting the appropriate approach. A transoral approach is indicated if the lesion is situated in the midline extradurally. If it extends more laterally or appears to be located intradurally, alternatives, such as the far lateral or extreme lateral transcondylar approaches, are considered. Preoperatively, the superior extent of the exposure is estimated by drawing an imaginary line in the plane of the lower teeth and hard palate toward the cranio-vertebral junction on a sagittal CT scan with an open mouth (Fig. 2). The inferior limit is an imaginary line in the plane of the upper teeth and retracted posterior limit of the tongue. If the lesion is in midline and is situated above this line, an extended trans-sphenoidal approach may be suitable. If, however, the lesion is situated below the plane of the hard palate, a transoral approach alone may be sufficient.

Preoperatively, dynamic, plain cervical radiographs in flexion and extension views are obtained to evaluate pre-existing instability at the cranio-vertebral junction. Even in the absence of instability, most cases will require stabilization after resection of the odontoid process and the involved ligaments because of postoperative iatrogenic instability. Either occipito-cervical or atlantoaxial stabilization can be performed. A high resolution CT scan of the cranio-vertebral junction (Figs 3a and b) is generally obtained.

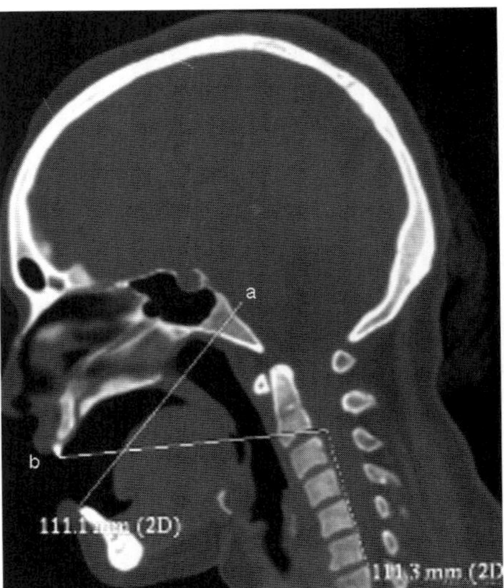

Fig. 2. Preoperative mid-sagittal CT scan used to estimate superior and inferior limit of exposure. Tongue can be retracted inferiorly during surgery. The superior extent of the exposure is determined by an imaginary line in the plane of lower teeth and hard palate toward the cranio-vertebral junction (a). The inferior limit is an imaginary line in the plane of upper teeth and retracted posterior limit of the tongue (b).

Reduction of dislocation preoperatively is achieved with cervical traction. MRI is better than CT scan to visualize soft tissue details (Fig. 3c).

The patient is placed in the supine position with the head resting on a headrest or a ring. The neck is normally extended slightly to facilitate a direct line of sight to the cranio-vertebral junction. The patient can be placed in a neutral position in the endoscopic technique. Cervical traction is placed preoperatively for reduction. The patient is intubated orally. Topical corticosteroid cream is applied to the tongue to minimize postoperative tongue swelling. We apply the Dingman retractor system. The patient's tongue is retracted inferiorly using a wide and rigid retractor blade. The endotracheal tube is placed to the left side in the oral cavity. It exits from the left corner of the patient's mouth and does not obstruct the surgical exposure. This provides adequate exposure and eliminates the need for a preoperative tracheostomy. A tracheostomy is generally reserved for those patients who have pre-existing bulbar or respiratory dysfunction. The soft palate and uvula can be retracted superiorly with a small retractor blade that attaches to the transoral retractor. We do not incise the soft palate, which can result in dysphagia, dysphonia, and nasal regurgitation of fluids. Adjustable lateral retractors are attached to the retractor frame to retract the pharyngeal soft tissues laterally. The tongue is inspected carefully to confirm that it is free from compression between the retractor blade and the teeth after application of the retractor system. Failure to recognize this compression can result in necrosis or swelling of the tongue. After final positioning of the retractors, the mouth, oropharynx and retractors

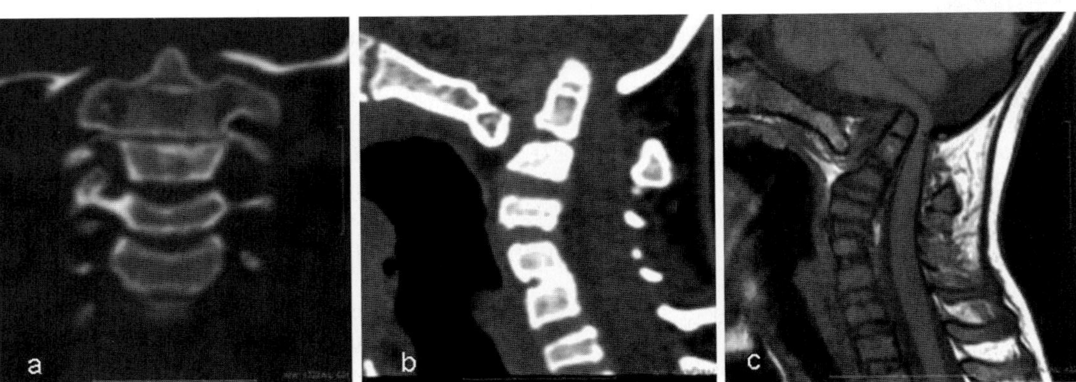

Fig. 3. Preoperative CT (a, b) and MRI scans (c) of a patient showing basilar invasion

are again prepped with betadine solution. Prophylactic antibiotics are administered intra-operatively. The surgeon operates from the head end or the right side of the patient using a 0° or 30°, 30 cm long 4 mm telescope with sheath. In our experience, a 30 cm long endoscope is more convenient to use than an 18 cm scope. Camera and light source cables are placed away from the instruments used in surgery.

The uvula is retracted into the nasopharynx with the help of an infant feeding tube; it is fixed to the end of infant feeding tube by a suture and is pulled back gently into the nasal cavity (Fig. 4). This helps increase the exposure. The posterior pharyngeal wall is infiltrated with 0.5% lidocaine with 1:200,000 epinephrine solution. A midline incision is made on the posterior pharyngeal wall, which is retracted using a pharyngeal retractor. The procedure must remain in the midline, which can be located by palpating the tubercle of C1 and by the position of the teeth. Shielded monopolar cautery with a fine-tip, set at low cutting power, is used to cut and dissect the posterior pharyngeal muscles and the anterior longitudinal ligament. The lateral retractors help in exposing the tissues as the incision is deepened.

The tip of a regular monopolar cautery, bent to a near-right angle, is used to detach the ligaments from the bone in a sub-periosteal fashion. This technique greatly reduces bleeding from these richly vascularized tissues. The longus colli and the longus capitis muscles are mobilized laterally and held in place with tooth-bladed lateral pharyngeal retractors. This exposes the inferior clivus, C1 arch and C2 vertebral body.

All soft tissues are cleared with electrocautery before removal of the anterior C1 arch and the odontoid process. Bone cuts are made through the arch of C1 on both sides of the odontoid process using a high-speed drill and Kerrison punch. The upper border of the odontoid process and the intervertebral disc between C2 and C3 are identified using fluoroscopy. Before performing an odontoidectomy, the edges of the odontoid are clearly defined and freed from any ligamentous attatchments. The apical and alar ligaments are detached from the odontoid using sharp curettes. A right-angled curette is used to free the posterior cortex of the odontoid from the underlying soft tissues and ligaments. The centre of the odontoid process is hollowed out using a high-speed drill, copious irrigation and suction,

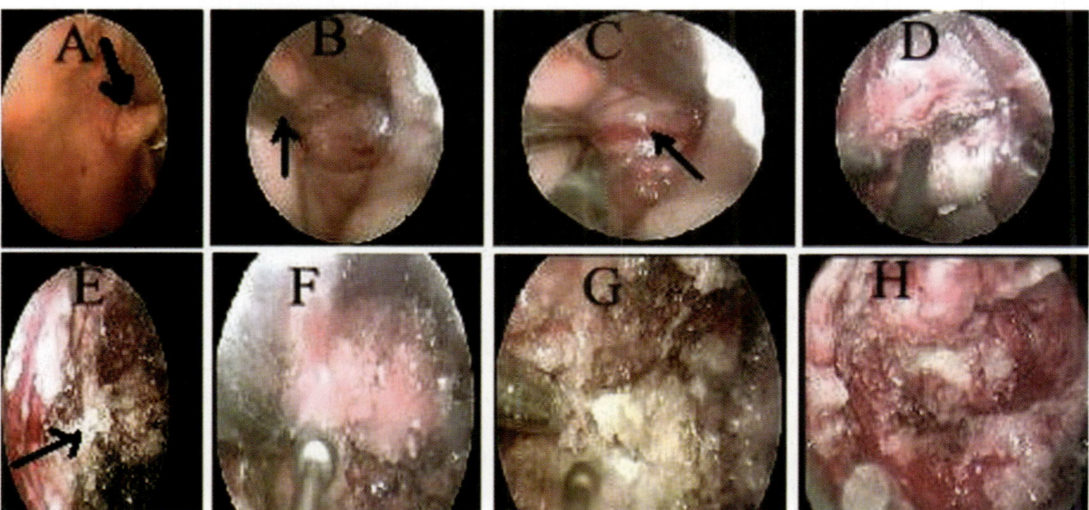

Fig. 4. Various steps of operation. The uvula (arrow in A and B) has been retracted. The posterior pharyngeal wall has been cut (arrow) and dissected (C and D). The anterior arch of atlas (arrow) is seen (E). The anterior arch of atlas and odontoid is being drilled (F and G). The spinal cord is well decompressed after odontoidectomy (H).

leaving an eggshell-thin layer of outer cortical bone. The remaining eggshell-thin bone is removed with either the drill or Kerrison rongeurs. Upward retraction of the odontoid tip toward the clivus is prevented by systematically detaching the odontoid from its associated ligaments before removing the odontoid or its base. After the anterior arch of C1 and the odontoid process are removed, the transverse ligament can be identified. Removal of the transverse ligament, tectorial membrane, and any residual ligaments may be required in some cases. All the compressive pathologies are resected to decompress the underlying cranio-vertebral junction dura mater adequately. If necessary, the inferior clivus is removed with a high-speed drill.

Performing an adequate closure in a deep wound after a transoral operation can be challenging. It can be facilitated using long, thin needle holders with a curved tip and instrument tying techniques (similar to those used in microvascular anastomosis). The wound closure is done in two layers. The muscle layer is approximated in a horizontal mattress with 3-0 vicryl sutures. The mucosal layer is sutured with simple interrupted 3-0 vicryl sutures. Care must be taken not to pull the sutures too tightly to prevent strangulating the delicate mucosal tissues. The mucosal layer incision heals quite rapidly. If the dura mater has been violated, reconstruction of the posterior pharyngeal wall is followed by temporary lumbar drainage to prevent a CSF leak. Autologous fascia lata, fat (harvested from the thigh) and tissue glue are used to repair the dural tear. The dural defect is reconstructed by a piece of fascia lata in an onlay fashion followed by fibrin glue, fat, Surgicel® and additional fibrin glue. Broad-spectrum antibiotic coverage is given for 10 days.

All the instruments are passed by the side of the endoscope. Palatal splitting or a self-retracting retractor was not required in any of our cases. The palate could be further pushed upwards by suction, drill or any other instrument used in dissection. The lower clivus was drilled in 4 patients. Posterior fixation was done in the same sitting after carefully turning the patient on traction. For posterior fixation, stainless steel, contoured rod implants were used in 16 patients because of financial constraints, but in the other 6 titanium implants were used.

We prefer to perform a posterior stabilization immediately after the transoral resection. In most cases, the cranio-vertebral junction becomes unstable after odontoidectomy and removal of ligaments. We usually perform an occipito-cervical stabilization using the occipital ring and autologous bone graft. The patient is positioned prone with the head placed in cervical traction. A cervical collar is used to augment stability while carefully turning the patient. The cranio-vertebral junction is placed in anatomical alignment under fluoroscopic visualization for subsequent stabilization. We perform an occipito-axial fusion; however, only a C1–C2 stabilization can also be done.

In most cases, routine extubation is attempted immediately after surgery, unless there is concern about a difficult airway. Topical corticosteroid is applied to the tongue to minimize postoperative swelling. A nasogastric feeding tube is placed postoperatively. Oral feedings are withheld for 5 days, after which the patient is started on clear fluids and later advanced to a mechanical, soft diet, as tolerated. Postoperatively, CT/MRI is done in all cases (Fig. 5).

Results

During the study period 22 patients, ranging from 15 to 56 years in age (mean 42 years), underwent transoral endoscopic odontoidectomy. Fifteen of the patients were male. The duration of the presenting symptoms ranged from 6 to 18 months (mean 14 months). All patients had quadriparesis at presentation. Three patients also had cranial nerve X paresis. Preoperatively, 17 patients were in Ranawat scale 3A and 5 in Ranawat scale 3B. Indications for surgery included AAD in 14 patients, basilar invasion in 7, and tubercular with retro-

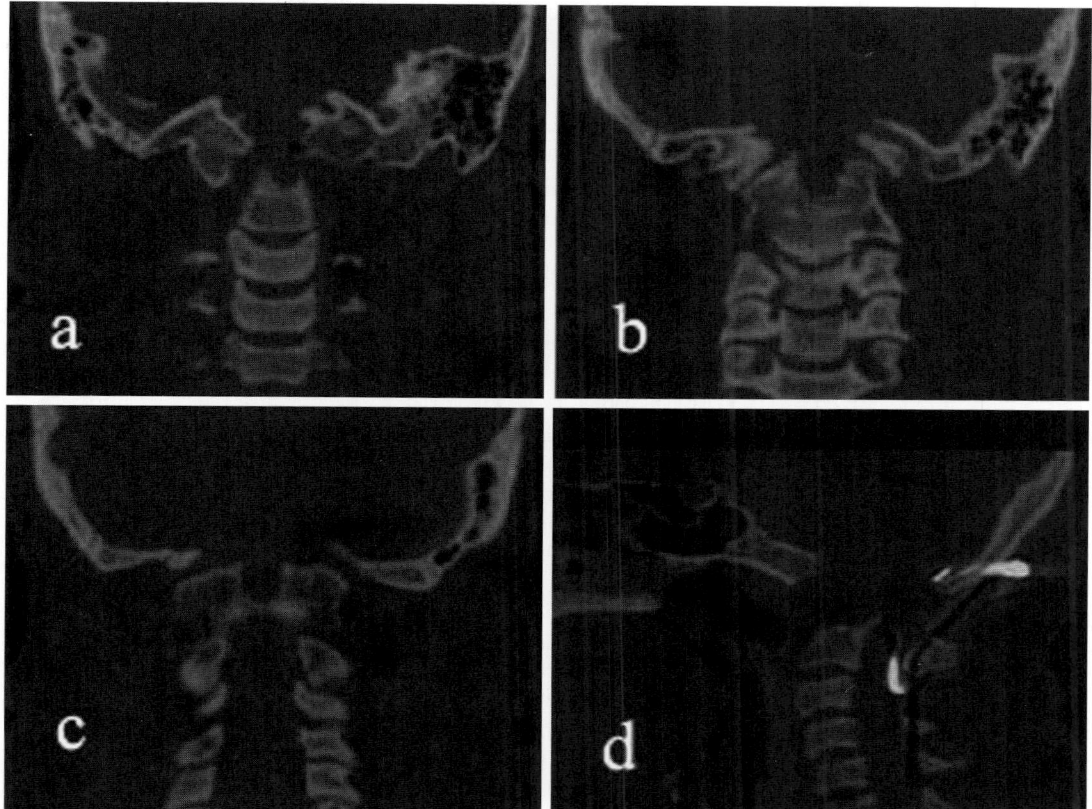

Fig. 5. Postoperative coronal and sagittal CT scans of tubercular atlanto-axial dislocation showing good bony decompression

pharangeal abscess and subluxation in 1 patient. All patients improved after surgery. There were 18 and 4 patients in Ranawat scales 1 and 2, respectively, at a follow up of 1 year. No deaths occurred. One patient had a CSF leak that stopped after external lumber drainage.

Discussion

Results after decompression and stabilization of the cranio-cervical junction depend on the preoperative neurological status of the patient. Our results compare well with other reports. Successful decompression was achieved in all 7 patients by Frempong-Boadu *et al.*[7] No adverse neurological sequelae were noted. One patient died from a peri-operative myocardial infarction. At a mean clinical follow up of 6.16 months, neurological status was noted to be stable or improved in all remaining patients in their series.[7] Husain *et al.* also reported good results after endoscopic transoral excision of the odontoid.[6]

Transoral microscopic excision of the odontoid exposure is generally limited by the extent to which the patient can open his or her mouth (Table 1). The location of the hard palate relative to the cranio-vertebral junction limits superior exposure, whereas the mandible and base of tongue limit the inferior exposure.[2]

The disadvantage is that the extension of these approaches to adjoining areas requires excision of the palate, tongue and mandible. Velopharyngeal

Table 1. Comparison of endoscopic transoral, microscopic and endonasal endoscopic excision of the odontoid process

Endoscopic transoral	Endoscopic endonasal	Microscopic transoral
Advantages		
• This is the most direct minimally invasive technique which is effective and safe. • Palatal splitting or prolonged retraction, required in microsurgical technique, can be avoided. • Another advantage is that it can be done when oral opening is as small as 1.0 cm as compared with at least 2.5–3 cm opening needed for microscopic excision. • Surgery can be done in any neck position (flexion or extension). It gives good exposure from lower clivus to C2–C3 disc space.	• It is a minimally invasive technique. • Feeding can be started early, palatal splitting not required and there is no tongue oedema. • Can be done in patients where mouth opening is <2.5 cm, can be done even with the head immobilized or in a halo jacket. • It can be done in any neck position (flexion or extension). • There is theoretically a reduced risk of infection as the incision in endonasal approach is above oropharynx and the wound is not constantly bathed in saliva.	• Most neurosurgeons are familiar with this approach.
Limitations		
• Water-tight dural closure is difficult. • There is a risk of infection as the operation is done through a contaminated route.	• There is narrow exposure and the lower body of C2 cannot be reliably removed. • Caudal exposure is limited by the nasal bones anteriorly and the hard palate posteriorly. • The line connecting the nasal bones anteriorly and the hard palate posterior is known as the nasopalatine line (NPL). It is very difficult to access the structure inferior to this line which is base of the body of axis. • Water-tight dural closure is difficult.	• Odontoid exposure is generally limited by the extent to which the patient can open mouth. Superior exposure is limited by the location of the hard palate, whereas the mandible and base of the tongue limit the inferior exposure. • Palate need to split especially in basilar invasion resulting in velopharyngeal insufficiency. Palatal dehiscence, upper airway obstruction, ischaemic necrosis of the tongue, swallowing difficulties, and meningitis could be other complications. • Another limitation of this procedure is that at least 2.5–3 cm opening is needed.

insufficiency is a recognized complication in up to 50% of patients in the immediate postoperative period. Other potential complications include palatal dehiscence, upper airway obstruction, ischaemic necrosis of the tongue, swallowing difficulties, and meningitis. Another limitation of this procedure is that at least a 2.5–3 cm opening is needed for microscopic excision of the odontoid.

The endoscopic transnasal approach is also minimally invasive. Messina *et al.* using fresh cadaver heads to study access to the craniovertebral junction found that this was possible by endoscope, using a lower trajectory, when compared with that necessary for the sellar region.[3] Leng *et al.* treated one patient by an endonasal endoscopic approach to the cervicomedullary junction; they suggested this minimally invasive technique as an alternative for anterior decompression of irreducible cervicomedullary junction pathology and found it to be effective.[4] Feeding is initiated early, palatal splitting is not required, tongue oedema is absent, and this approach can be used in patients in whom the mouth opening is <2.5 cm—a requirement for transoral excision. This approach can be performed even with the head immobilized or in a halo jacket, or with the neck in any position (flexion or extension). Another advantage is that the incision in the endonasal approach is above the oropharynx; this may theoretically reduce the risk of infection, as the wound is not constantly bathed in saliva. Nayak *et al.*, however, reported good results with no peri-operative complications with transnasal endoscopic odontoidectomy in rheumatoid disease.[13] Water-tight closure of wound is difficult, especially in intradural surgeries. Limitations of this procedure are a narrow exposure and unreliability in removing the lower body of C2.[14] Caudal exposure is limited by the nasal bones anteriorly and the hard palate posteriorly. The line connecting the nasal bones anteriorly and the hard palate posteriorly is known as the nasopalatine line (Fig. 6). It is very difficult to access the structure inferior to this line, which is the base of the body of axis.

Endoscopic transoral excision of the odontoid process has been found to be direct, effective and safe. Palatal splitting or prolonged retraction, required in the microsurgical technique, can be avoided in this minimally invasive technique of endoscopic transoral excision of the odontoid.[5–7,15] Other advantages of this procedure are that it can be done when the oral opening is as small as 1.5 cm, compared with the 2.5–3 cm opening needed for microscopic excision. Furthermore, surgery can be done in any neck position (flexion or extension). The procedure gives good exposure from the lower clivus to C2–C3 disc space. Nevertheless, many difficulties and complications are encountered, such as the risk of contamination by bacterial flora, difficulties in closing the dura mater, and early oral feeding. We encountered one complication of a CSF leak in

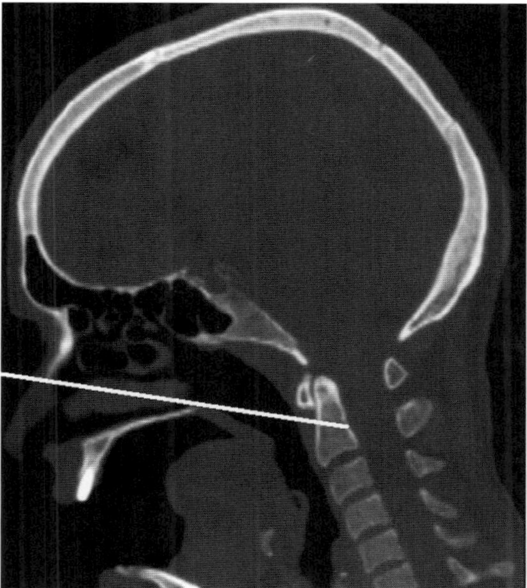

Fig. 6. Nasopalatine line showing inferior limit of exposure. It is difficult to excise the inferior part of C2 body in endonasal odontoidectomy

this study, which could have been avoided. Such problems should be anticipated and prevented, esspecially when the dens is dislocated too much and the dura protrudes between the tip of the dens and the lower end of the clivus.

Pillai *et al.* examined four cadaveric specimens to compare the surgical working area and surgical freedom associated with an endoscopic and a microscopic approach to the ventral cranio-vertebral junction.[5] The exposure of the clivus provided by the endoscope and by the operating microscope without splitting the soft palate was also measured and compared between the specimens. They found that the surgical area exposed over the posterior pharyngeal wall was significantly improved using the endoscope (606.5 ± 127.4 mm^3) compared with the operating microscope (425.7 ± 100.8 mm^3), without any compromise of surgical freedom ($p < 0.05$). The extent of the clivus exposed with the endoscope (9.5 ± 0.7 mm) without splitting the soft palate was significantly improved compared with that associated with the microscopic approach ($2.0 \pm$

0.4 mm) (p<0.05). They concluded that the endoscope aided the approach to the ventral cranio-vertebral junction transorally, with minimal tissue dissection, no palatal splitting, and no compromise of surgical freedom.[5] In addition, the use of an angled-lens endoscope can significantly improve the exposure of the clivus without splitting the soft palate. Husain *et al.* also managed 11 patients of irreducible osseous dislocations with cranio-vertebral junction abnormality by a transoral endoscopic approach; good decompression was achieved in all patients.[6] Frempong-Boadu *et al.* concluded that the endoscopically assisted transoral surgery represents an emerging alternative to standard microsurgical techniques for transoral approaches to the anterior cervico-medullary junction, which provides a safe method for anterior decompression without the need for extensive soft palate splitting, hard palate resection, or extended maxillotomy.[7] Lee *et al.* also opined that the management of benign disease via endoscopic methods is largely accepted now, but more data are needed before the controversy on the role of endoscopic management of malignant disease of the cranio-vetebrae is decided.[15]

Wu *et al.* performed an anterior release with microendoscopic technique.[8] Anterior transarticular screw fixation and grafting using morselized autologous bone grafts was used after reduction. Percutaneous microendoscopic anterior release, transarticular (C1–C2) fixation and bone graft fusion has been described by Chi *et al.*[16]

The transcervical approach accesses the odontoid for resection from the body of C2 to the lip of the basion. The angles of attack in the transcervical approach when centred on the surgical target are limited, but this approach offers a clean, sterile operative field.[17] A comparison of endonasal, transoral, and transcervical approaches concluded that the endonasal and transoral approaches allow wider exposure with larger working angles to the cranio-cervical junction.[18] Clinical investigations are required to determine the optimal indications for each approach.

Conclusion

Endoscopic transoral odontoidectomy is a direct minimally invasive technique that is safe and effective in the surgical management of irreducible AAD and basilar invagination. Angled scopes improve exposure of the clivus. With this technique palatal splitting is not required even in basilar invasion.

References

1. Narayan P, Rodts GE, Haid RW. C1–C2 Brooks fusion. In: Fessler RG, Sekhar LN (eds). *Atlas of neurosurgical techniques: Spine and peripheral nerves.* New York, NY: Thieme; 2006:139–52.
2. Liu JK, Couldwell WT, Apfelbaum RI. Transoral approach and extended modifications for lesions of the ventral foramen magnum and craniovertebral junction. *Skull Base* 2008;**18**:151–66.
3. Messina A, Bruno MC, Decq P, *et al.* Pure endoscopic endonasal odontoidectomy: Anatomical study. *Neurosurg Rev* 2007;**30**:189–94; discussion 94.
4. Leng LZ, Anand VK, Hartl R, *et al.* Endonasal endoscopic resection of an os odontoideum to decompress the cervicomedullary junction: A minimal access surgical technique. *Spine (Phila Pa 1976)* 2009;**34**:E139–E143.
5. Pillai P, Baig MN, Karas CS, Ammirati M. Endoscopic image-guided transoral approach to the craniovertebral junction: An anatomic study comparing surgical exposure and surgical freedom obtained with the endoscope and the operating microscope. *Neurosurgery* 2009;**64** (Suppl 2):437–42; discussion 42–4.
6. Husain M, Rastogi M, Ojha BK, *et al.* Endoscopic transoral surgery for craniovertebral junction anomalies. Technical note. *J Neurosurg Spine* 2006;**5**:367–73.
7. Frempong-Boadu AK, Faunce WA, Fessler RG. Endoscopically assisted transoral-transpharyngeal approach to the craniovertebral junction. *Neurosurgery* 2002;**51**(5 Suppl):S60–S66.
8. Wu YS, Chi YL, Wang XY, *et al.* Microendoscopic anterior approach for irreducible atlantoaxial dislocation: Surgical techniques and preliminary results. *J Spinal Disord Tech* 2010;**23**:113–20.

9. Ranawat CS, O'Leary P, Pellicci P, *et al.* Cervical spine fusion in rheumatoid arthritis. *J Bone Joint Surg Am* 1979;**61**:1003–10.

10. Di Lorenzo N. Craniocervical junction malformation treated by transoral approach. A survey of 25 cases with emphasis on postoperative instability and outcome. *Acta Neurochir (Wien)* 1992;**118**:112–16.

11. Frankel HL, Hancock DO, Hyslop G, *et al.* The value of postural reduction in the initial management of closed injuries of the spine with paraplegia and tetraplegia. *I Paraplegia* 1969;**7**:179–92.

12. Hukuda S, Mochizuki T, Ogata M, *et al.* Operations for cervical spondylotic myelopathy. A comparison of the results of anterior and posterior procedures. *J Bone Joint Surg Br* 1985;**67**:609–15.

13. Nayak JV, Gardner PA, Vescan AD, *et al.* Experience with the expanded endonasal approach for resection of the odontoid process in rheumatoid disease. *Am J Rhinol* 2007;**21**:601–6.

14. de Almeida JR, Zanation AM, Snyderman CH, *et al.* Defining the nasopalatine line: The limit for endonasal surgery of the spine. *Laryngoscope* 2009; **119**: 239–44.

15. Lee SC, Senior BA. Endoscopic skull base surgery. -*Clin Exp Otorhinolaryngol* 2008;**1**:53–62.

16. Chi YL, Xu HZ, Lin Y, *et al.* Percutaneous micro-endoscopic anterior release, fixation and fusion for irreducible atlanto-axial dislocation. *Zhonghua Wai Ke Za Zhi* 2007;**45**:383–6.

17. Wolinsky JP, Sciubba DM, Suk I, *et al.* Endoscopic image-guided odontoidectomy for decompression of basilar invagination via a standard anterior cervical approach. Technical note. *J Neurosurg Spine* 2007;**6**: 184–91.

18. Baird CJ, Conway JE, Sciubba DM, *et al.* Radiographic and anatomic basis of endoscopic anterior craniocervical decompression: A comparison of endonasal, transoral, and transcervical approaches. *Neurosurgery* 2009;**65** (6 Suppl):158–63; discussion 63–4.

14

A comparative outcome analysis of 3-dimensional (3D) and 2-dimensional (2D) endoscopic trans-sphenoidal surgery in the treatment of pituitary adenomas in a series of 115 patients*

VLADIMIR DADASHEV, ELINA KARI, SARAH WISE, ADRIANA IOACHIMESCU, NELSON OYESIKU

ABSTRACT

Introduction: Two-dimensional (2D) endoscopes are limited by poor depth perception, lack of stereoscopic vision, and image distortion. Recently, a new 3-dimensional (3D) endoscopic system that provides improved stereoscopic vision has been developed. No data exist comparing the results and outcomes of 2D vs 3D endoscopy in treatment of a large cohort of pituitary adenoma patients. We compared the results of transnasal endoscopic pituitary surgery using the 2D and 3D endoscopy systems.

Methods: A total of 115 patients underwent endoscopic transnasal trans-sphenoidal pituitary adenomectomy at Emory University Hospital. In all cases, pituitary tumour resection was performed by a single neurosurgeon (NMO). The endoscopic transnasal approach and closure was performed by the otolaryngology service. The 3D endoscopic system was used for pituitary adenomectomy in 72 patients (63%), and the 2D system was used in 43 patients (37%) over a 2-year period. A retrospective analysis included preoperative, perioperative and postoperative metrics. The statistical comparison was completed using t-test and chi-square test.

Results: The preoperative data for the two groups (3D vs 2D) are presented: the average age 49.5 vs 45.9 years, tumour size (all tumours) 6.9 vs 5.8 cm^3, and tumour size (macroadenomas) (94/115) 8.3 vs 7.1 cm^3. The perioperative data (3D vs 2D) include: median operative time 145 vs 168 minutes, EBL 200 vs 200 ml, LD placement 35/72 (49%) vs 21/43 (49%). The

---

* A complete version of this paper has been submitted for publication to the journal *Neurosurgery.*

postoperative data (3D vs 2D) include: hospital stay 5 vs 5 days, endocrine complications 7/72 (10%) vs 5/43 (12%), CSF leak rate 5/72 (7%) vs 4/43 (9%), remission for functioning tumours was 20/30 (67%) vs 12/21 (57%), re-admission rate 15/72 (21%) vs 10/43 (23%), re-operation rate for all 4/72 (6%) vs 8/43 (19%), and trans-sphenoidal CSF leak repair 0/72 (0%) vs 3/43 (7%). The re-operation rate and the CSF leak repair rate were statistically different (p<0.03, chi-square). The other parameters were not statistically different.

Conclusions: Three-dimensional endoscopy improves the depth of field and provides stereoscopic vision. This improvement resulted in a statistically significant decrease in overall re-operation and CSF leak repair rate in our series.

TECHNICAL DETAILS

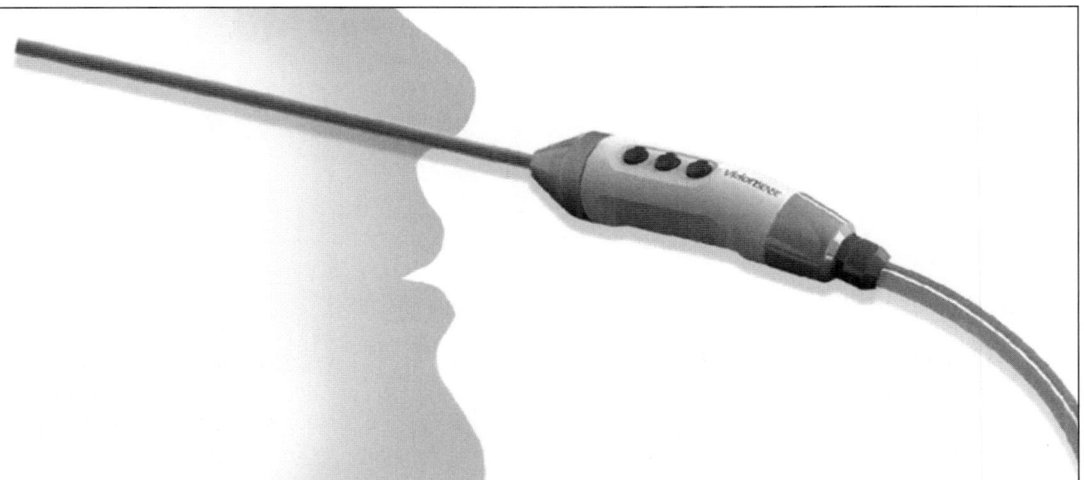

Fig. 1. The 2D system used was the Storz endoscope system (Karl Storz GmbH and Co. KG, Tuttlingen, Germany) with both straight 0° and angled (30° and 45°) endoscopes. The endoscopes used were 30 cm in length and 4 mm in diameter. The 3D system used was the newly designed single chip stereoscopic camera endoscope (Visionsense Corp., Orangeburg NY). The camera divides the input into left and right images (inter-pupillary distance 0.8 mm, *see* Fig. 2). The dual aperture generates two slightly offset images in a single device (at the tip of the scope) and is essential in recreating a stereoscopic image (binocular vision). The light from each aperture then passes through a single lens, with a large spread function. The light next passes through an array of micro-lenses that each focus on the sensors and the light is digitized. The processed stereoscopic image is reconstructed. The endoscope diameter is 4.9 mm and the lengths come as 20 cm or 30 cm with the viewing angle or 0° and 30°. The surgeon must wear polarized 3D lenses to view the images on a video screen intraoperatively (*see* Fig. 2).

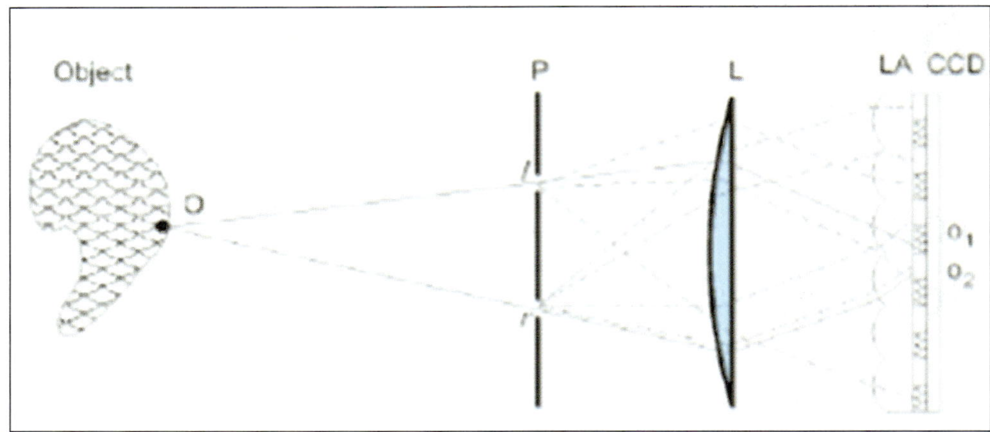

Fig. 2. Visionsense camera scheme: Light enters into a focal plane P dual aperture plane, followed by a lens (L) and microarray.

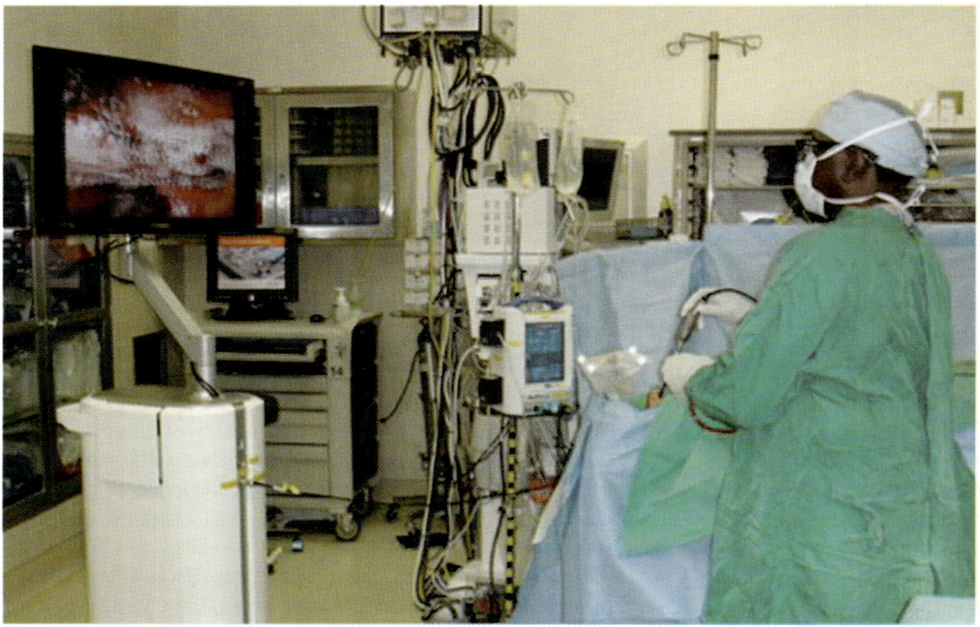

Fig. 3. The senior surgeon (Dr Nelson Oyesiku) is using 3D endoscope for a pituitary adenoma resection. The scope cable is a small diameter (as light gets digitized by the scope microchip) and no light source is needed. The surgeon is also wearing 3D glasses.

15

Percutaneous transforaminal endoscopic discectomy

SUSHIL PATKAR

Relief of severe back and radicular pain continues to remain as the main indication of surgery in prolapsed lumbar intervertebral disc (PVD).

Progress of surgical treatment lies in its self annihilation. Surgeons continuously struggle to find a less invasive solution to a given surgical problem till ultimately they succeed in a non-surgical solution for a given surgical problem. Lumbar disc surgery since the original description by Mixter and Barr has also seen the same course from wide laminectomy to hemilaminectomy to fenestration and finally microlumbar discectomy. All the procedures attempt to decrease the surgical wound, hasten the postoperative convalescence, reduce complications and minimize recurrence.

Cochrane review 2007 showed at the end of 4 years no benefit between surgical and medical management of lumbar PVDs for pain relief. Cochrane review 2009 concluded that surgical treatment can hasten pain relief and return to productive life. Also long-term reviews of results of disc surgery always show a considerable baggage of back pain old and new. Various theories from biomechanical micro-instability and surgical scar have been incriminated.

Endoscopic discectomy has been attempted since 1975, but MRI, new research and better instrumentation has renewed a paradigm shift in understanding and treating lumbar PVD.

New concepts

- MRI examination revealed no correlation between size of prolapse and severity of pain. Thus compression of the root is not the only cause of pain in acute PVD, a new chemical theory of root inflammarion secondary to exposure of the root to degenerated neucleus pulposus has been widely accepted.
- Provocative discography is a good test to identify the culprit disc, especially when the MRI of a patient shows more than one PVD.
- Endoscopic discectomy is performed under local anaesthesia, thus giving the surgeon a chance to identify the pain-producing structures, confirm pain relief during surgery, avoid root injury under vision and avoid general anaesthesia, all through a small port of 7 mm.
- A safe zone exists between the exiting root and traversing root known as the triangle of Pervez Kambin through which most disc prolapses can be accessed.

Indications

- Unilateral contained disc prolapse
- Leg pain more than backache
- Nucleosus in continuity with the prolapsed component
- Minor neurological deficit

Of course, after completion of an adequate trial of conservative treatment

Contraindications

- Sequestrated migrated disc prolapse
- Canal stenosis
- Calcified disc
- Osteophyte pressing the root
- Cauda equina syndrome
- Instability

Operative technique

Operation is performed under local anaesthesia in the standard prone position over bolsters with a radiolucent table top.

'C' arm guidance is used throughout the operation and therefore protective lead apron and thyroid cover has to be used by the theatre personnel (prone position).

Mild sedation and analgesia

Continuous dialogue with an awake patient is mandatory to identify and remove the offending pathology.

Marking entry point

- Draw midline AB along spinous processes with the pedicles equidistant to the midline.
- Identify disc in antereo-posterior plane with end plates parallel to the floor and draw horizontal line CD perpendicular to AB
- In lateral image identify centre of disc and measure up to CD distance-X
- On the line CD mark distance X from midline on the side of pain, this is the 'entry point' (Figs 1–5).
- Infiltrate local anaesthetic with adrenaline with a long no. 18 G needle at 45° to the surface at the 'entry point', advance the needle till posterior vertebral body line (lateral view)

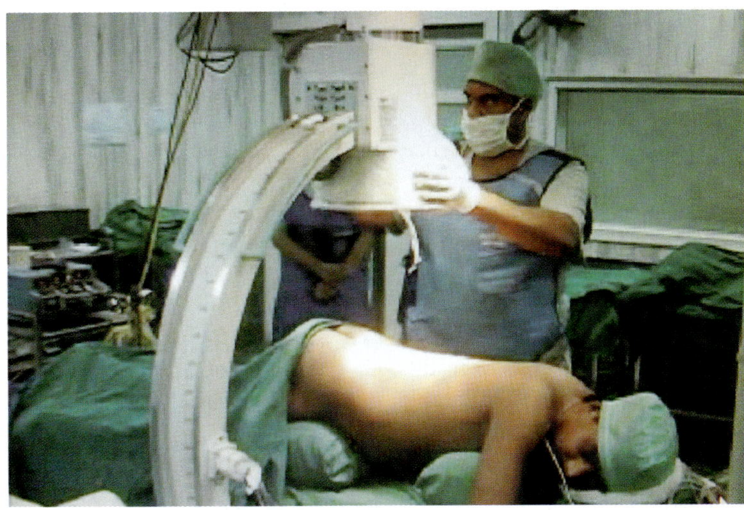

Fig. 1. Entry point marked under C arm

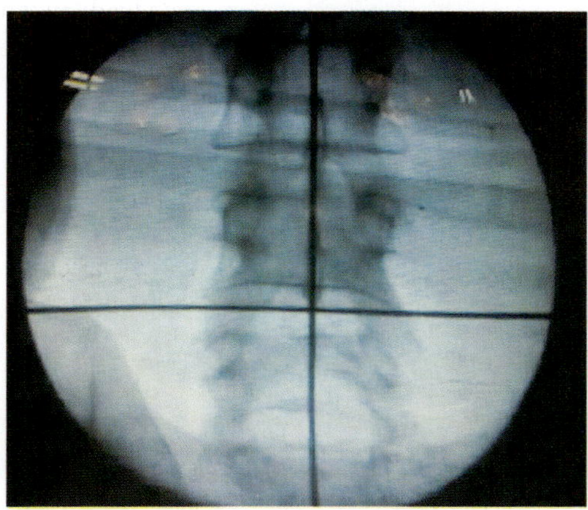

Fig. 2. Marking disc centre

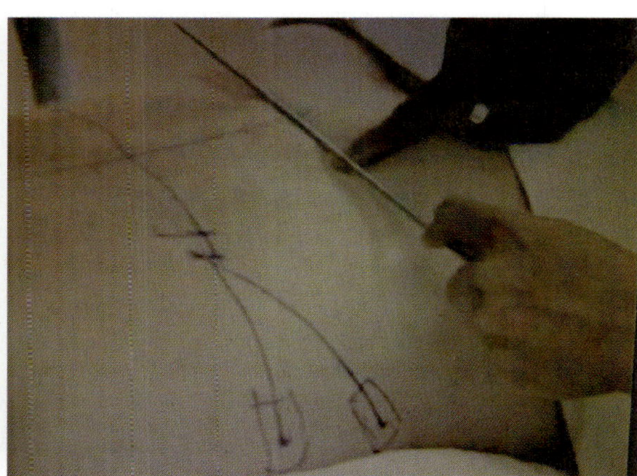

Fig. 3. Yeung A—technique of marking the entry point

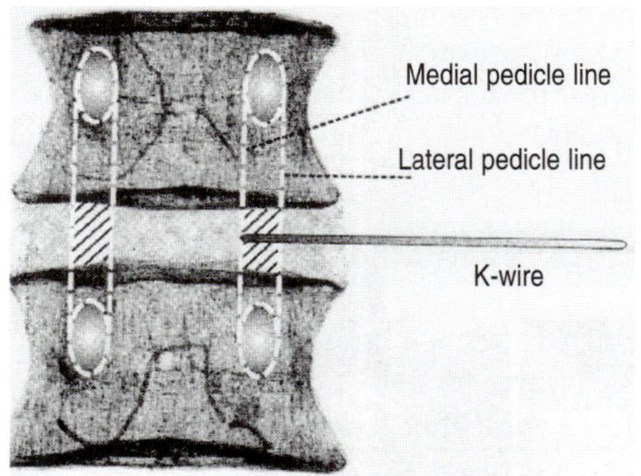

Fig. 4. Identifying the pedicular lines

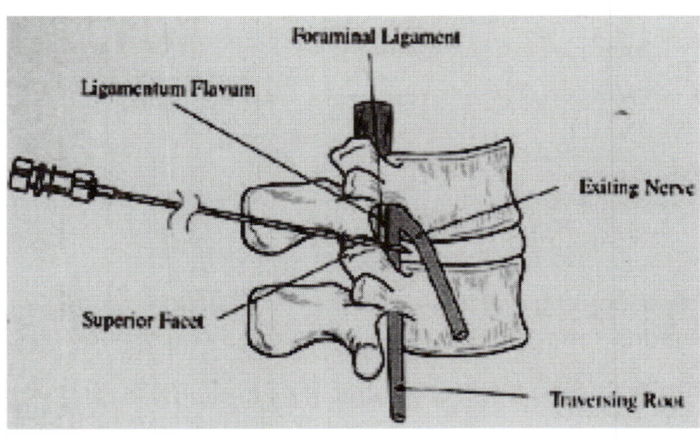

Fig. 5 Safe zone for entry into the disc

and lateral to the medial pedicular line (antereo-posterior view).

- Watch for radicular symptoms while advancing the needle and reposition if required.
- Advance the needle into the fdisc always remaining lateral to medial pedicular line on the antereo-posterior image
- Perform epidurogram in the safe zone (2 cc of omnipaque with saline) (Fig. 6)
- Advance needle into the disc while remaining lateral to the medial pedicular line. Once in the disc centre perform discogram (2–3 cc of omnipaque with saline), provocative pain confirms the offending disc (Fig. 7).
- Pass a guide-wire through the needle and

remove the needle
- Insert dilator over the wire after making a small stab incison
- With twisting movements advance the dilator to the annulus

Inject local anaesthetic through the dilator for the annulus.

Pass the beveled operating sheath over the dilator (bevel facing dorsally) and tap it into the annulus (Figs 8–10).

Remove dilator and pass trephine to cut window into the annulus Fig. 11.

Pass the disc scope (length 20 cm; outer diameter 6.5 mm; operating channel 3.7 mm with irrigation and suction channels) through

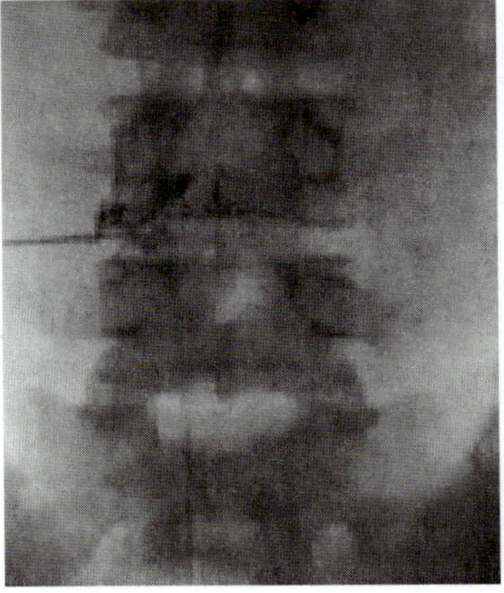

Fig. 6. Epidurogram of the exiting root

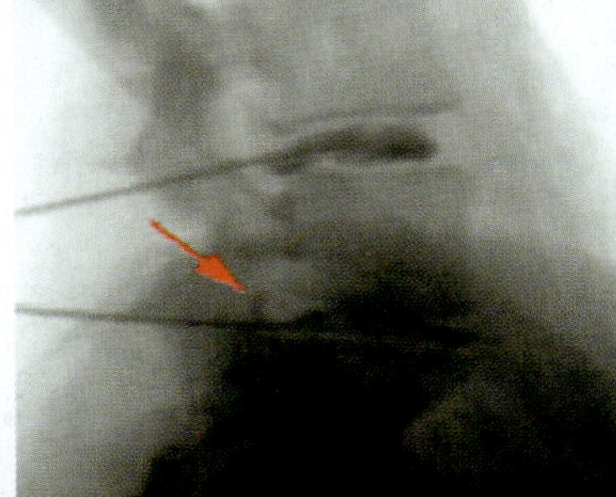

Fig. 7. Discogram

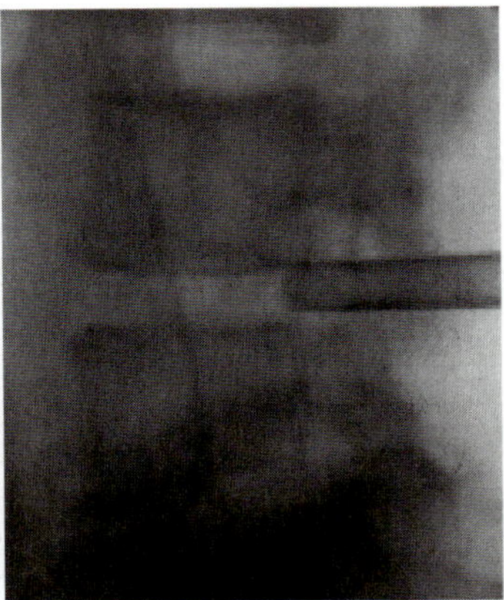

Fig. 9. Position of sheath—lateral view

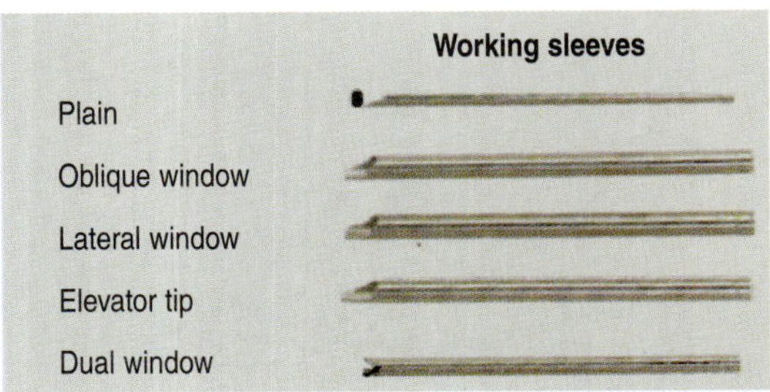

Fig. 8. Operating sheaths—length 7.5 cm, outer diameter 7.5 mm through which the endoscope is passed

the sheath and start high flow irrigation (1 L cold saline with 1 g chloramphenicol).

Tilt scope dorsally and decompress nuclear material from within the disc towards the dorsally situated dural tube (Figs 12–14).

End-point of decompression

- Identification of annular defect and impulse on coughing through the defect
- Sudden relief of the patient when the offending fragment is removed
- Identifying dural pulsations through the defect.

End of procedure

- After removing the scope inject 40 mg of methylprednisone through the sheath before removing
- Two skin sutures at entry point
- Bed rest for 6 hours, antibiotics and analgesics for 2 days

Postoperative management

- Mobilzed after 6–8 hours
- Rest at home for 3–6 day
- Resume work after 1 week
- Sports after 3 weeks

Complications

- Discitis 1%–1.5%
- Dural tears and CSF leak 1%–3%
- Nerve root injury 3%–5%
- Dysesthesia 8%–10%
- Psoas haematoma 1%
- Residual disc 15%–20%

Personal series

- 96 patients
- M 50 years, F 46 years (18–56 years)
- Good and excellent results in 80% (89/96)
- 2 conversion to open

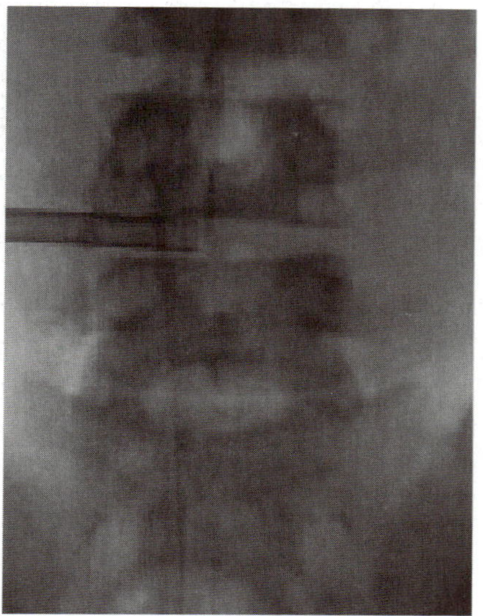

Fig. 10. Position of sheath—antereo-posterior view

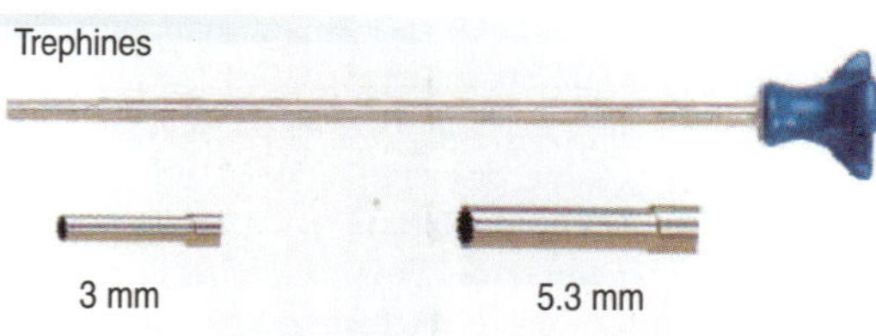

Fig. 11. Trephine which is passed through the operating sheath to cut a window into the annulus at the safe zone

Fig. 12. Spine endoscope (length 20 cm; outer diameter 6.5 mm; operating channel 3.7 mm)

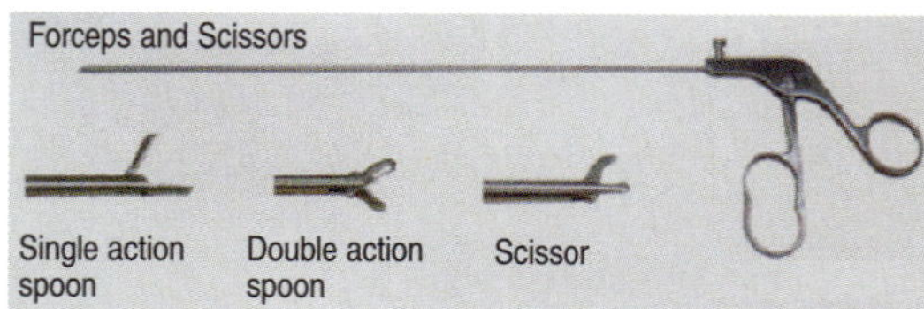

Fig. 13. Instruments used through the operating channel (length: 250 mm to 300 mm, diameter 3.5 mm)

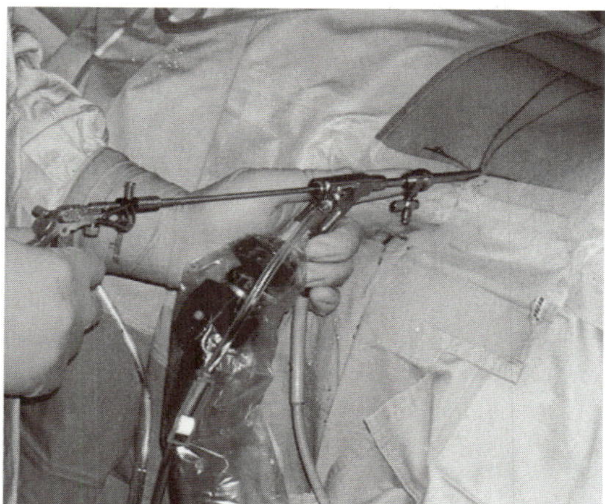

Fig. 14. Discectomy through endoscope

- 1 re-surgery
- No deficits, no CSF leaks
- 6 patients postoperative radicular dysesthesia

Excellent—complete relief, Good—some pain but back to work without medication.

Conclusion

Microlumbar discectomy remains the gold standard of surgical treatment in a given case of lumbar PVD that requires surgery.

Percutaneous transforaminal endoscopic discectomy is a therapeutic option between open surgery and conservative management. The procedure is performed under local anaesthesia providing an opportunity to remove only that which is offending and confirming pain relief on

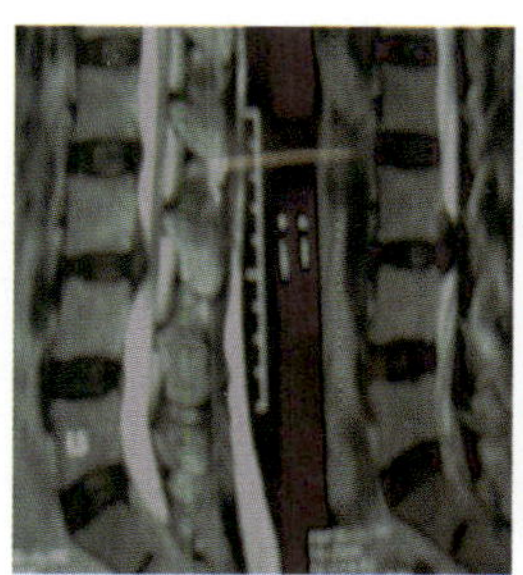

Fig. 15. Preoperative MRI

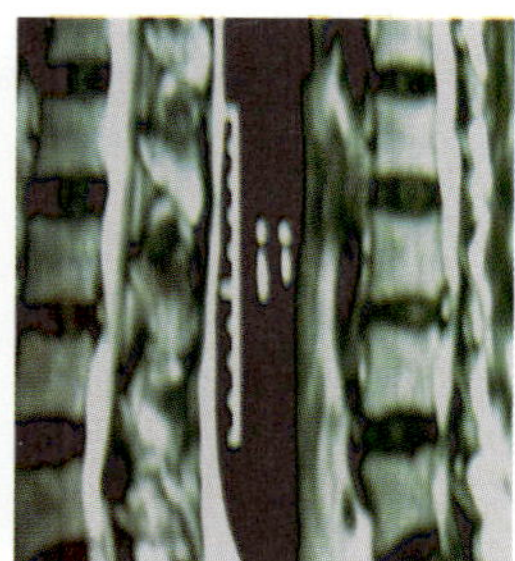

Fig. 16. Postoperative MRI

operation table in addition to being minimally invasive and avoiding the access-related problems of open surgery. There is no doubt that lesser disc tissue is removed, thus inviting an increased recurrence rate but this is traded off with faster recovery, no added back pain and preserved spinal biomechanics. With improvements in equipment (lasers, radiofrequency and endoscopic drills) surgical outcomes will improve and this procedure will eventually become a standard of care.

Suggested reading

1. Boden SD, Davis DO, Dina TS, *et al.* Abnormal magnetic-resonance scans of the lumbar spine in asymptomatic subjects. A prospective investigation. *J Bone Joint Surg [Am]* 1990;**72**:403–8.

2. Boos N, Rieder R, Schade V, *et al.* 1995 Volvo Award in clinical sciences. The diagnostic accuracy of magnetic resonance imaging, work perception, and psychosocial factors in identifying symptomatic disc herniations. *Spine* 1995;**20**:2613–25.

3. Kambin P. Arthroscopic and Endoscopic Micro-diskectomy via Posterolateral access. In: Fessler RG, Sekhar L (eds). *Atlas of neurosurgical techniques spine and peripheral nerves.* NY: Thieme Medical Publishers; 2006:816–25.

4. Kambin P. History of minimally invasive spine surgery: Emerging spine surgery technologies. In: Corbin TP, Connolly PJ, Yuan HA, *et al.* (eds). *Evidence and framework for evaluating new technology.* St. Louis, MO: Quality Medical Publishing, Inc; 2006;263–71.

5. Mayer HM, Brock M. Percutaneous endoscopic discectomy: Surgical technique and preliminary results compared to microsurgical discectomy. *J Neurosurg* 1993;**78**:216–25.

6. Onik G, Helms G. Percutaneous lateral discectomy using a new aspiration probe. *AJNR Am J Neuroradiol* 1985;**6**:290.

7. Yeung AT, Tsou PM. Posterolateral endoscopic excision of lumbar disc herniation: Surgical technique, outcome, and complications in 307 consecutive cases. *Spine* 2002;**27**:722–31.

8. Bernard TN Jr. Lumbar discography followed by computed tomography. Refining the diagnosis of low-back pain. *Spine* 1990;**15**:690–7.

9. Bogduk N, Tynan W, Wilson AS. The nerve supply to the human lumbar intervertebral discs. *J Anat* 1981;**132**:39–56.

10. Buirski G, Silberstein M. The symptomatic lumbar disc in patients with low-back pain. Magnetic resonance imaging appearances in both a symptomatic and control population. *Spine* 1993;**18**:1808–11.

11. Ruetten S, Komp M, Merk H, *et al.* Full-endoscopic interlaminar and transforaminal lumbar discectomy versus conventional microsurgical technique: A prospective, randomized, controlled study. *Spine (Phila Pa 1976)* 2008;**33**:931–9.

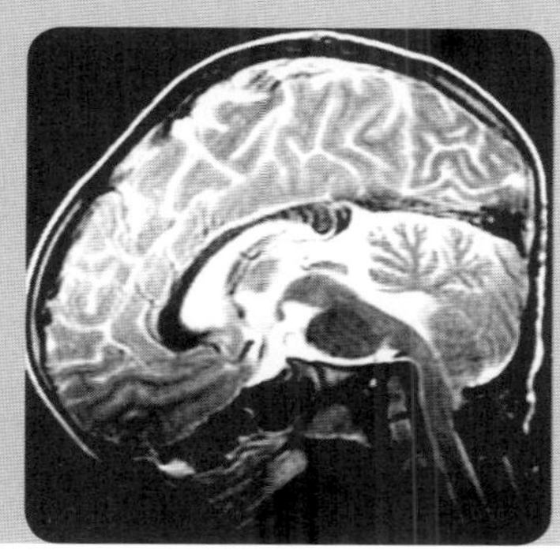

Spinal surgery

16

The trans-spinous mini-open approach for resection of intradural spinal neoplasms: Cadaveric feasibility study and report of 3 clinical cases

DANIEL C. LU, SANJAY S. DHALL, PRAVEEN V. MUMMANENI

ABSTRACT

Study design: Cadaveric feasibility study and clinical case reports

Objective: To demonstrate the feasibility and initial clinical experience with a new minimally invasive approach for resection of intradural tumours.

Summary of background data: Standard approaches to thoracic intradural tumours often involve a large incision and significant tissue destruction. Minimally invasive techniques have been applied successfully for a variety of surgical decompression procedures, but have rarely been used for the removal of intradural thoracic tumours.

Methods: Initially, 12 procedures were performed on six cadavers to determine the feasibility of the trans-spinous mini-open approach (using an expandable tubular retractor), and to compare this approach to a standard open approach. We noted the body mass index (BMI) of all specimens. Measurements were taken to compare the mini-open approach with the open approach in terms of the number of laminae accessed and the length of the incision. Subsequently, the trans-spinous mini-open approach was used to biopsy one clinical case of intradural, intramedullary tumour (glioblastoma multiforme), and to remove two intradural, extramedullary tumours (meningiomas) in 2 other patients.

Results: The BMI of the cadavers ranged from 18–43. Regardless of the BMI, we found that we could perform up to 3-level laminectomies in all the 6 cadavers via a mini-open approach. In specimens with a BMI of <22, an additional half-level was accessed. The incision length did not exceed 4.5 cm in all cadavers undergoing the mini-open approach. In the same cadavers, we found that with the standard open approach, the incision length increased with increasing BMI, from 8.0 cm to 15 cm. The three clinical cases were performed successfully through a mini-open trans-spinous approach without any complications. The mean operative time was 3½ hours (range 3–4 hours). The mean blood loss was 133 cc (range 100–150 cc). The mean hospital stay was 5½ days (range 4–7 days).

Conclusions: The mini-open approach allows complete dorsal access to the spinal canal with less tissue disruption than with a standard open procedure. This is especially true in obese patients in whom the incision length may be three times smaller compared with a standard open approach. The mini-open trans-spinous resection of thoracic intradural tumours can be performed safely.

Introduction

Surgical access and resection of intradural thoracic tumours typically requires a long midline incision (two levels rostral and caudal to the involved pathology), muscle dissection, removal of posterior spinal elements, and partial facetectomy. This approach allows for a large exposure of the dorsal surface of the spinal cord and has demonstrated safety and efficacy in resection of intradural tumours.[1–4] However, traditional open approaches are associated with significant tissue trauma and allow a large space for the accumulation of a pseudomeningocele.

In this chapter, we propose a new mini-open approach to access intradural spinal pathology by using an expandable, tubular retractor. We first performed an anatomical feasibility cadaveric study of this mini-open midline trans-spinous process approach, and we subsequently used it to access tumours in 3 patients.

Materials and methods

Cadaveric study design

Twelve procedures were performed on 6 fresh cadavers. For the cadaveric study, a mid-line trans-spinous approach using a minimally invasive, expandable retractor (Pipeline, DePuy Spine, Raynham, MA, USA) was performed in the mid-thoracic spine of the cadavers. Measurements were taken of the length of incision; the number of laminae that were accessible through the retractor was noted. Next, the procedure was converted in all 6 cadavers to a standard open approach utilizing standard retractors. This conversion typically required an extension of the incision to 2 levels above and below the region of interest. Final measurements of the incision length were made. The cadaveric BMI was assessed.

Surgical technique

Under fluoroscopic guidance, a 3–4 cm long incision was made in the midline. The bovie was used to dissect the paraspinal muscle off of the base of the spinous process. The muscle was not dissected free from the lamina. The spinous processes were then amputated at their base with a rongeur. Serial muscle dilatation was performed in the midline with dilatation tubes (Fig. 1) and the pipeline expandable retractor was placed in the midline over the remaining base of the spinous process. The tube was then expanded and fixed to the operating table. With the use of the expandable retractor, minimal tissue dissection was necessary and the muscle attachments were not removed from the lateral lamina or facets (Fig. 2). A high-speed drill was used to perform a bilateral laminectomy to expose the dorsal aspect of the spinal cord. The facet joints were left completely intact. Undercutting of the lateral ledges of the lamina with 2 mm rongeurs allowed for a near pedicle-to-pedicle exposure of the entire dorsal spinal cord with minimal tissue disruption. A midline

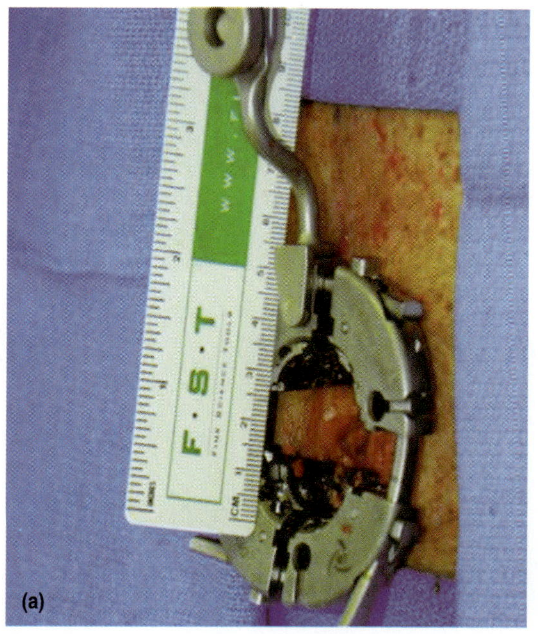

(a)

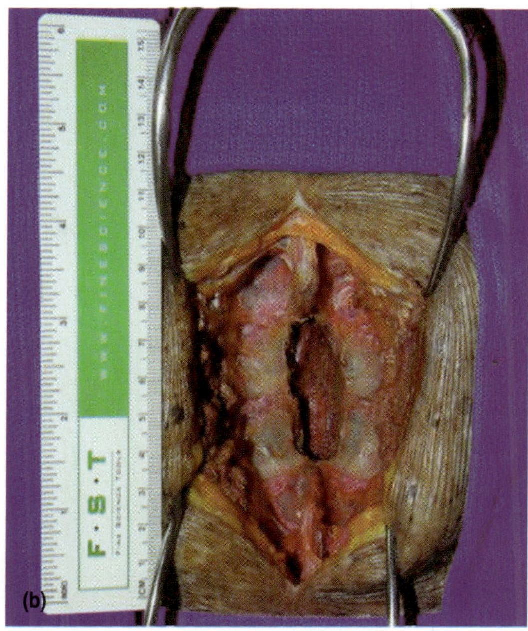

(b)

Fig. 1. Cadaveric study of minimally invasive trans-spinous approach. **(a)** A 4.5 cm midline incision is needed to place an expandable tubular retractor (Pipeline, DePuy Spine, Raynham MA, USA) which allows access to up to 3 levels of thoracic lamina. **(b)** A traditional open approach requires approximately an 8 cm incision to access the same three lamina.

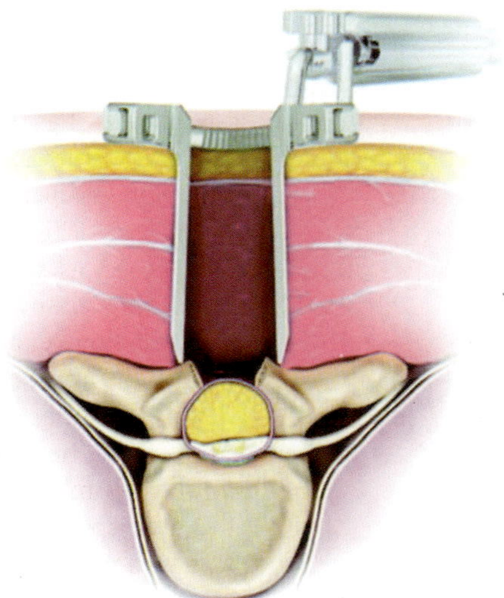

Fig. 2. Illustration of the mini-open approach. Artist s illustration of an axial view of an intradural thoracic meningioma accessed via a midline, trans-spinous, mini-open approach with an expandable tubular retractor. The surgeon s visualization of the dorsal tumour is complete with a pedicle-to-pedicle view.

incision of the dura was performed and the dural edges were retracted with sutures. Intradural tumour biopsy and/or removal were then accomplished with standard microsurgical techniques.

Clinical cases

Case 1

A 46-year-old woman with a history of Hodgkin lymphoma diagnosed and treated with thoracic radiation 20 years previously, developed back pain, leg weakness, and bowel and bladder incontinence. On examination, the patient was functionally paraplegic with a T4 sensory level (ASIA B). Magnetic resonance imaging (MRI) revealed a large enhancing lesion in the thoracic spinal cord extending from T2 to T10. A T5–T6 mini-open trans-spinous biopsy with partial resection of the tumour was performed. We did not attempt a gross total removal of this lesion, which spanned 8 segments. Pathology revealed glioblastoma multiforme. At 1-year follow up, the patient's neurological examination was unchanged (ASIA B).

Case 2

A 40-year-old woman presented with a 3-month history of bilateral thoracic radiculopathy and progressive paraparesis with urinary incontinence. Neurological examination revealed 2 out of 5 strength in the bilateral lower extremities with hyper-reflexia and clonus (ASIA C). An MRI revealed a 2 cm intradural, extramedullary dorsal mass centred at the T4 region (Fig. 3). A T3–T5 mini-open trans-spinous removal of the tumour was performed. Pathology revealed meningioma. A postoperative MRI revealed gross-total

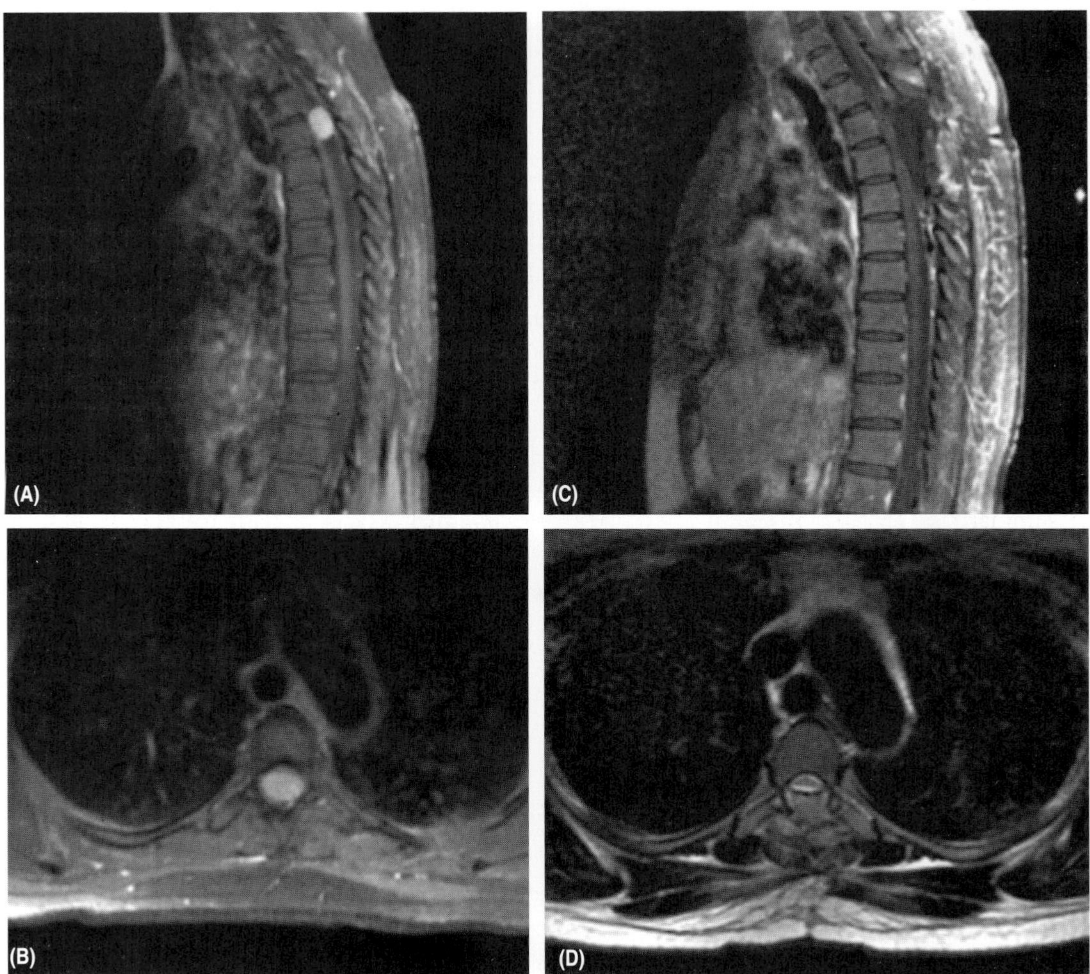

Fig. 3. Preoperative and postoperative imaging of representative case 2. Preoperative (A, B) T$_1$-weighted MR imaging with contrast demonstrating a 2 cm, intradural, homogeneously-enhancing lesion (intradural meningioma) at the T4 region. A mini-open, trans-spinous approach was performed to resect this mass. Postoperative (C, D) T$_1$-weighted MR imaging demonstrated gross total resection of the tumour.

resection of the tumour (Fig. 3). Upon discharge, the patient had improved strength and at 1-year follow up, she was ambulatory with a cane and had regained bladder control (ASIA D).

Case 3

A 67-year-old man presented with progressive lower extremity paraparesis and was unable to stand unassisted for 1 minute. On physical examination, he had 2–3 out of 5 lower extremity strength and clonus (ASIA C). An MRI revealed a T7 intradural lesion with significant cord compression.

A T6–T8 mini-open trans-spinous resection of tumour was performed. Pathology revealed meningioma. Postoperative MRI demonstrated a gross-total resection of the tumour. At 1-year follow up, the patient ambulated independently (ASIA D).

Results

Cadaveric study

As summarized in Table 1, the BMI for each cadaver was recorded (mean 29.5, range 18–43). The incision lengths of the mini-open and standard open approaches required to access three laminae were compared. The average length of the incision for the mini-open approach (mean

4.4 cm) differed significantly from the open approach (mean 11.7 cm, $p < 0.001$, paired t-test). Interestingly, the incision length remained essentially unchanged (range 4.2–4.5 cm) in these 6 cadavers, regardless of the BMI, when a mini-open trans-spinous approach with an expandable retractor was used. However, in these same cadavers, we found that the incision length required to expose the same three laminae via the standard open approach increased with a bigger BMI (range 8–15 cm).

Clinical cases

The average age for the three clinical cases was 51 years with an average BMI of 28.9 (Table 2). Preoperatively, a small fiducial screw localizer was placed into the lamina at the level of intended surgery by interventional radiology using computed tomography (CT) guidance (in order to avoid wrong-level surgery).

In each case, two thoracic laminectomies were performed to access the intradural tumour. The laminectomized levels ranged from T3–T8. The average estimated blood loss was 133 cc, the average operative time was 210 minutes, the average length of the incision was 4.4 cm, and the average length of hospitalization was 136 hours (Table 3). Gross total tumour removal was performed in 2 patients (cases 2, 3). In the third patient (case 1), we did not attempt a gross total removal as the lesion spanned 8 levels; we performed an intradural tumour biopsy and partial resection only. All patients have either stable (case 1) or improved neurological function

Table 1. Cadaver findings

Case no.	BMI	MIS incision length (cm)	Open incision length (cm)	Levels of thoracic lamina accessed
1	18	4.2	8.0	3.0
2	22	4.2	10.0	3.0
3	28	4.5	11.0	3.0
4	30	4.5	12.0	3.0
5	36	4.5	14.0	3.0
6	43	4.5	15.0	3.0

Table 2. Patient profile

	Age (year)/ Sex	Duration of symtoms (months)	Level	BMI
1	46/F	24	T5–T6	28.0
2	40/F	6	T3–T5	23.2
3	67/M	3	T6–T8	35.5

Table 3. Operative statistics

	Pathology	Laminectomy levels	EBL (cc)	OR time (min)	Length of incision (cm)	Length of hospital stay (h)
1	GBM*	T5–T6	100	180	4.0	96
2	Meningioma	T3–T5	150	240	4.2	168
3	Meningioma	T6–T8	150	210	5.0	146

*GBM=gliobastoma multiforme

Table 4. Pre- and Postoperative neurological function

	Preoperative ASIA score	Postoperative ASIA score
1	B	B
2	C	D
3	C	D

Table 5. Cadaver findings

	Follow-up period	Preoperative modified Prolo score	Postoperative modified Prolo score
1	1 year	P3F1E2M4	P4F2E2M5
2	1 year	P3F1E1M3	P4F4E2M4
3	1 year	P5F1E1M5	P5F2E3M5

(ASIA score and modified prolo score) (cases 2 and 3) at medium term follow up (Tables 4 and 5). Postoperative complications (no spinal fluid leaks, no wound infections, no pseudo-meningoceles, etc.) did not occur.

Discussion

Intradural spinal cord tumours are rare lesions with an incidence of up to 10 per 10,000 people.[5,6] Traditionally, a midline open surgical procedure consisting of a laminectomy with intradural resection has been performed for intradural spinal tumours with excellent outcomes.[1-4] In open cases in patients with low BMI and small intradural tumours, many surgeons have used relatively small incisions without facet removal. However, in patients with a BMI of >35, an open surgical exposure typically requires a relatively large incision and dissection and destruction of paraspinal musculature 2 levels above and 2 levels below the target lamina in order to avoid creep of adipose tissue and musculature into the operative field.

Some authors have tried to minimize this paraspinal muscle trauma in the past by using an open hemi-laminectomy approach to access intradural tumours.[7-15] In an effort to further minimize tissue destruction and destabilization, a minimally invasive, tubular, muscle splitting, hemilaminar approach has been utilized by Fessler and colleagues in the resection of intradural, extramedullary tumours.[16] However, such a minimally invasive hemi-laminectomy technique may not be ideal for resection of large intradural tumours on account of the limited access to the full, bilateral aspect of the dorsal spinal cord. In addition, in cases of intra-medullary lesions, a truly midline myelotomy is difficult through a unilateral, hemi-laminectomy approach, as the surgeon has only an oblique view of the central spinal canal.

To have a midline, dorsal access to intradural tumours while minimizing muscle dissection, other authors have tried an open split laminotomy technique.[17] However, visualization of the bilateral, dorsal spinal cord is still difficult with this technique because of the overhanging laminae. In a prior report, 37% of the patients undergoing a split laminotomy had subtotal tumour resections and 16% of the patients suffered from neurological decline after this approach was utilized.

We have described our experience with resection of intradural lesions through a mini-open trans-spinous process approach with the use of an expandable tubular retractor system. This approach allows direct midline access to the entire dorsal aspect of the spinal cord with decreased disruption of paraspinal tissues compared with traditional open techniques. In addition, unlike the minimally invasive unilateral hemi-laminectomy techniques, our approach allows for a direct, dorsal, midline access for a myelotomy in cases of intramedullary lesions (Fig. 2).

In our cadavers, we demonstrated an incision length for our mini-open approach to be nearly 3 times smaller than a traditional open approach (Fig. 1). Furthermore, whereas the incision length increased with increasing BMI in the standard open technique, this was not observed in the mini-open trans-spinous approach. We found that the incision size was at a maximum of 4.5 cm regardless of BMI in the mini-open approach compared with up to 15 cm for a standard open approach (to access the same three laminae in the same cadavers). This highlights a particular advantage of the mini-open approach in obese patients. Expandable tubular retractors secure adipose tissue away from the surgical exposure and allow for a smaller initial incision and less tissue dissection compared with standard open retractors.

As with all minimally invasive procedures, inadequate exposure that compromises visualization of vital structures is a concern. However, in our experience, safe and complete resection of intradural spinal tumours that span 3 segments or less can be accomplished with this mini-open technique.

In our case of intramedullary tumour (case 1), we selected the mini-open trans-spinous approach with the intention only to perform a biopsy. Due to the extensive preoperative spinal cord involvement (T2–T10) and lack of tissue diagnosis, complete resection was not our goal. However, case 1 does highlight a limitation of this mini-open approach. This technique is not suitable for complete resection of tumours that extend beyond 3 levels on account of the limitations of retractor expansion. Furthermore, it is important to be aware of the rostral-caudal boundaries of the tumour. To ensure that tumour is resected, regions rostral and caudal to the tumour should be explored with an instrument such as the Woodson dissector or with imaging via an intraoperative ultrasound.

Whereas dural closure is tedious with this and other minimally invasive approaches, no post-operative cerebrospinal fluid leak or pseudo-meningocele was seen in any of our cases. We suspect that an additional advantage of less invasive surgery is the reduced space available for accumulation of a postoperative pseudomeningocele.

In our clinical study, all patients exhibited stable or improved neurological function (ASIA and Modified Prolo scores). Our experience supports the safety and efficacy of this new technique.

None of our patients underwent fusion, and none of them had delayed post-laminectomy kyphosis 1 year after their tumour removals. Post-laminectomy kyphosis is unlikely in the mid-thoracic region where there is robust structural support involving the rib cage. Additionally, with less tissue destruction, the likelihood of kyphosis is possibly further minimized. However, longer follow up is necessary to assess adequately the incidence of this phenomenon.

Conclusion

On the basis of this study, we conclude that the mini-open trans-spinous resection of mid-thoracic intradural tumours can be performed safely. This approach allows complete dorsal access to the midline spinal canal while minimizing the tissue disruption associated with a standard midline, open procedure, especially in patients with a large BMI.

References

1. McCormick PC. Anatomic principles of intradural spinal surgery. *Clin Neurosurg* 1994;**41**:204–23.

2. McCormick PC, Post KD, Stein BM. Intradural extramedullary tumors in adults. *Neurosurg Clin N Am* 1990;**1**:591–608.

3. McCormick PC, Stein BM. Miscellaneous intradural pathology. *Neurosurg Clin N Am* 1990;**1**:687–99.

4. Tobias ME, McGirt MJ, Chaichana KL, *et al.* Surgical management of long intramedullary spinal cord tumors. *Childs Nerv Syst* 2008;**24**:219–23.

5. Kurland L. The frequency of intracranial and intraspinal neoplasms in the resident population of Rochester, Minnesota. *J Neurosurg Spine* 1958;**15**:627–41.

6. Stein B, McCormick P. *Spinal intradural tumors.* New York: McGraw-Hill; 1996.

7. Balak N. Unilateral partial hemilaminectomy in the removal of a large spinal ependymoma: Case report and technical review. *Spine J* 2007.

8. Bertalanffy H, Mitani S, Otani M, *et al.* Usefulness of hemilaminectomy for microsurgical management of intraspinal lesions. *Keio J Med* 1992;**41**:76–9.

9. Kanemoto Y, Ohnishi H, Koshimae N, *et al.* Ventral T-1 neurinoma removed via hemilaminectomy without costotransversectomy: Case report. *Neurol Med Chir (Tokyo)* 1999;**39**:685–8.

10. Koch-Wiewrodt D, Wagner W, Perneczky A. Unilateral multilevel interlaminar fenestration instead of laminectomy or hemilaminectomy: An alternative surgical approach to intraspinal space-occupying lesions. Technical note. *J Neurosurg Spine* 2007;**6**:485–92.

11. Oktem IS, Akdemir H, Kurtsoy A, *et al.* Hemilaminectomy for the removal of the spinal lesions. *Spinal Cord* 2000;**38**:92–6.

12. Pompili A, Caroli F, Cattani F, *et al.* Unilateral limited laminectomy as the approach of choice for the removal of thoracolumbar neurofibromas. *Spine* 2004;**29**:1698–702.

13. Pompili A, Caroli F, Telera S, *et al.* Minimally invasive resection of intraduralextramedullary spinal neoplasms. *Neurosurgery* 2006;**59**:E1152.

14. Sario-glu AC, Hanci M, Bozkus H, *et al.* Unilateral hemilaminectomy for the removal of the spinal space-occupying lesions. *Minim Invasive Neurosurg* 1997;**40**:74–7.

15. Sridhar K, Ramamurthi R, Vasudevan MC, *et al.* Limited unilateral approach for extramedullary spinal tumours. *Br J Neurosurg* 1998;**12**:430–3.

16. Tredway TL, Santiago P, Hrubes MR, *et al.* Minimally invasive resection of intradural-extramedullary spinal neoplasms. *Neurosurgery* 2006;**58**:ONS52–58; discussion ONS52–58.

17. Banczerowski P, Vajda J, Veres R. Exploration and decompression of the spinal canal using split laminotomy and its modification, the "archbone" technique. *Neurosurgery* 2008;**62**:ONS432–440; discussion ONS440–431.

17

Multilevel cervical compressive myelopathy: Posterior approach—Laminectomy/laminoplasty

SHASHANK SHARAD KALE

Cervical spondylotic myelopathy frequently causes slow, progressive neurological deterioration.[1–7] The patients with moderate-to-severe involvement warrant operative intervention to alter the natural history.[2,4–10] The surgical treatment is decompression of the spinal cord. Anterior and posterior procedures have been developed to halt further deterioration and ameliorate present symptoms. Anterior decompression, corpectomy and arthrodesis is an excellent treatment alternative, but not without substantial complications.[9,11–15] The anterior approach may be particularly difficult in patients with multilevel involvement and underlying congenital or developmental stenosis. The posterior approach offers simplicity, less potential operative risk, and allows decompression away from the offending abnormalities including osteophytes, ossified or buckling ligaments, and disc protrusions. The traditional posterior surgical operation for decompression has been laminectomy, and laminoplasty has developed as an attractive alternative and is gaining wide acceptance. Both procedures allow for dorsal cord migration, decreasing axial tension and improving vascular perfusion. Late complications, in particular post-laminectomy kyphosis or instability in multilevel procedures, are well-known complications, although the prevalence varies. Laminoplasty was introduced as a potentially motion-sparing technique for the treatment of cervical stenosis. This procedure was first described by Hirabayashi[16] and Hirabayashi and Satomi[17] in the Japanese literature, primarily as a treatment for myelopathy resulting from ossification of the posterior longitudinal ligament (OPLL).[18] This procedure attempts to avoid the above-mentioned complications. In the western hemisphere, laminoplasty has been used primarily to treat cervical spondylotic myelopathy. Different techniques have been described, and the results of several large clinical series are available for review.

Techniques

Hirabayashi's initial description of laminoplasty was an open-door technique, with sutures used to maintain the opening of the spinal canal.[14,17] The open-door technique has been modified by several authors[19–27] and has been applied to a number of patient populations, including those suffering from OPLL, spondylosis, rheumatoid arthritis, and intradural pathology. The open-door laminoplasty and its variations are the most commonly used techniques reported.

Other laminoplasty techniques have also been described. Casha *et al.*[28] described a suspended laminoplasty procedure as a means of reconstructing the posterior tension band after intradural surgery. Replacement of laminae after a laminectomy, performed following intradural surgery has been described by other authors; however, not all authors specifically reconstruct the dorsal tension band. Edwards *et al.*[29] described the 'T-saw' laminoplasty in the western literature. This technique involves splitting the spinous processes using a wire saw. Some authors have referred to this technique as the 'French-window' technique and have described long-term results.[30] *En bloc* removal of the posterior elements and reconstruction with hydroxyapatite spacers and titanium plates was described by Goto *et al.*[31] Other authors have described the use of titanium plates, allograft bone, locally harvested autograft, and resorbable plates to accomplish the same end-point.[25] There has been no published comparison of clinical results achieved using the various techniques. It would make sense that preservation of the interspinous

and yellow ligaments would have less of a destabilizing influence on the cervical spine compared with techniques that sacrifice these structures; however, the clinical significance of this assumption has only been addressed through the comparison of retrospective case series.[32]

In AIIMS the use of laminoplasty is limited to patients with symptomatic multilevel stenosis with retained cervical lordosis, young and active patients. Laminoplasty is not recommended when there is instability or deformity of the spine and when there is short segment stenosis—typically less than 3 levels. These patients are treated with ventral decompression and fusion.

Preoperative work-up

Clinical history and examination should prove myelopathy. Neck pain is not a good indication for this procedure. MRI is the most commonly used imaging study to confirm the diagnosis, occasionally mylography may be useful. Standing X-rays of the cervical spine are useful for evaluating the degree of lordosis, and help demonstrate the presence of OPLL. Both these factors may influence the decision to treat the

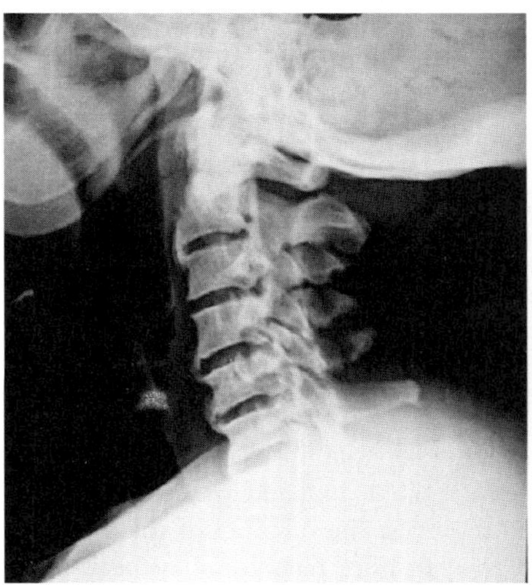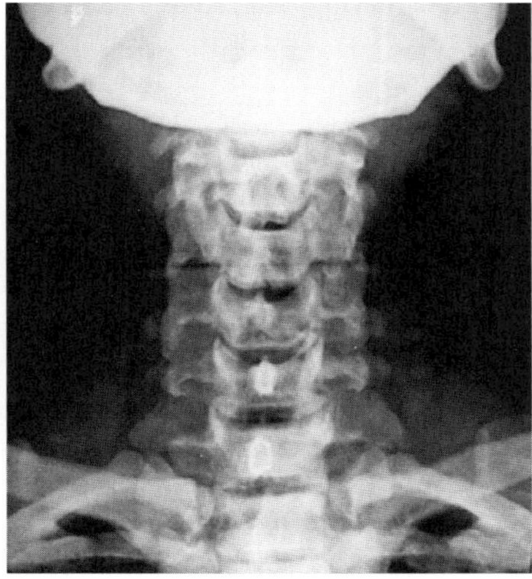

Fig. 1. Preoperative Plain X-ray C Spine AP and Lat of a patient treated with open-door cervical laminoplasty. Note the OPLL at the level of C_2/C_3 and C_5/C_6, and the bridging anterior osteophytes. The lordosis though reduced is present.

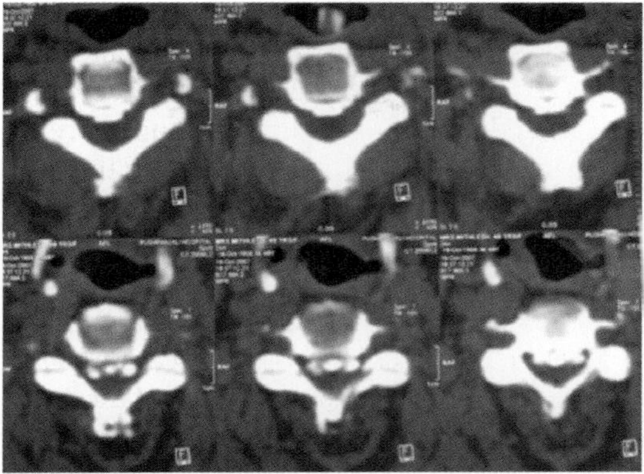
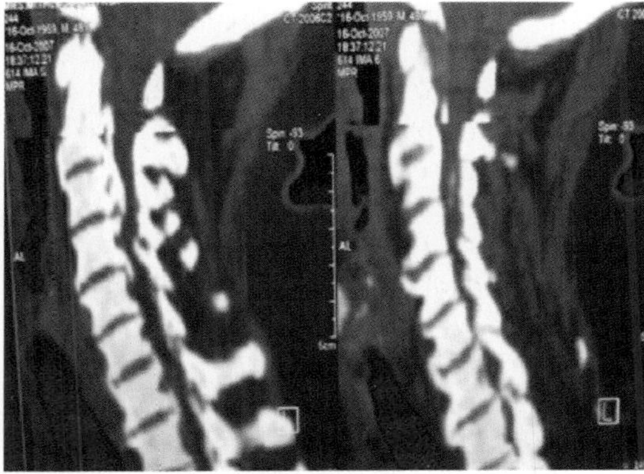

Fig. 2. Preoperative CT Scan of the cervical spine in the same patient. The OPLL is clearly seen in the axial and the sagittal images. Note the extent of spinal stenosis in the axial images.

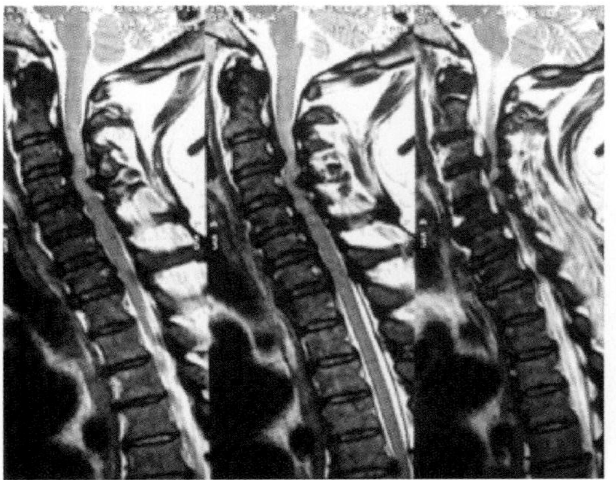
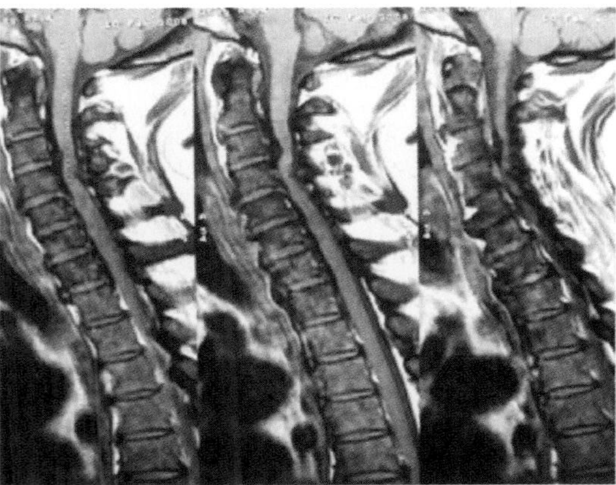

Fig. 3. Preoperative MRI of the same patient. T_2-weighted sagittal image on the left and the T_1-weighted sagittal image on the right demonstrate the multilevel stenosis due to disc bulges and OPLL.

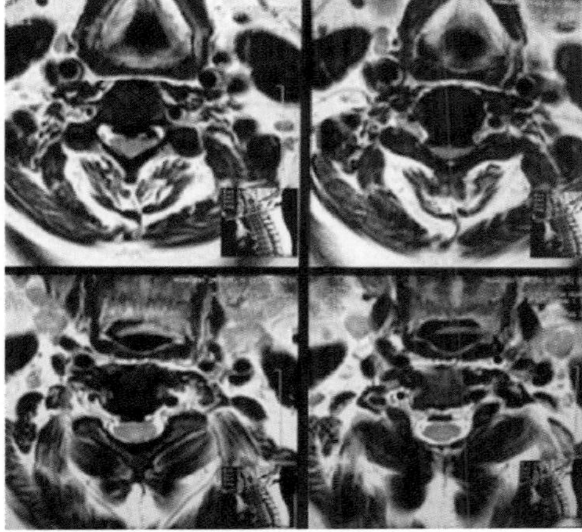

Fig. 4. Axial T_2-weighted images of the same patient demonstrating the extent of spinal cord compression.

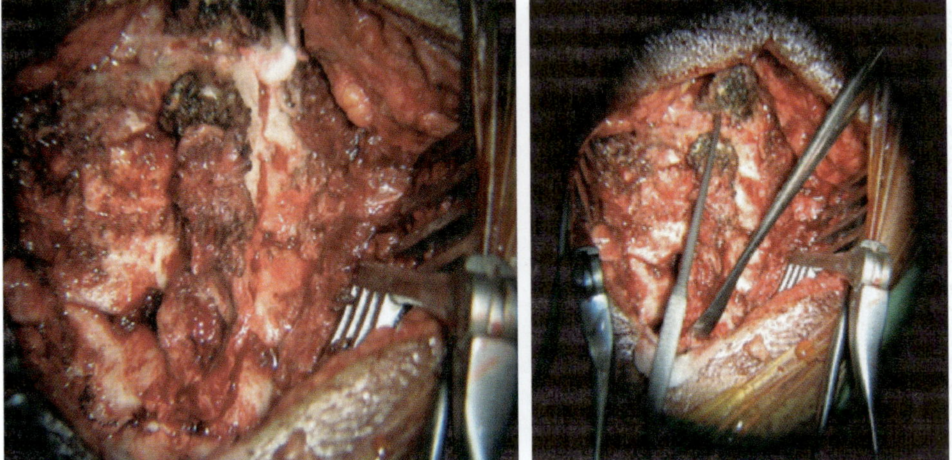

Fig. 5. Intraoperative photograph demonstrating the trough made on one side. Note that the lateral masses have not been completely exposed and the joint capsules saved.

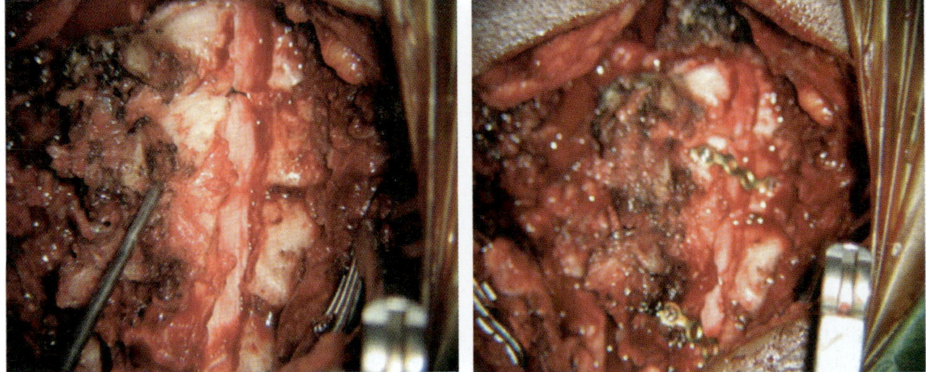

Fig. 6. Intraoperative photograph showing the gentle lifting of the laminae on the open door side. The photograph on the right shows the titanium miniplates bent in a lazy 'S' fixed to the lamina and the lateral mass. Note alternate levels have been used for the fixation.

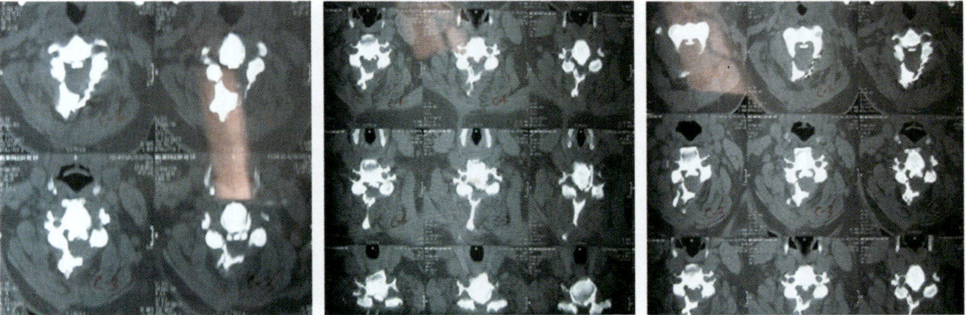

Fig. 7. Postoperative CT scan axial images of the same patient demonstrate acceptable positions of the troughs, excellent decompression at C_2, C_3 levels. the door seems to have closed somewhat at C_5 level. The patient demonstrated good neurological recovery and is back to doing her house work, so no further surgery was recommended.

patient with laminectomy/laminoplasty. Finally the number of levels involved determines the surgical treatment.

The next step is the determination of the number of levels to be decompressed, which side is to be opened and which side is to be fractured to make the hinge of the 'open-door'. The most common procedure performed is a C₃–C₆ laminoplasty. The more symptomatic side is chosen for the open-door procedure. If there is no laterality a right-handed surgeon would do well to choose the left side for the open door, but it may vary according to the surgeons ease. Electrophysiological monitoring is usually not employed as there is no deformity correction; all manipulation is under direct visualization of the laminae and the dura.

Key steps of technique

- Decompress the abdomen
- Midline dissection of the cervical spine dorsally, minimize disruption of facet joints and interspinous ligaments.
- Use high-speed drill, create troughs bilaterally at lateral edge of the lamina, hinge side first.
- Decompress all affected segments typically C₃–C₆
- Divide yellow ligament at the C₂/C₃ and the C₆/C₇ level
- Push spinous processes towards hinge side to create a fracture of the laminae and to open the spinal canal
- Control epidural bleeding
- Use titanium miniplates and 4–6 mm screws at, at least every other level to hold laminae open
- Irrigate and close

An open-door laminoplasty is preferred because it preserves the interspinous ligaments and is technically less demanding. The patient is positioned prone and strict control of spinal alignment/traction is not mandatory as no fixation is being performed. It is important to decompress the abdomen as this decreases the

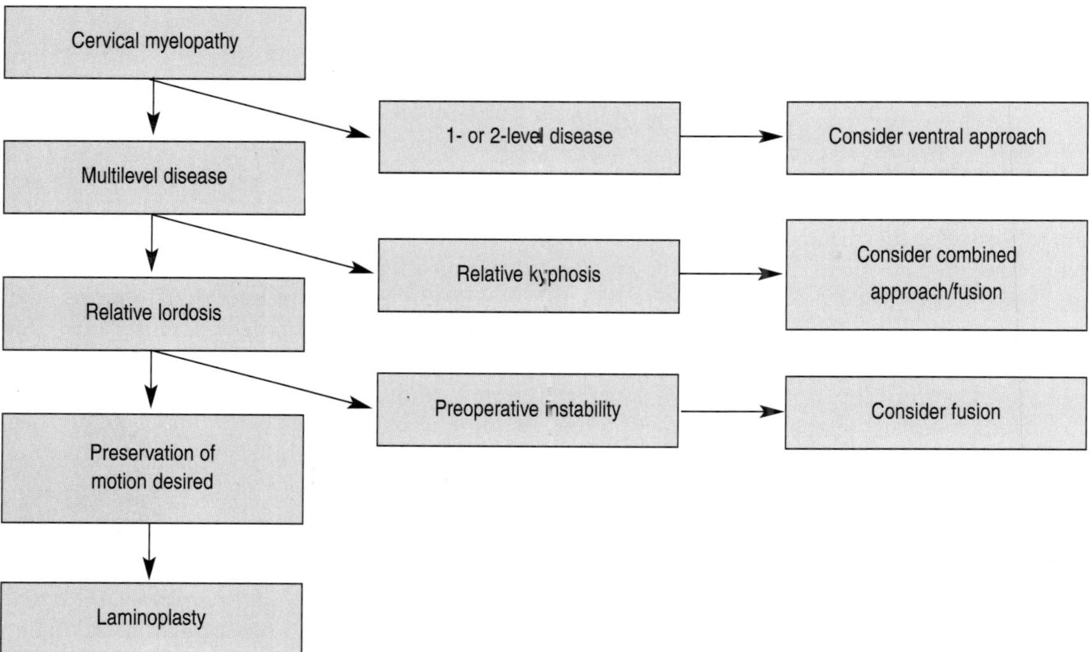

Fig. 8. Algorithm for decision-making[33]

venous pressure and consequently extradural venous bleeding which sometimes may be difficult to control. A midline dissection is performed, the entire lateral masses may not be exposed, and care is taken to minimize disruption of the facet joints. A high speed drill with a matchstick head is used to create troughs bilaterally at the lateral edge of the laminae just medial to the lateral masses. Typically the levels C_3 to C_6 are used. A 1 mm or a 2 mm Kerrison rongeur may be used to complete the trough on the open door side. The spinous processes are pushed towards the hinge side to create a greenstick fracture of the lamina and the spinal canal is thus opened. Haemostasis is achieved using bipolar or surgical or gelfoam. Titanium miniplates 1 mm thickness are used and are bent in the 'lazy S' shape required to maintain the open door and fixed with 5 or 6 mm titanium screws. One end of the plate is fixed to the lateral mass and the other to the raised lamina. The wound is copiously irrigated and closed in multiple layers.

Postoperatively patient is encouraged to begin normal activities as soon as possible. Imaging is performed at 6 weeks. Simple X-rays or a CT scan may be used.

Published results of laminoplasty

Iwasaki et al.[34] reported an improvement rate of 64% using the assessment method of Hirabayashi and Satomi[17] and a 14% incidence of deterioration most frequently caused by progression of OPLL after following 92 patients for 10 years. They observed kyphosis development in 8% patients; however, none of these had any symptoms attributable to kyphosis. Ogawa et al.[35] reported 5-year follow-up in 72 patients with an improvement rate of 63%. Satomi et al.[36] in a large series of 204 patients reported overall improvement in 64% patients, 88 of these had cervical Spondylotic myelopathy. Edwards et al.[29] reported in Western patients that 67%–83% reported improvement and none had loss of

lordosis. Martin–Benlloch et al.[37] reported good outcomes and no loss of cervical lordosis in any patient after 2 years of follow-up, in Spondylotic myelopathy patients treated with T-saw laminoplasty. Laminoplasty has also been shown to be an effective treatment modality for patients with stenosis resulting from rheumatoid disease of the subaxial cervical spine.[38,39]

Laminoplasty and cervical range of motion

Morio et al.[40] noted an overall straightening of the spine and a decrease in the range of motion in a group of 51 patients operated on for cervical myelopathy. However in their series the loss of lordosis was in no case symptomatic. Similar results were reported by Suda et al.[39]—a decrease in cervical range of motion in a series of patients with rheumatoid arthritis. Kawaguchi et al.[41] reported that skipping levels between reconstructed laminae and encouragement of neck movements early in the postoperative period improved the cervical range of motion and decreased the neck pain.

Neck stiffness following laminoplasty may serve a protective function. Hirabayashi and Yoshida,[14,42] and Kaminsky et al.[43] found a limitation of approximately 50% in range-of-motion. The stability of the spine following laminoplasty has been examined in biomechanical studies comparing cervical laminoplasty with laminectomy.[6,44] Nowinski et al.[45] examined nine cadaveric specimens after multilevel laminoplasty or laminectomy had been performed. Cervical spine levels 2 to 7 were tested with physiological loading. Cervical laminectomy with 25% or more facetectomy resulted in highly significant increase in cervical motion for all motions compared to the intact controls. With the numbers available, cervical laminoplasty was not significantly different from the intact control, except for a marginal increase in axial rotation. This limitation of mobility can prevent late instability and neurological deterioration.

Pre- and Post -laminectomy kyphosis

The prevalence of post-laminectomy kyphosis, a challenging problem to treat because of the lack of posterior elements, varies in the available literature.[8,15,46–56] The aetiology of post-laminectomy kyphosis is primarily mechanical, from loss of posterior support. As little as 25% facetectomy significantly increases motion in all directions,[45] and 50% facetectomy allows visualization of 3–5 mm of the nerve roots.[42,57]

Suda *et al.*[58] evaluated the effect of pre-existing kyphosis on outcome after laminoplasty. These authors followed 114 patients for just over 2 years after laminoplasty and noted an average of 60% improvement in neurological problems. They did a multivariate analysis of sorts, and were able to demonstrate that local kyphosis of 13 degrees or more was associated with poor outcomes.

Kawakami *et al.*[59] found that the presence of postoperative kyphosis was a negative predictor of resolution of symptoms, regardless of surgical approach (anterior or posterior), and stressed the importance of promoting lordosis when performing any sort of surgery on patients with cervical stenosis. Kawakami *et al.*[60] later suggested that the inclusion of C_2 in the decompression may improve outcomes after laminoplasty in selected patients without preoperative lordosis. Overall, the consensus of most authors is that laminoplasty is best performed on patients with an intact cervical lordosis or at least without a significant kyphosis.

Comparison with laminectomy

Kaminsky *et al.*[43] compared the results achieved in a group of 28 patients with spondylotic myelopathy who underwent laminoplasty with results achieved in a similar group of 22 patients treated with laminectomy alone. They noted similar neurologic improvements between the groups (using a modified Nurick scale); however, patients in the laminoplasty group had significant reduction in neck pain compared with patients in the group that underwent laminectomy alone.

Herkowitz, using his own grading system, compared anterior cervical arthrodesis, laminectomy, and laminoplasty for multilevel Spondylotic radiculopathy in 45 patients with a minimum 2-year follow-up and concluded that laminoplasty was an effective alternative to anterior cervical fusion and laminectomy.[61] The complications of anterior arthrodesis and laminectomy could be avoided with laminoplasty. Patients with laminectomy had the poorest results.

Yoshida *et al.*[32] studied axial neck pain before and after laminoplasty in a group of 173 patients and found that axial symptoms were largely unaffected by the procedure. It appears that whatever benefit laminoplasty offers versus laminectomy in terms of axial symptoms is related more to a worsening of symptoms caused by laminectomy than to a beneficial effect of laminoplasty.

Complications

Wound complications are the most frequently reported complication, along with (generally transient) motor deterioration.[15,55,62,63] Satomi *et al.*[36] reviewed a series of 204 patients treated with laminoplasty and described an incidence of complications of 10.8% with a 7.8% incidence of (primarily axial) muscle weakness. Other authors have described the occurrence of C_5 root palsies, the proposed mechanism being identical to that seen with cervical laminectomy (that is, traction on the upper cervical nerve roots, particularly C_5, caused by dorsal migration of the spinal cord).[64,65]

Conclusion

Laminoplasty is a safe and efficacious procedure in the management of selected patients with multiple level cervical Spondylotic myelopathy or radiculopathy, cervical stenosis resulting from CPLL, rheumatoid arthritis, or other multilevel processes.[66] Various outcome measures including modified nurick grades, pain scores and gait alterations demonstrated more substantial improvements in laminoplasty patients, with fewer late complications, than laminectomy.[1,7,14,16,17,23,54,61,63,67–70,72–77] This must be balanced with the potential loss of cervical range of motion, neck stiffness, and the potential for transient neurological injury encountered with laminoplasty. Laminoplasty is a valuable procedure that should be in the armamentarium of surgeons treating patients with cervical myelopathy.

References

1. Clark CR. Indications and surgical management of cervical myelopathy. *Sem Spine Surg* 1989;**1**:254–61.
2. Clark E, Robinson PK. Cervical myelopathy: A complication of cervical spondylosis. *Brain* 1956;**79**:483–7.
3. Emery SE, Smith MD, Bohlman HH. Upper-airway obstruction after multiple level corpectomy for myelopathy. *J Bone Joint Surg* 1991;**73-A:**544–51.
4. Gregorius FK, Estrin T, Crandall PH. Cervical spondylotic radiculopathy and myelopathy. A long-term follow-up study. *Arch of Neurology* 1976;**33**:618–25.
5. Lees F, Aldren JW. Natural history and prognosis of cervical spondylosis. *Br Med J* 1972;**95**:1607–10.
6. Nurick S. The natural history and the results of surgical treatment of the spinal cord disorder associated with cervical spondylosis. *Brain* 1972;**95**:101–8.
7. Symon L, Lavender P. The surgical treatment of cervical spondylotic myelopathy. *Neurology* 1967;**17**:117–27.
8. Cattell HS, Clark GL. Cervical kyphosis and instability following multiple laminectomies in children. *J Bone Joint Surg* 1967;**49A:**713–20.
9. Emery S, Bohlman HH, Bolesta M, Jones P. Anterior cervical decompression and arthrodesis for the treatment of cervical spondylotic myelopathy: Two to seventeen-year follow-up. *J Bone Joint Surg* 1998;**80-A:**941–51.
10. Herkowitz HN. The surgical management of cervical spondylotic radiculopathy and myelopathy. *Clin Orthop* 1989;**239**:94–108.
11. Aita I, Hayashi K, Wadano Y, *et al.* Posterior movement and enlargement of the spinal cord after cervical laminoplasty. *Spine* 1998;**80B:**33–37.
12. Farey ID, McAfee PC, Davis RF, *et al.* Pseudo- arthrosis of the cervical spine after anterior arthrodesis: Treatment by posterior nerve-root decompression, stabilization, and arthrodesis. *J Bone Joint Surg* 1990;**72-A:**1171–7.
13. Fernyhough JC, White JI, LaRocca H. Fusion rates in multilevel cervical spondylosis comparing allograft fibula with autograft fibula in 126 patients. *Spine* 1991;**16**:561–4.
14. Hiarabayashi K, Bohlman HH. Multilevel cervical spondylosis. Laminoplasty versus anterior decompression. *Spine* 1995;**20**:1732–34.
15. Yonenobu K, Hosono N, Iwasaki M, *et al.* Laminoplasty versus subtotal corpectomy. *Spine* 1992;**17**:1281–4.
16. Hirabyashi K. Expansive open-door laminoplasty for cervical spondylotic myelopathy. *Shujutu* 1978;**32**:1159–63.
17. Hirabyashi K, Satomi K. Operative procedure and results of open-door laminoplasty. *Spine* 1988;**13**:870–6.
18. Kawai, Sunago K, Doi K, *et al.* Cervical laminoplasty (Hattori's Method): Procedure and follow-up results. *Spine* 1998;**13**:1245–50.
19. Itoh T, Tsuji H. Technical improvements and results of laminoplasty for compressive myelopathy in the cervical spine. *Spine* 1985;**10**:729–36.
20. Lee TT, Manzano GR, Green BA. Modified open-door cervical expansive laminoplasty for cervical spondylotic myelopathy: Operative technique, outcome, and predictors for gait improvement. *J Neurosurg* 1997;**86**:64–8.
21. Nakano N, Nakano T, Nakano K. Comparison of the results of laminectomy and open-door laminoplasty for cervical spondylotic myeloradiculopathy and ossification of the posterior longitudinal ligament. *Spine* 1988;**13**:792–94.
22. O'Brien MF, Petersen D, Casey AT, *et al.* A novel technique for laminoplasty augmentation of spinal canal area using titanium miniplate stabilization: A computerized morphometric analysis. *Spine* 1996;**21**:474–83.
23. Tomita K, Nomura S, Umeda S, *et al.* Cervical laminoplasty to enlarge the spinal canal multilevel ossification of the posterior longitudinal ligament with myelopathy. *Arch Orthop Trauma Surg* 1988;**107**:148–53.
24. Mochida J, Nomura T, Chiba M, *et al.* Modified expansive open-door laminoplasty in cervical myelopathy. *J Spinal Disord* 1999;**12**:386–91.
25. Patel CK, Cunningham BJ, Herkowitz HN.

Techniques in cervical laminoplasty. *Spine J* 2002;2: 450–5.

26. Shaffrey CI, Wiggins GC, Piccirilli CB, *et al*. Modified open-door laminoplasty for treatment of neurological deficits in younger patients with congenital spinal stenosis: Analysis of clinical and radiographic data. *J Neurosurg* 1999;**90**:170–7.

27. Tani S, Isoshima A, Nagashima Y, *et al*. Laminoplasty with preservation of posterior cervical elements: Surgical technique. *Neurosurgery* 2002;**50**:97–101; discussion 101–102.

28. Casha S, Engelbrecht HA, DuPlessis SJ, *et al*. Suspended laminoplasty for wide posterior cervical decompression and intradural access: Results, advantages, and complications. *J Neurosurg Spine* 2004;**1**:80–6.

29. Edwards CC II, Heller JG, Silcox DH III. T-Saw laminoplasty for the management of cervical spondylotic myelopathy: Clinical and radiographic outcome. *Spine* 2000;**25**:1788–94.

30. Saruhashi Y, Hukuda S, Katsuura A, *et al*. A long-term follow-up study of cervical spondylotic myelopathy treated by 'French window' aminoplasty. *J Spinal Disord* 1999;**12**:99–101.

31. Goto T, Ohata K, Takami T, *et al*. Hydroxyapatite laminar spacers and titanium miniplates in cervical laminoplasty. *J Neurosurg* 2002;**97**:323–9.

32. Yoshida M, Tamaki T, Kawakami M, *et al*. Does reconstruction of posterior ligamentous complex with extensor musculature decrease axial symptoms after cervical laminoplasty? *Spine* 2002;**27**:1414–8.

33. Resnick DK. Cervical laminoplasty. In: Mummaneni PV, Lenke LG, Haid RW (eds). *Spinal deformity. A guide to surgical planning and management*. Quality medical Publishing, Inc; 2008.

34. Iwasaki M, Kawaguchi Y, Kimura T, *et al*. Long-term results of expansive laminoplasty for ossification of the posterior longitudinal ligament of the cervical spine: More than 10 years follow-up. *J Neurosurg* 2002;**96**:180–89.

35. Ogawa Y, Toyama Y, Chiba K, *et al*. Long-term results of expansive open door laminoplasty for ossification of the posterior longitudinal ligament of the cervical spine. *J Neurosurg Spine* 2004;**1**:168–74.

36. Satomi K, Ogawa J, Ishii Y, *et al*. Short-term complications and long-term results of expansive open-door laminoplasty for cervical stenotic myelopathy. *Spine J* 2001;**1**:26–30.

37. Martin-Benlloch JA, Maruenda-Paulino JI, Barra-Pla A, *et al*. Expansive laminoplasty as a method for managing cervical multilevel Spondylotic myelopathy. *Spine* 2003;**28**:680–4.

38. Mukai Y, Hosono N, Sakura H, *et al*. Laminoplasty for cervical myelopathy caused by subaxial lesions in rheumatoid arthritis. *J Neurosurg* 2004;**100**:7–12.

39. Suda Y, Saitou M, Shioda M, *et al*. Cervical laminoplasty for subaxial lesions in rheumatoid arthritis. *J Spinal Disord* 2004;**17**:94–101.

40. Morio Y, Yamamoto K, Teshima R, *et al*. Clinicoradiologic study of cervical laminoplasty with posterolateral fusion or bone graft. *Spine* 2000;**25**:190–6.

41. Kawaguchi Y, Kanamori M, Ishiara H, *et al*. Preventive measures for axial symptoms following cervical laminoplasty. *J Spinal Disord* 2003;**16**:487–501.

42. Yoshida M, Otani K, Shibasaki K, *et al*. Expansive laminoplasty with reattachment of spinous process and extensor musculature for cervical myelopathy. *Spine* 1992;**17**:491–7.

43. Kaminsky SB, Clark CR, Traynelis VC. Operative treatment of cervical spondylotic myelopathy and radiculopathy. A comparison of laminectomy and laminoplasty at five year average follow-up. *Iowa Orthop J* 2004;**24**:95–105.

44. Yonenobu K, Fuji T, Okada K, *et al*. Causes of neurologic deterioration following surgical treatment of cervical myelopathy. *Spine* 1986;**11**:818–22.

45. Nowinski GP, Vesarius H, Dipl-Ing, Nolte LP, *et al*. A biomechanical comparison of cervical laminaplasty and cervical facetectomy with progressive facetectomy. *Spine* 1993;**18**:1995–2004.

46. Alvisi C, Borromei A, Cerisoli M, *et al*. Long-term evaluation of cervical spine disorders following laminectomy. *J Neurosurgical Sciences* 1988;**32**:109–12.

47. Callahan RA, Johnson RM, Margolis RN, *et al*. Cervical facet fusion for control of instability following laminectomy. *J Bone Joint Surg* 1977;**59A**:991–1002.

48. Herman JM, Sonntag VKH. Cervical corpectomy and plate fixation for post-laminectomy kyphosis. *J Neurosurg* 1994;**80**:963–70.

49. Inoue A, Ikata T, Katoh S. Spinal deformity following surgery for spinal cord tumors and tumorous lesions: Analysis based on an assessment of spinal functional curve. *Spinal Cord* 1996;**34**: 53–62.

50. Kamioka Y, Yamamoto H, Tani T, *et al*. Postoperative instability of cervical OPLL and cervical radiculo-myelopathy. *Spine* 1989;**14**:1177–83.

51. Lonstein JE. Postlaminectomy kyphosis. *Clin Orthop* 1977;**128**:93–100.

52. Lonstein JE, Winter RB, Moe JH, *et al.* Neurologic deficits secondary to spinal deformity: A review of the literature and report of forty-three cases. *Spine* 1980;**5**:551–5.

53. Mikawa Y, Shikara J, Yamamuro T. Spinal deformity and instability after multilevel cervical laminectomy. *Spine* 1987;**12**:6–11.

54. Sim FH, Svien HJ, Bickel WH, *et al.* Swan-neck deformity following extensive cervical laminectomy. *J Bone Joint Surg* 1974;**56-A**:564–80.

55. White AA, Panjabi MM. Biomechanical considerations in the surgical management of cervical spondylotic myelopathy. *Spine* 1988;**7**:856–60.

56. Zdelblick TA, Bohlman HH. Cervical kyphosis and myelopathy. *J Bone Joint* 1989;**71-A**:170–82.

57. Raynor RB, Pugh J, Shapiro I. Cervical faccetectomy and its effect on spine strength. *J Neurosurg* 1985;**63**:278–82.

58. Suda K, Abumi K, Ito M, *et al.* Local kyphosis reduces surgical outcomes of expansive open-door laminoplasty for cervical spondylotic myelopathy. *Spine* 2003;**28**:1258–62.

59. Kawakami M, Tamaki T, Iwasaki H, *et al.* A comparative study of surgical approaches for cervical compressive myelopathy. *Clin Orthop Relat Res* 2000;**381**:129–36.

60. Kawakami M, Tamaki T, Ando M, *et al.* Relationships between sagittal alignment of the cervical spine and morphology of the spinal cord and clinical outcomes in patients with cervical spondylotic myelopathy treated with expansive laminoplasty. *J Spinal Disord Tech* 2002;**15**:391–7.

61. Herkowitz HN. A comparison of anterior cervical fusion, cervical laminectomy, and cervical laminoplasty for the surgical management of multiple level spondylotic radiculopathy. *Spine* 1988;**13**:774–80.

62. Hosono N, Yonenobu K, Ono K. Neck and shoulder pain after laminoplasty: A noticeable complication. *Spine* 1996;**21**:1969–73.

63. Torg JS, Pavlov H, Genuario SE, *et al.* Neuropraxia of the cervical spinal cord with transient quadriplegia. *J Bone Joint Surg* 1969;**68-A**:1354–70.

64. Chiba K, Toyama Y, Matsumoto M, *et al.* Segmental motor paralysis after expansive open-door laminoplasty. *Spine* 2002;**27**:2108–15.

65. Minoda Y, Nakamura H, Konishi S, *et al.* Palsy of the C5 nerve root after midsagittal splitting laminoplasty of the cervical spine. *Spine* 2003;**28**:1123–7.

66. Hukudu S, Ogata M, Mochizuki T, *et al.* Laminectomy versus laminoplasty for cervical myelopathy: Brief report. *J Bone Joint Surg* 1988;**70B**:325–6.

67. Baba H, Uchida K, Maezawa Y, *et al.* Three-dimensional computed tomography for evaluation of cervical spinal canal enlargement after en-bloc open-door laminoplasty. *Spinal Cord* 1997;**35**:674–9.

68. Hase H, Watanabe T, Hirasawa Y, *et al.* Bilateral open laminoplasty using cervical laminas for cervical myelopathy. *Spine* 1991;**16**:1269–76.

69. Herkowitz HN. Surgical management of cervical disc disease: 'Open-Door' laminoplasty. *Seminars in Spine Surgery* 1989;**1**:245–53.

70. Kimura I, Oh-Hama M, Shingu H, *et al.* Cervical myelopathy treated by canal-expansive laminoplasty. *J Bone Joint Surg* 1984;**66-A**:914–20.

71. Kimura I, Shingu H, Nasu Y, *et al.* Long-term follow-up of cervical spondylotic myelopathy treated by canal-expansive laminoplasty. *J Bone Joint Surg* 1995;**77B**:956–61.

72. Kohno K, Kumon Y, Oka Y, *et al.* Evaluation of prognostic factors following expansive laminoplasty for cervical spinal stenotic myelopathy. *Surg Neurology* 1997;**48**:237–45.

73. Nagata K, Ohashi T, Abe J, *et al.* Cervical myelopathy in elderly patients: Clinical results and MRI findings before and after decompression surgery. *Spinal Cord* 1996;**34**:220–26.

74. Prolo DJ, Oklund SA, Butcher M. Toward uniformity in evaluating results of lumbar spine operations. A paradigm applied to postoperative lumbar interbody fusions. *Spine* 1986;**11**:601–6.

75. Satomi K, Nishu Y, Kohno T, *et al.* Long-term follow-up studies of open-door expansive laminoplasty for cervical stenotic myelopathy. *Spine* 1994;**19**:507–10.

76. Tsuji H. Laminoplasty for patients with compressive myelopathy due to so-called spinal canal stenosis in cervical and thoracic regions. *Spine* 1982;**7**:28–34.

77. Yonenobu K, Hosono N, Iwasaki M, *et al.* Neurologic complications of surgery for compressive myelopathy. *Spine* 1991;**16**:1277–82.

18

Multilevel cervical compressive myelopathy: Anterior approach—corpectomy and fusion

DEEPU BANERJI

Multilevel cervical compressive myelopathy (MCCM) is usually due to cervical canal stenosis secondary to cervical spondylosis (CS) or ossification of the posterior longitudinal ligament (OPLL), especially in the Oriental population.[1,2] The pathogenesis ranges from osteophyte formation, ligamentous hypertrophy or ossification leading to canal narrowing and/or lysthesis secondary to instability of the degenerating spine. This causes direct and repeated injury to the spinal cord during cervical motion and/or vascular damage due to any of the above-mentioned causes.[3–5,7–8] MCCM can be associated with radiculopathy at various levels, depending on the level of compression of the cervical root from the laterally directed osteophytes or facetal hypertrophy.[1,2,6]

Once myelopathy sets in, the natural course is progressive and the majority of patients with moderate-to-severe compressive myelopathy require some form of spinal decompression. In 80%–90% of patients, the cause of compression is due to an anterior lesion.[1–3,7] However, congenital spinal stenosis may predispose a patient to early symptoms and signs. Hypertrophy (or ossified) and often buckling of the ligamentum flavum, especially in extension, compromises the spinal canal from behind. In a narrow canal, flexion causes the spinal cord to stretch leading to a few millimetres of lengthening, causing anterio–posterior thinning and side-to-side broadening. This stretching of the spinal cord in flexion presses the cord against posteriorly protruding osteophytes and ridges, or the posterior borders of the vertebral body at the point of maximal hypermobility (degenerative) leading to temporary demyelination or permanent damage, seen as cord signal changes on MRI. Similarly, extension of the cervical spine leads to shortening of the spinal cord in a superior-inferior direction and increase in anterio–posterior diameter. In a narrow spinal canal this leads to further compression of the spinal cord, which may get aggravated by buckling of a hypertrophied ligamentum flavum from behind. In addition, in a narrow canal with hypermobility, the cord may get pinched between the posterior inferior ridge of the superior vertebrae and the superior border of the inferior lamina—known as dynamic narrowing.[5,9–15] Spinal decompression is planned keeping all these abnormalities in perspective.

For a century, laminectomy has been the standard treatment modality for decompression of MCCM with a good outcome. However, on long-term review, it is associated with persistent neck pain, post-laminectomy membrane formation causing progressive neurological deficit, and progressive kyphotic deformity and/or instability due to damage to the posterior support structures, also called tension band.[16–22] Anterior cervical decompression has been practised since the 1950s, initially for discoidectomy as well as for multilevel decompression, either as multilevel segmental decompression or multilevel corpectomy in cases of MCCM, along with various fusion and stabilization techniques.[23–30] However, significant complications associated with the multilevel anterior approach such as dysphagia, hoarsness of voice, graft dislodgement pseudoarthrosis, vascular injuries and implant failure restricted its use in MCCM. It is also technically very demanding when three or more levels of decompression are needed.[34,35] Laminoplasty was introduced to replace laminectomy and anterior decompression for MCCM to reduce the complications associated with laminectomy and the anterior cervical approach. It provided adequate spinal decompression, maintained spinal alignment and range of motion (ROM), and protect the dura from behind.[37,38] However, long-term reviews do not share this optimism. While it is still a useful technique for decompression of more than three levels of the cervical spine, it is associated with long-term neurological or symptomatic worsening, and progressive kyphotic deformity and canal restenosis.[16,38–45]

The ideal approach to MCCM is still a subject of debate, with many proponents and opponents for each approach. However, these new approaches and conflicting reviews emphasize the complexity of managing the cervical spine, especially when dealing with MCCM. Each of the above approaches has been in practice for many years, with refinement of techniques and technologies, and better understanding of diseases of the cervical spine and its biomechanics. We review the current literature regarding the benefits and outcomes these approaches.

Neurological improvement

Various reports reviewing the outcome have found that the anterior approach has definite advantages over the posterior approach in MCCM.[23,26,27,30,40,41,43,44,46,47] Neurological improvement ranges from 68% to 98% (recovery rate 68%)[26,30,40,46–49] for the anterior approach versus 50%–70% (recovery rate 52%–55%)[26,39–41] for the posterior approach in the short-term. There are conflicting reports about the long-term outcome, with some reports suggesting no advantage of either approach at the end of a decade, and others reporting further deterioration (10%– 33%) following the posterior approach after 7–14 years, especially with laminectomy.[16,18,20] Segmental motor deficits are observed in posterior decompression on both short- and long-term follow up.[50] This is due to cord movement over the anterior bony osteophytes/ ridges. The anterior approach can decompress both the spinal cord and nerve roots, if these are compressed. However, in the posterior approach, to decompress the nerve root, often 25%–50% of facetectomy is required, which adds to spinal instability in case of laminectomy. With laminoplasty, lateral access is difficult on the side of the hinge.[16,41] OPLL is known to grow both vertically and transversely following both laminectomy and laminoplasty, leading to further neurological worsening.[16,41,51,52] The neurological outcome is better with the anterior approach in young patients and the elderly, i.e. above 75 years of age.[16,41] Overall, the neurological recovery rate is better with anterior decompression.

Pain relief

Axial pain relief is significantly better with the anterior approach than laminectomy. This is because of immediate stabilization of the degenerative segments with the anterior approach. Though axial pain is supposed to be less with laminoplasty, in view of preservation of the posterior tension band, long-term follow up reveals a high incidence of neck pain ranging from 40% to 60%.[16,39,44,53] Some reviews found that the frequency of neck pain was the same in both the laminectomy and laminoplasty groups.[44] Neck pain and radiculopathy have also been reported after anterior decompression and fusion on long-term follow up due to adjacent segment degeneration, though at a lesser frequency.[16,41,54]

Loss of alignment and kyphosis

The anterior approach addresses the cervical alignment better and can correct kyphosis, although over the long term there may be a small reduction in correction. Ratlif and Cooper reported a 35% incidence of post-laminoplasty loss of cervical alignment and 10% incidence of development of kyphosis in a meta-analysis of laminoplasty in the English literature.[39,55,56] Kyphotic deformity or loss of lordosis is a contraindication for the posterior approach. At least 10° of lordosis is advocated for undertaking posterior decompression. Although the incidence of progressive kyphotic deformity is higher with laminectomy, it is seen even in those undergoing laminoplasty in the long-term, though at a lesser frequency.[16,39,41] This is due to denervation injury to the latissimus dorsi and paraspinal muscles resulting from retraction injury when they are retracted beyond the medial facets.

Range of motion (ROM)

While anterior decompression and fusion significantly reduces the ROM of the cervical spine, it is well preserved in cases of laminectomy, often adding to kyphosis and instability in the long-term.[16,41] Laminoplasty, though advocated to preserve the ROM, has been shown to lead to progressive reduction in ROM on long-term follow up, indirectly giving better stability to the spine.[39,41,44,45,53] Ratliff and Cooper, in a meta-

analysis, found a progressive decrease in the ROM in 50% of patients (range 20%–80%).[39] Wada *et al.* in their comparison of the anterior versus the posterior approach reported a decrease in the ROM from 40% to 20% in the anterior group compared with 40% to 11% in the posterior group.[53]

OPLL progression

It has been well documented that in the long run both laminectomy and laminoplasty are associated with progression of OPLL in both the vertical and horizontal direction leading to neurological worsening. This is possibly due to preservation of motion in these segments. It is recommended that if OPLL is more than 7 mm in anterio–posterior depth or the spinal canal occupancy is more than 60%, the neurological outcome or recovery rate is poor. Also, if OPLL is of the hill type rather than the plateau type, the outcome in posterior decompression is poor.[16,41–44,51]

Complications of surgery

Complications of surgery are certainly higher with the anterior approach due to close proximity to important neurovascular structures. Common complications with the anterior approach are dysphagia, hoarseness of voice, pseudoarthrosis, implant failure, vascular injury, CSF leak, excessive bleeding from engorged veins, tracheo-oesophageal fistula and neurological worsening, especially C_5 radiculopathy.[34,57] Boayke *et al.* in a prospective 30-day review of data on cervical corpectomy from the Veterans Affairs National Surgical Quality Improvement program database of the USA comprising 1560 patients, found a hospital mortality of only 1.6%. Graft/implant-related complications accounted for 5.4%. Multivariate analysis showed that age more than 80 years, type I diabetes, American Association of Anesthesiologists' class >3 were significantly associated with the complications.

Corpectomy ≥3 levels too had a higher incidence of complications.[31] However, with increase in experience, refinement of techniques and low profile (i.e. thin cervical plates with good strength) and advanced (dynamic) cervical plating systems, complications are mostly avoidable or have fallen to 5%–7%.[16,23,41,48,57] Complications associated with the posterior approach, though fewer, include haematoma, infection, worsening of neck pain, neurological worsening in the form of radiculopathy due to cord shift or posterior instrumentation especially lateral mass or pedicle screws, progressive kyphosis, progression of OPLL and canal stenosis.[16,39–42,44,45]

Long-term, good functional outcome with the anterior approach especially with median corpectomy in various series and personal experience has led me to undertake anterior decompression routinely for up to 3 levels or occasionally 4 levels (Fig. 1), especially when there is a very thick OPLL or loss of lordosis (Figs 2, 3) or instability.[23,33,40,43,46–49,57] Corpectomy up to C_7 and fusion with D1 is likely to be unstable because of increased stress, as it is a junction between the mobile cervical and fixed dorsal spine. In such situations, a posterior fusion and stabilization is recommended. There are reports suggesting that combining 3 or more levels of corpectomy with posterior stabilization or what is called 360° fixation because of altered biomechanics or laminectomy with posterior stabilization for MCCM provides optimum decompression with good stabilization.[49,58,59] However, there is no consensus or clinical evidence to support 360° stabilization except in selected cases with probable instability. In experienced hands and by following certain surgical principles to avoid complications, the rate of complications has certainly come down over the years. The principle of the surgical technique I follow for anterior median corpectomy is given below.

Surgical steps for anterior median cervical corpectomy

Anaesthesia

Ideally, endoscope-assisted intubation should be given to avoid too much flexion, more so in an unstable spine. Cuff pressure should not be above

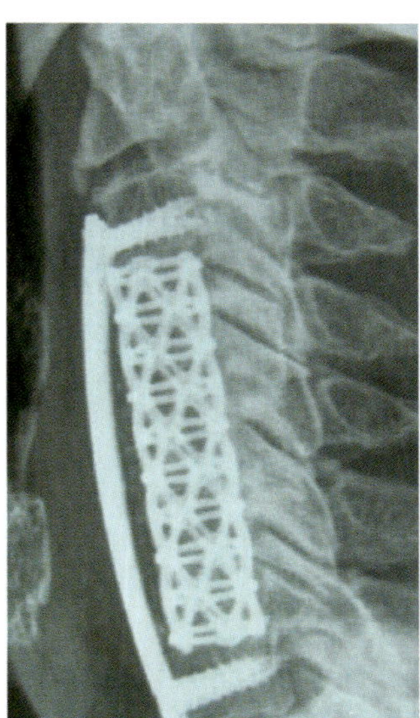

Fig. 1. Three-level corpectomy with TMC

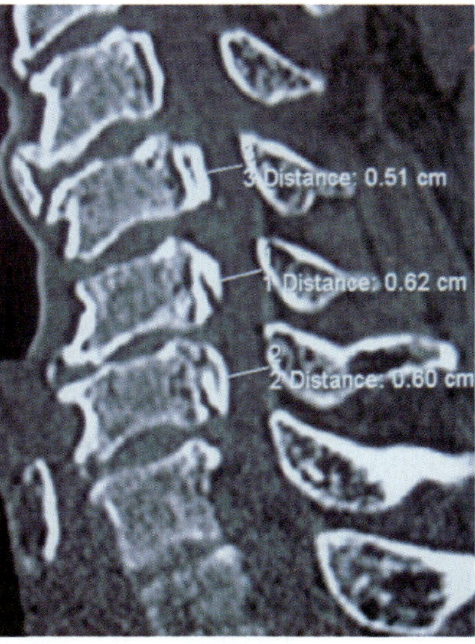

Fig. 2. Segmental OPLL with loss of lordosis

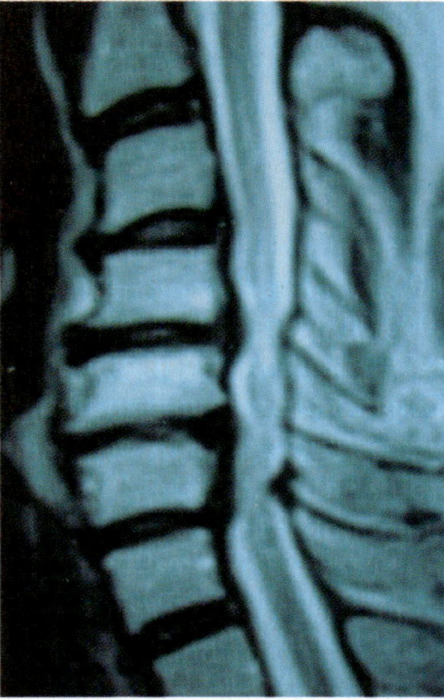

Fig. 3. Anterior compression with loss of lordosis

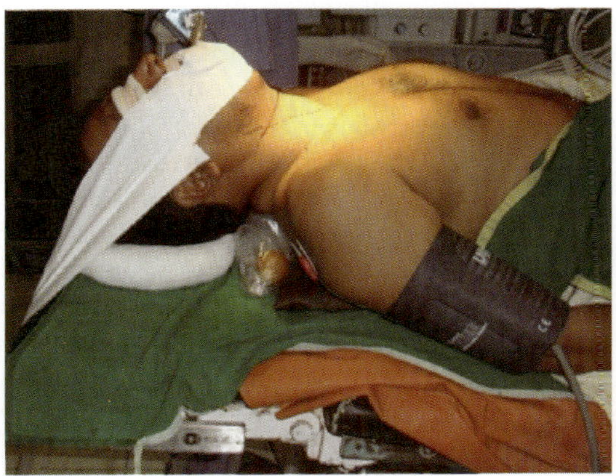

Fig. 4. Operative position

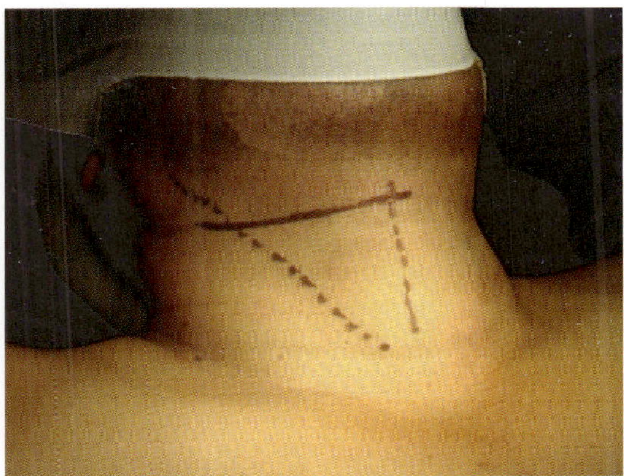

Fig. 5. Horizontal incision. Vertical line—midline; Oblique line —anterior border of sternocleidomastoid muscle

20 mm. After application of retractors, once deflate and re-inflate the cuff up to 15–20 mm to avoid traction injury to the recurrent laryngeal nerve (RLN).

Position (Fig. 4)

The patient should be supine with a roll between the shoulders, i.e. the cervico-dorsal junction and chin should be extended to give a lordotic extension to the cervical spine and increase the operative field, especially in those with a short neck. If there is gross instability, skull traction is applied to stabilize the spine during surgery. The chin can be maintained in position by adhesive straps. The shoulder is pulled down with adhesive tapes for better C-arm visualization of the lower cervical vertebrae. Too much skin traction is to be avoided as it can impair venous return and cause engorgement bleeding.

Incision and exposure (Fig. 5)

A horizontal cervical crease incision is made for up to 2-level corpectomy with 4-level fusion. A vertical–oblique incision is made medial to the sternocleidomastoid muscle in case of 3 or more

levels of exposure. The literature recommends a left-sided incision to avoid injury to the RLN. However, many reviews have not found any significant correlation between injury to the RLN and side of incision. I prefer a right-sided approach. The skin and platysma should be incised in the same plane for better cosmetic results. Undermine the skin flap for 1–2 cm on either side to increase exposure. The omohyoid muscle is divided for exposure below C_5. The RLN is more likely to be damaged at around the C_6 level and to avoid this it is advisable to remain in the pre-vertebral plane. The inferior thyroid artery and vein cross at C_6 and can be dissected and mobilized. If needed, they should be divided away from the thyroid gland. Exposure at C_4 and above carries a risk of damage to the superior laryngeal nerve. It runs from lateral to medial in juxtaposition with and behind the superior thyroid artery. It needs to be identified micro-scopically if the approach is above C_4 or remain in prevertebral plane. If the neck is short and in the lateral skiagram the angle of the mandible is seen at the lower level of the C_4 vertebra, then exposure of the C_2–C_3 disc space is difficult. In such situations, an anterior extrapharyngeal approach with mobilization of the submandi-bular gland, diagastric muscle and hypoglossal nerve is useful for exposure of C_2/C_3.[60]

Cervical retraction

Once the prevertebral fascia is exposed, it is divided longitudinally according to the extent of exposure needed. The vertebrae are identified and marked under the C-arm with a needle in the disc space. Both the longissimus colli muscles are identified and the centre of their medial borders is the midline. Both the longissimus colli muscles are stripped from the bone laterally with cautery and sharp dissection for a distance of approximately 5–7 mm. It is recommended to limit use of cautery beyond 5 mm and use sharp periosteal elevators instead to avoid damage to the vertebral artery, which is usually 9 mm away from the medial border of the longissimus colli at the level of the disc, but can be closer and tortuous in the elderly and if it is atherosclerotic. Cervical retractors are then placed with their inferior and outwardly directed jaws under these muscles and fixed to the retraction system (Fig. 6). The teeth of the blades should not be sharp and the retraction should be released intermittently as often as possible to avoid dysphagia and hoarseness.

Corpectomy

Discoidectomy is done at the desired levels. Initially, the vertebral bodies can be nibbled with roungers to create a gutter and also save bone for filling titanium mesh cages (TMC), if so desired. The gutter also prevents slippage of the drill from the smooth anterior surface of the bodies and prevents injury to important structures. Using a high-speed drill, vertebrectomy is done initially with 3 mm cutting burrs and then with diamond burrs once near the posterior surface of the bodies. It is important to remember that the depth is more at the disc level (because of osteophytes) than at the mid-body level. The side-to-side dimension of the gutter should be trapezoid, i.e. anterior approximately 12 mm wide and reaching 15–16 mm in depth (Fig. 7). The last millimetre of the posterior portion of the bodies should be removed with 1 mm karrison punches to avoid drill-related inadvertent injury to the spinal cord. In OPLL with dural involvement, it is better to thin the bone maximally and then make it float in the centre by freeing it from the side and superior–inferiorly with the help of punches. Thus, dural opening can be avoided.

Fusion and stabilization

For a tricortical strut graft of up to 8 cm, bone can be harvested from the anterior superior iliac spine. For larger segments, a fibular graft is used. After initially using these bones, I have changed to bone-filled TMC to avoid graft-related

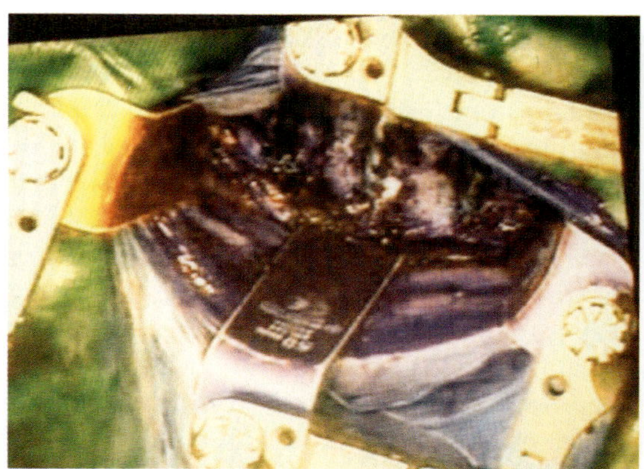

Fig. 6. Retractors placed under the longismuss muscle (red)

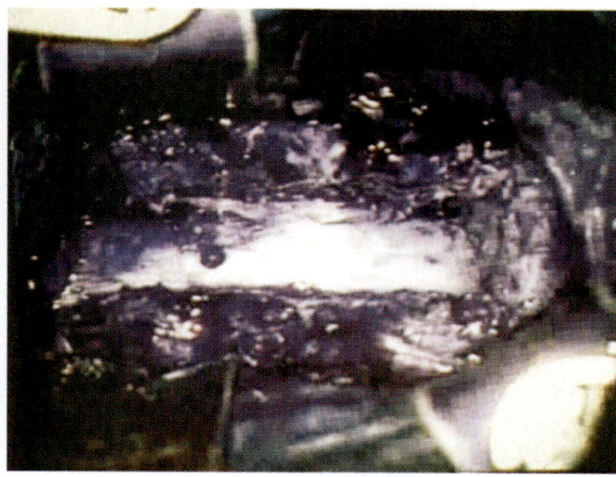

Fig. 7. Three-level corpectomy with dural exposure

complications (20%–30%). Since fusion with tricorticate cancellous bone is excellent, the use of a cervical plate and screws is optional. I have not used instrumentation when using a strut graft; graft-related complications are 5.5%. Use of a titanium plate still can prevent this complication and avoid subsidence. However, with TMC, a plate and screws are used for stabilization and the process of fusion can take a long time (Fig. 1). Finally, closure is always done with an external drain for 24 hours to avoid any haematoma collection.

Discussion

MCCM is a debilitating neurological problem. Once established, it usually progresses. Early intervention and decompression within 6 months to 1 year have shown good recovery rates.[2,3,5,9] Decompression of up to two levels is usually undertaken anteriorly with fusion, and has shown excellent results with few complications. There is no consensus on what is the best approach when more than 2 levels of decompression are required. The advent of laminoplasty in the eighties and further refinements in technique held the promise of providing equally good results with fewer complications than laminectomy and anterior decompression.[37,38] However, recent reports of long-term results and a meta-analysis show that it has fallen short of this promise. A recent review by Ratliff and Cooper of a meta-analysis failed to establish any advantage of laminoplasty over laminectomy over a long follow-up period.[39] Epstien in his review article recommended the posterior approach only for the geriatric population with a normally aligned spine and stated that in the young and elderly (above 75 years) with significant anterior compression, the posterior approach will fail to achieve good results. With significant OPLL, the posterior approach is likely to be associated with progressive neurological deterioration.[16,41] Iwasaki *et al.* from Osaka did only expansive

laminoplasty for OPLL from 1986 to 1996, and both anterior decompression and expansive laminoplasty from 1996 onwards. In their series up to 2003, they reported that with hill-type OPLL and an occupation ratio of >60% the results of anterior decompression were superior, while laminoplasty patients had either a fair or poor outcome.[42,43] There are other series reporting better outcomes with laminoplasty than the anterior approach. Recent reports have also recommended anterior decompression with posterior stabilization or laminectomy, and posterior stabilization with lateral mass screw and rod fixation for MCCM.[58,59] Ultimately, it is the experience of the surgeon and a customized approach to each patient that will provide the best outcome in each case. It is better to have experience with all approaches and apply them as per requirement than persist with one only approach.

In summary, the anterior approach is preferable for up to 3 levels or occasionally 4 levels when there is significant anterior compression, loss of cervical sagittal alignment, instability or for patients in the age group of ≤65 years. One may additionally do a posterior stabilization when the anterior construct spans ≥3 levels. Posterior decompression can be recommended for any compression, anterior or posterior, extending for more than 3 levels, and in the geriatric population that has a preserved lordotic alignment. However, there is a definite advantage of doing extensive laminectomy instead of laminoplasty with posterior stabilization for these indications in more than 3 levels of compression.

References

1. Clark C. In: Frymoyer JW (ed). *The Adult Spine: Principles and Practice.* 2nd ed. Philadelphia: Lippincott-Raven, 1997:1323–48.
2. Clark E, Robinson PK. Cervical myelopathy: A complication of cervical spondylosis. *Brain* 1956;**79**: 483.
3. Montgomery DM, Brower RS. Cervical myelopathy: clinical syndrome and natural history. *Orthop Clin*

North Am 1992;**23**:487–93.

4. Hayashi H, Okada K, Hashimoto J. Cervical spondylotic myelopathy in the aged patient: A radiographic evaluation of the aging changes in the cervical spine and etiologic factors of myelopathy. *Spine* 1988;**13**:618–25.

5. Matsunaga S, Sakou T, Taketomi E *et al.* Clinical course of patients with ossification of the posterior longitudinal ligament: A minimum 10-year cohort study. *J Neurosurg* 2004;**100**(3 suppl):245–48.

6. Rowland L (ed). *Merritt's textbook of neurology.* 9th ed. Pennsylvania: Williams and Wilkins, Media, 1995:455–59.

7. Teresi LM, Lufkin RB, Reicher MA *et al.* Asymptomatic degenerative disk disease and spondylosis of the cervical spine: MR imaging. *Radiology* 1987;**164**:83–8.

8. Crandall PH, Gregorius FK. Long-term follow-up of surgical treatment of cervical spondylotic myelopathy. *Spine* 1977;**2**:139–46.

9. McCormack BM, Weinstein PR. Cervical spondylosis. An update. *West J Med* 1996;**165**:43–51.

10. Fehlings MG, Skaf G. A review of the pathophysiology of cervical spondylotic myelopathy with insights for potential novel mechanisms drawn from traumatic spinal cord injury. *Spine* 1998;**23**:2730–37.

11. Firooznia H, Ahn JH, Rafii M, *et al.* Sudden quadriplegia after a minor trauma: The role of preexisting spinal stenosis. *Surg Neurol* 1985;**23**:165–8.

12. Penning L. *Functional pathology of the cervical spine.* Baltimore: Williams and Wilkens, 1968.

13. Brieg A, Turnbull I, Hassler O. Effects of mechanical stresses on the spinal cord in cervical spondylosis: A studyof fresh cadaver material. *J Neurosurg* 1996;**25**:45–8.

14. Reed JD. Effects of flexion-extension movements of the head and spine upon the spinal cord and nerve roots. *J Neurol Neurosurg Psychiatry* 1960;**23**:214–6.

15. Shoda E, Sumi M, Kataoka O, *et al.* Developmental and dynamic canal stenosis as radiologic factors affecting surgical results of anterior cervical fusion for myelopathy. *Spine (Phila Pa 1976)* 1999;**24**:1421–4.

16. Epstein NE. Review: Laminectomy for cervical myelopathy. *Spinal Cord* 2003;**41**:317–27.

17. Epstein JA, Epstein NE. The surgical management of cervical spinal stenosis, spondylosis, and myeloradiculopathy by means of the posterior approach. In: Clark CR (ed). The Cervical Spine Research Society Editorial Committee (Ed). *The Cervical Spine.* 2nd ed. JB Lippincott: Philadelphia 1989:625–43.

18. Kato Y, Iwasaki M. Fuji T, *et al.* Long-term follow-up results of laminectomy for cervical myelopathy caused by ossification of the posterior longitudinal ligament. *J Neurosurg* 1998;**89**:217–23.

19. Snow RB, Weiner H. Cervical laminectomy and foraminotomy as surgical treatment of cervical spondylosis: A follow-up study with analysis of failures. *J Spinal Disord* 1993;**6**:245–50.

20. Ebersold MJ, Pare MC, Quast LM. Surgical treatment for cervical spondylotic myelopathy. *J Neurosurg* 1995;**82**:745–51.

21. Yonenobu K Hosono N, Iwasaki M, *et al.* Neurologic complications of surgery for cervical compression myelopathy. *Spine* 1991;**16**:1277–82.

22. Kaptain GJ, Simmons NE, Replogle RE, *et al.* Incidence and outcome of kyphotic deformity following laminectomy for cervical spondylotic myelopathy. *J Neurosurg (US)* 2000;**92**(2 Suppl):199–204.

23. Banerji D, Acharya R, Behari S, *et al.* Corpectomy for multilevel cervical spondylosis and ossification of the posterior longitudinal ligament. *Neurosurg Rev* 1997;**20**:25–31.

24. Epstein NE.The surgical management of ossification of the posterior longitudinal ligament in 51 patients. *J Spinal Disord* 1993;**6**:432–54.

25. Epstein NE. Advanced cervical spondylosis with ossification into the posterior longitudinal ligament and resultant neurological sequelae. *J Spinal Disord* 1996;**9**:477–84.

26. Kawano H, Handa Y, Ishii H, *et al.* Surgical treatment for ossification of the posterior longitudinal ligament of the cervical spine. *J Spinal Disord* 1995;**8**:145–50.

27. Saunders, RL, Bernini PM, Shirreffs TG Jr, *et al.* Central corpectomy for cervical spondylotic myelopathy: A consecutive series with long-term followup. *J Neurosurg* 2002;**97**(2 Suppl):176–9.

28. Emery SE, Bohlman HH, Bolesta MJ, *et al.* Anterior cervical decompression and arthrodesis for the treatment of cervical spondylotic myelopathy. Two to seventeen-year follow-up. *J Bone Joint Surg Am* 1998;**80**:941–51.

29. Williams KE, Paul R, Dewan Y. Functional outcome of corpectomy in cervical spondylotic myelopathy. *Ind J Orthopedics* 2009;**43**:205–9.

30. Saunders RL, Bernini PM, Shirreffs TG Jr, *et al.* Central corpectomy for spondylotic myelopathy: A consecutive series with long-term follow-up evaluation cervical. *J Neurosurg* 1991;**74**:163–70.

31. Boakye M, Patil CG, Ho C, *et al.* Cervical corpectomy:

Complications and outcomes. *Neurosurgery* 2008;**63** (4 Suppl 2):295–301; discussion 301–2.

32. Beutler WJ, Sweeney CA, Connolly PJ. Recurrent laryngeal nerve injury with anterior cervical spine surgery: Risk with laterality of surgical approach. *Spine* 2001;**26**:1337–42.

33. Saunders RL, Pikus HJ, Ball P. Four-level cervical corpectomy. *Spine (Phila Pa 1976)* 1998;**23**:2455–61.

34. Hiarabayashi K, Bohlman HH. Multilevel cervical spondylosis. Laminoplasty versus anterior decompression. *Spine* 1995;**20**:1732–34.

35. Yonenobu K, Hosono N, Iwasaki M, *et al.* Laminoplasty versus subtotal corpectomy. *Spine* 1992;**17**:1281–84.

36. Hirabyashi K. Expansive open-door laminoplasty for cervical spondylotic myelopathy. *Shujutu* 1978;**32**: 1159–63.

37. Hirabyashi K, Satomi K. Operative procedure and results of open-door laminoplasty. *Spine* 1988;**13**: 870–76.

38. Kawai S, Sunago K, Doi K, *et al.* Cervical laminoplasty (Hattori's method): Procedure and follow-up results. *Spine* 1998;**13**:1245–50.

39. Ratliff JK, Cooper PR. Cervical laminoplasty: A critical review. *J Neurosurg* 2003;**98**(3 Suppl):230–8.

40. Masaki Y, Yamazaki M, Okawa A, *et al.* An analysis of factors causing poor surgical outcome in patients with cervical myelopathy due to ossification of the posterior longitudinal ligament: Anterior decompression with spinal fusion versus laminoplasty. *J Spinal Disord Tech* 2007;**20**:7–13.

41. Epstein N. Posterior approaches in the management of cervical spondylosis and ossification of the longitudinal ligament. *Surg Neurol* 2002;**58**:194–207; discussion 207–8.

42. Iwasaki M, Okuda S, Miyauchi A, *et al.* Surgical strategy for cervical myelopathy due to ossification of the posterior longitudinal ligament, Part 1: Clinical results and limitations of laminoplasty. *Spine (Phila Pa 1976)* 2007;**32**:647–53.

43. Iwasaki M, Okuda S, Miyauchi A, *et al.* Surgical strategy for cervical myelopathy due to ossification of the posterior longitudinal ligament, Part 2: Advantages of anterior decompression and fusion over laminoplasty. *Spine (Phila Pa 1976)* 2007;**32**: 654–60.

44. Hale JJ, Gruson KI, Spivak JM. Laminoplasty: A review of its role in compressive cervical myelopathy. *Spine J* 2009;**9**:426; author reply 426–7.

45. Chiba K, Ogawa Y, Ishii K, *et al.* Long-term results of expansive open-door laminoplasty for cervical myelopathy—average 14-year follow-up study. *Spine (Phila Pa 1976)* 2006;**31**:2998–3005.

46. Chagas H, Domingues F, Aversa A, *et al.* Cervical spondylotic myelopathy: 10 years of prospective outcome analysis of anterior decompression and fusion. *Surg Neurol* 2005;**64** Suppl 1:S130–5.

47. Vedantam R, Kumar G, Sujith S. Functional outcome after central corpectomy in poor-grade patients with cervical spondylotic myelopathy or ossified posterior longitudinal ligament. *Neurosurgery* 2005;**56**:1279–85.

48. Mayr MT, Subach BR, Comey CH, *et al.* Cervical spinal stenosis: Outcome after anterior corpectomy, allograft reconstruction, and instrumentation. *J Neurosurg* 2002;**96**(1 Suppl):10–6.

49. Koller H, Hempfing A, Ferraris L, *et al.* 4- and 5-level anterior fusions of the cervical spine: Review of literature and clinical results. *Eur Spine J* 2007;**16**: 2055–71.

50. Chiba K, Toyama Y, Matsumoto M, *et al.* Segmental motor paralysis after expansive open-door laminoplasty. *Spine (Phila Pa 1976)* 2002;**27**:2108–15.

51. Hori T, Kawaguchi Y, Kimura T. How does the ossification area of the posterior longitudinal ligament thicken following cervical laminoplasty? *Spine (Phila Pa 1976)* 2007;**32**:E551–6.

52. Chiba K, Yamamoto I, Hirabayashi H, *et al.* Multicenter study investigating the postoperative progression of ossification of the posterior longitudinal ligament in the cervical spine: A new computer-assisted measurement. *J Neurosurg Spine* 2005;**3**:17–23.

53. Wada E, Suzuki S, Kanazawa, A, *et al.* Subtotal corpectomy versus laminoplasty for multilevel cervical spondylotic myelopathy: A long-term follow-up study over 10 years. *Spine* 2001;**26**:1443–47.

54. Edwards CC 2nd, Heller JG, Murakami H. Corpectomy versus laminoplasty for multilevel cervical myelopathy: An independent matched-cohort analysis. *Spine (Phila Pa 1976)* 2002;**27**:1168–75.

55. Cabraja M, Abbushi A, Koeppen D, *et al.* Comparison between anterior and posterior decompression with instrumentation for cervical spondylotic myelopathy: Sagittal alignment and clinical outcome. *Neurosurg Focus* 2010;**28**:E15.

56. Ryken TC, Heary RF, Matz PG, *et al.* Cervical laminectomy for the treatment of cervical degenerative myelopathy. *J Neurosurg Spine* 2009;**11**:142–9.

57. Jain SK, Salunke PS, Vyas KH, *et al.* Multisegmental

cervical ossification of the posterior longitudinal ligament: Anterior vs posterior approach. *Neurology India* 2005;**53**:283–5.

58. Houten JK, Cooper PR. Laminectomy and posterior cervical plating for multilevel cervical spondylotic myelopathy and ossification of the posterior longitudinal ligament: Effects on cervical alignment, spinal cord compression, and neurological outcome. *Neurosurgery* 2003;**52**:1081–7.

59. Yu Chen, Guo Y, Chen D, *et al.* Long-term outcome of laminectomy and instrumented fusion for cervical ossification of the posterior longitudinal ligament. *Int Orthop* 2009;**33**:1075–80.

60. Behari S, Banerji D, Trivedi P, *et al.* Anterior retropharyngeal approach to the cervical spine. *Neurol Ind* 2001;**49**:342–9.

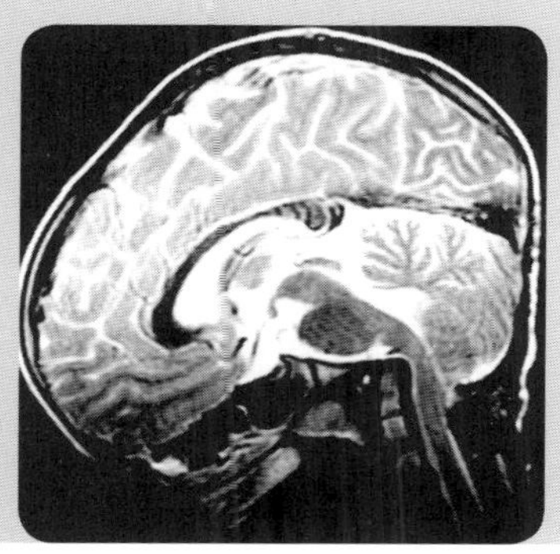

Clinical neurology

19

Tic disorders

PUNIT AGRAWAL

Introduction

Recurrent tics are most commonly associated with inheritable neuropsychiatric conditions that fall within a spectrum of classified disorders. These have a typical onset and prevalence during childhood and adolescence. Adult-onset tic disorders are far less frequent, and can sometimes be attributable to an exacerbation of a pre-existing condition. Individuals who are genetically predisposed and have a positive family history of tic disorders may develop tics themselves after an illness, increased life stresses, or toxin/drug exposure.

Even when there is a lack of family history, secondary causes of tics due to toxin/drugs, structural lesions and other causes are reported to occur at any age. Secondary tic disorders can also have similar neuropsychiatric features as primary tic disorder. At this time, there is no specific biomarker for the diagnosis of a primary tic disorder, and thus the diagnosis is based on history and clinical findings. Differentiating tics from other abnormal movements is also sometimes difficult, particularly if due to a secondary aetiology that has other concurrent abnormal movements or other neuropsychiatric overlay. However, there are certain aspects to an individual's history and presentation of tics that will help with the diagnosis, as discussed later in this chapter.

Every individual with a tic disorder varies with regard to the severity of the tic, its frequency, location and the degree of impairment it causes. In many cases of primary tic disorders, the tics themselves may be mild and minimally bothersome, and often require no major pharmacological intervention. However, there is an increased risk of concurrent psychiatric and behavioural problems in individuals with primary tic disorders, particularly those reported with Tourette syndrome. It is it not uncommon for these psychiatric and behavioural aspects of an individual's presentation to be more disabling than the actual tics. Early identification of any concurrent issues is important as this allows for prompt initiation of psychiatric or behavioural therapy, which can lead to a marked improvement in function and quality of life. With this in mind, it is now being increasingly accepted that a multidisciplinary team approach to the treatment of tic disorders and co-morbid behavioural/ psychiatric conditions tends to provide the best possible outcomes. This team should include the primary care physician, neurologist, psychiatrist, psychologist, the family and teachers.

Definitions

Tics are described as intermittent sudden, rapid, repetitive, non-rhythmic, purposeless abnormal movements (motor tic) or vocalization (phonic tic).[1-3] These can be classified into simple or complex. *Simple motor* tics are repeated partial or brief movements without a purpose, and commonly involve only one muscle group. Some examples of simple motor tics include head turning, facial grimacing, mouth opening, tongue movement, eye blinking or closure, shoulder shrugging, arm jerking and abdominal tightening. *Complex motor* tics appear as stereotypical normal activities or a sequence of movements done at random times, again with no purpose. Some examples include head shaking, throwing, kicking or jumping. There are a few specific complex motor tics. Mimicking someone else's movement is termed *echopraxia*, and inappropriate or obscene gestures are termed *copropraxia*. *Dystonic tics* are described as prolonged motor tics that cause a sustained posturing, and may be attributed to interruption and blocking of further tics.

Simple vocal tics are commonly meaningless sounds such as grunts. They may include sniffing, snorting, throat clearing, yelling or sucking noises. These can be further described as the simple passage of air through the vocal cords, pharynx, larynx, mouth or nasal passages. Linguistically meaningful syllables, partial words, full words or phrases are considered *complex vocal tics*. Some forms of complex vocal tics also have specific terminology such as repeating someone else's words (*echolalia*), repeating one's own words (*palilalia*) or making verbal obscene or socially inappropriate utterances (*coprolalia*). Coprolalia is rare and occurs in less than 10% of individuals with Tourette syndrome.[4]

Tics can initially appear to be similar to other movements or disorders such as compulsions, stereotypical behaviour, fidgeting, myoclonus, chorea or dystonia. Differentiating tics from these can sometimes be difficult, but there are certain distinguishing features. The characteristic abnormal movement or vocalization described as a tic is usually associated with *premonitory sensory phenomena*. These are commonly described as an irresistible urge, tension, build-up or other discomfort that is alleviated by the performance of the tic.[1,3,5] The occurrence of sensory phenomena is reported in 90% of adolescents, but this sensation may not be obvious to all patients initially as awareness of premonitory urges increases with age.[6] The premonitory sensation is often localized in the same region as the tic, but can sometimes be a more diffuse, unpleasant feeling.

With the preceding sensation, tics can often be voluntarily suppressed temporarily. However, the suppression can lead to a build-up reported as a rebound, which leads to an exaggerated performance of the abnormal movement or vocalization.[5] Further, it has been noted that the concentration needed to suppress tics during school can lead to reduced attention to performing well in school.[7,8] Tics are also usually less frequent during periods of attention and activities. Tics performed at home may be worse due to the daytime suppression during school hours. During the summer vacation there is less overall tic performance. The presence of this rebound effect is under continuing debate, with a few studies finding no obvious evidence of the phenomenon.[3,9]

It is also common for tics to be highly suggestible, with an increase in tic performance when they are the main topic of conversation, such as during visits to a physician's office. Another interesting aspect of tics that set these movements aside from other movement disorders is that these may persist during sleep.[9] Overall, tics have a natural tendency to wax and wane within an hour, day and week.

Classification

Though tics are part of the spectrum of a disorder, they have certain features that are used to classify and diagnose primary tic disorders as described in the *Diagnostic and Statistical Manual of Mental Disorders*, 4th edition (DSM-IV). Important aspects include the presence or absence of both motor and vocal tics, and the onset and duration the tic disorder. Further, when diagnosing a primary tic disorder, it must be ensured that a secondary cause such as drugs or a neurodegenerative condition has been ruled out.

The most common and well known tic disorder is *Tourette syndrome*. This neuropsychiatric condition is defined by a duration of tics for over 12 months, and must include the presence of both multiple motor tics and at least one vocal tic at some period during the duration of tic symptoms. The age of onset is before the age of 18 years.[1,10]

The other syndromes described in the DSM-IV represent the spectrum of tic disorders that do not reach the diagnostic criteria of Tourette syndrome, and may also not encompass the severity or co-morbid issues more commonly associated with it. In *chronic motor tic disorder*, there is an absence of vocal tics during the course of the disease and with onset before the age of 18 years. Similarly, in *chronic vocal tic disorder*, there is an absence of motor tics and also with the onset before the age of 18 years. Again, this diagnosis requires tics to be present for >12 months. Tic disorders lasting for <1 year and >4 weeks are diagnosed as *transient motor tic disorder, transient vocal tic disorder*, or *transient motor and vocal tic disorder*. Any tic disorder falling outside the criteria for age of onset or duration <4 weeks is diagnosed as *tic disorder, not otherwise specified*.

Secondary tic disorders

Though far less common than primary tic disorders, an increasing number of case studies are reporting secondary causes of tics. In several of these studies, there were associated co-morbid psychobehavioural issues such as attention deficit or obsessive compulsion similar to that seen in primary tic disorders (*discussed below*).

Deep brain lesions that include damage to the basal ganglia due to ischaemia from stroke, hypoxia and carbon monoxide have been found to cause tics as well as psychobehavioural symptoms.[11–15]

The development of neuropsychiatric symptoms following these specific lesions is similar to those seen with primary tic disorders. This has led to the basal ganglia being considered as the primary site of pathology in all tic disorders. However, the symptoms of both transient and chronic tic disorder have been identified following traumatic brain injury, with lesions in both the basal ganglia and frontal lobe areas.[16–17]

In addition, more diffuse lesions in the brain involving the deep brain structures including the basal ganglia have also been reported to cause sequelae of chronic tic disorders. This was particularly seen in post-mortem studies identifying involvement of the basal ganglia and other areas from brains of individuals with tic disorders following the 1916–1927 pandemic of encephalitic lethargica.[18–19]

Other infectious causes for encephalitis associated with case reports of subsequent tic disorders include varicella zoster, *Mycoplasma pneumoniae*, herpes simplex, Lyme disease and human immunodeficiency virus.[20–22] There is also ongoing debate and investigation with regard to the development of tic disorders, particularly Tourette syndrome, in association with group A beta-haemolytic streptococci.[23,24]

Immune disorders with symptoms that can lead to primary central nervous system involvement, such as antiphospholipid antibody syndrome, have been reported in association with symptoms of tic disorders.[25,26] It has been theorized that these infectious and immunological disorders may primarily target the basal ganglia. This can lead to tic disorder with both neurological and psychiatric involvement, and has prompted investigation to identify antibodies against the basal ganglia with positive results.[27]

This suggests that the primary target of dysfunction in both primary and secondary tic disorders is the basal ganglia. This would help explain the reports of tics that appear in certain neurodegenerative conditions with specific basal ganglia pathology such as neuroacanthocytosis, Huntington disease, Wilson disease, and neurodegeneration with brain iron accumulation (previously termed Hallervorden–Spatz disease).[21,28–33]

Numerous drugs that may have an increased risk for causing or exacerbating tic disorders have been identified. These include cocaine, heroin, amphetamines, methylphenidate, caffeine, antidepressants, dopamine-blocking drugs, levodopa, pemoline, carbamazepine, phenytoin, phenobarbitol and lamotrigine. Though many of these have a diffuse central nervous system effect, it can be theorized that they can also alter primary function within the basal ganglia, which can lead to features of tic disorder.[21,34–42]

Epidemiology and history of primary tic disorders

The onset of primary tic disorders with motor tics is most common between the ages of 3 and 8 years, with peak severity between 8 and 12 years of age in chronic disorders.[43] The location of the tic at onset is most commonly in the eyes (blinking), face, head and neck.[43] The age of onset of tics associated with transient tic disorders and chronic tic disorders including Tourette syndrome is similar. It is estimated that over 90% of tics due to Tourette syndrome start by the age of 11 years.[44,45] Transient tic disorders is the most common childhood tic syndrome present in about 1 out of 10 children,[46] with some studies finding an average prevalence of 20% in the community.[47,48] There is commonly a rostrocaudal progression of tics in those individuals who go on to develop tics of the trunk or limb.[43]

Tics that persist and become chronic often have a peak occurrence between the ages of 8 and 12 years, followed by a slow decline until early adulthood. The development of complex motor tics is usually preceded by simple motor tics and, with time and brain development, may turn into more elaborate, involved motor movements descriptive of complex motor tics. Vocal tics also may develop in the early years of childhood. In Tourette syndrome, vocal tics are typically not seen for 1–2 years after the onset of motor tics; these have an average age of onset of around 8 years. Similar to complex motor tics, simple vocal tics develop first and, over time, change to complex vocal tics in later adolescence in those predisposed.[43] Coprolalia is not common and is usually only associated with Tourette syndrome. The age of onset is around 15 years.[49] Observational studies have estimated the prevalence of chronic motor or vocal tic disorders (excluding Tourette syndrome) to be about 5%. Less than 5% of patients with chronic tic disorders have isolated vocal tics.[46]

Progression of a tic disorder to both multiple motor and vocal tics to a diagnosis of Tourette syndrome has an estimated worldwide prevalence of 1–30 per 1000 children and adolescents.[48,50] Tourette syndrome is more common in males than females with a ratio of 4:1.[48,50,51] Throughout the course of Tourette syndrome and other chronic tic disorders, the tics tend to wax and wane in frequency and severity during the course of the day, week and month. This variability can be attributed to stress, anxiety, excitement, fatigue and engagement in activities. It is also often noted that individuals with tic disorders have fewer tics during activities involving fine motor skills such as playing video games and instruments, and during sports.

The natural development of compensatory mechanisms with modification, along with continued brain development, may lead to attenuation of tic performance over time, but with periods of exacerbation due to other factors. As individuals with chronic tic disorders reach adulthood, there is a marked reduction in the frequency and severity of tics, and only 50%

persist into adulthood. However, the majority of tics are mild and often not recognized by affected individuals.[50–54]

Co-morbid psychiatric and behavioural symptoms

Over time, Tourette syndrome is increasingly being recognized as a neuropsychiatric condition. It is estimated that three-fourths of children with Tourette syndrome have mild tics, and that the presence of concurrent psychiatric or behavioural problems can often be the primary cause of functional impairment.[48,51,55] The other primary tic disorders, in particular, chronic motor tic disorders, are also associated with a higher incidence of co-morbid psychiatric and behavioural problems.[56,57]

The most commonly reported co-morbid psychobehavioural problems include attention deficit hyperactivity disorder (ADHD), obsessive–compulsive disorder (OCD), learning difficulties, impaired executive function, rage attacks, emotional problems, mood and anxiety symptoms, oppositional defiant disorder, and other disruptive behaviours.[58,59] These co-morbid issues can cause markedly more problems, extending from poor peer acceptance, low self-esteem, decreased academic performance, and overall impaired psychosocial function.[58–61] If not recognized and addressed early, these psycho-behavioural issues can lead to significant impairment that can persist into adult life.

The two most commonly recognized co-morbid psychobehavioural problems seen in the spectrum of Tourette syndrome are ADHD and OCD.[62] OCD occurs in about half the individuals with Tourette syndrome, and becomes more severe several years after the peak age of tics.[63] Compulsions due to OCD (repetitive intrusive thoughts leading to performance of a purposeful movement or action to alleviate the associated anxiety) can be sometimes mistaken for tics (pre-monitory urge with associated non-purposeful movement), which can confound treatment. It is also not uncommon for individuals with both tics and compulsive disorders to have a mix of both in an abnormal movement, such as performance of specific tic a certain number of times. One interesting aspect in treating OCD and tic disorders associated with Tourette syndrome is that these both tend to lessen with dopamine-blocking agents, suggesting a common pathological neurochemical process for these two problems. The response to selective-serotonin reuptake inhibitors in those with OCD symptoms and Tourette syndrome is not as good as in those without Tourette syndrome.[64,65]

ADHD is seen in more than half the individuals with Tourette syndrome.[59] It is usually present before the onset of tic symptoms.[55] Treatment of ADHD with psychostimulants has been contro-versial, as they have the potential to exacerbate tics.[42] However, other studies have provided conflicting data, suggesting that psychostimulants such as methylphenidate do not worsen tics.[66] Combination treatment with methylphenidate for the ADHD plus the alpha-2 agonist clonidine for the tics is an effective strategy for treating individuals with Tourette syndrome and ADHD.[67] Along with attention problems, children and adolescents with Tourette syndrome have a higher incidence of learning problems,[60,61] and an increased need for special education classes.[4,68] Difficulty with school performance may have multiple causes, including the direct effects of the tics and concurrent psychological/behavioural abnormalities in addition to learning disabilities.[69–74]

These concurrent co-morbid issues in Tourette syndrome and other primary tic disorders emphasize the need for a team approach to treating these syndromes. Such a team would consist of experts from several medical disciplines, the family and teachers.

Adult tic disorders

The most likely cause of tic disorders in adult life is the extension of a tic disorder originally present during childhood or adolescence, or a due to secondary aetiology (as discussed above).[15,33,75,76] In most individuals with primary tic syndromes, there is a marked reduction in tic severity and frequency through late adolescence and early adult life. Thus, the tics are less persistent and troublesome in adults. The true prevalence of primary tic disorders that persist into adult life is not well established, partially due to compensatory mechanisms and improved ability to suppress tics as adulthood approaches.[43] However, an estimated one-third of children with Tourette syndrome reported freedom from tics by early adulthood, with about half reporting mild persisting tics, and less than a quarter reporting moderate or severe tics.[77]

Individuals in whom severe tics persist into adult life may have had lower academic qualifications, which may affect the attainment of higher levels of education or employment.[60,61] Further, individuals who have persistent, debilitating tics or co-morbid behavioural/psychiatric issues may also find it difficult to hold on to a job, leading to increased rates of unemployment or disability.[61]

The onset of a primary tic disorder during adult life is rare, and it is suspected that individuals reporting an adult onset without an identifiable cause may have had milder unrecognized tics as a child.[43,78,79]

Pathophysiology of tic disorders

The pathophysiology of tic disorders remains unclear, though it is now more widely accepted that these are genetic disorders with a mixed pattern of inheritance. An estimated 10–100-fold risk of developing Tourette syndrome has been seen in first-degree relatives of those with a tic disorder.[80–83]

No single gene or chromosome has been identified, but reports suggest that several different genetic loci may be involved including areas on chromosomes 2, 5, 6, 8, 10, 11, 13, 14, 20, 21 and X.[84–89]

Continued investigation supports involvement of the corticostriatothalamocortical pathways with primary dysfunction of the basal ganglia and frontal cortex.[90,91] The corticostriatothalamocortical pathway has different circuit patterns concerned with both motor and behavioural modification:[92–94]

- Motor—supplementary motor cortex to the putamen
- Oculomotor—premotor frontal cortex (frontal eye fields) to the central caudate
- Dorsolateral prefrontal (planning and executive function)—Dorsolateral prefrontal cortex (Brodmann's area 9) and anterior prefrontal cortex (Brodmann's area 10) to dorsolateral caudate
- Anterior cingulate (limbic)—anterior cingulate cortex to ventral striatum (nucleus accumbens, ventromedial caudate/putamen and olfactory tubercle)
- Lateral orbitofrontal circuit-inferolateral prefrontal cortex to ventromedial caudate.

Integration of these circuits could provide an explanation for the sensory phenomena and motor symptoms of tic disorders, as well as associated co-morbid psychological and behavioural issues. Further, it has been proposed that the inability to adequately inhibit unwanted sensory input due to changes in function of the basal ganglia within these circuits could be a common link that may contribute to the development of the tics, OCD, impulse control, and even ADHD, as seen in individuals with Tourette syndrome.[95]

The clinical improvement seen with dopamine-blocking agents and findings on PET scan of increased striatal dopaminergic activity in Tourette syndrome[96] suggest that the primary area of dysfunction could be increased striatal interneurons leading to excessive activity in the direct pathway of the basal ganglia, leading to an abnormal increase in thalamocortical activity.[97]

However, volumetric MRI studies provide data that contradict this hypothesis. MRI findings include loss of volume of the caudate and lenticular nuclei, which can be correlated with increased tic severity. In addition, the lesser volume of the lenticular nuclei also correlate with OCD symptoms in children and persistence of Tourette syndrome into adulthood.[98,99] Other pathological studies have shown that individuals with Tourette syndrome lose cells from the caudate nuclei and globus pallidus externus, as well as an increase in the cells of the globus pallidus internus. This is consistent with the findings of an increase in parvalbumin-positive gamma-aminobutyric acidergic neurons in the globus pallidus internus.[90]

Apart from the basal ganglia, imaging studies have identified cortical changes. These include an increase in volume of the dorsal prefrontal and parieto-occipital areas, smaller inferior occipital areas,[100] and thinning of the sensorimotor cortical areas.[101,102] The severity of tics has been found to increase in those with more volume loss in the orbitofrontal and sensorimotor cortical areas.[100] An increase in size of the white matter tracts under the pre- and post-central gyri and changes in the size of the corpus callosum have also been associated with an increase in tic severity.[103–105]

It is not certain which of these changes are due to direct pathology and which are due to changes in brain activity over time. Much emphasis has been placed on functional imaging in recent years and these may help in identifying areas of the brain active during different components of tic production and performance. Premonitory sensory phenomena that occur before the onset of a tic have been found to correlate with increased activity in the sensory association, anterior cingulate and supplemental motor cortical areas.[106] Tic suppression has been found to be associated with some cortical areas with increased activity and other areas with decreased activity.[107] The performance of tics has been associated with increased activity in the primary motor and Broca's cortical areas, in addition to diminished activity in the anterior cingulate and sup-plemental motor areas.[106,108–110] A longitudinal study on these increased areas of activities may provide further insight and help delineate the sequence of early versus late changes associated with tic disorders.

Treatment of tics

An abnormal history or findings on clinical examination should provoke further investigation to find a secondary cause, especially in those individuals who present with initial symptoms after the second decade of life. This may include brain imaging, electroencephalography, serological, urine or cerebral spinal fluid studies depending on individual cases.[111]

In addition to assessing tics, it is also important to ask about features suggestive of the presence of any co-morbid psychobehavioural or learning disability. There should be a multi-disciplinary treatment team comprising the primary care doctor, neurologist, psychiatrist, psychologist and teacher. Implementing proper therapy and a teaching environment early may result in better ability to overcome some of the obstacles that could lead to future impairment and dysfunction. It is also important to educate patients and the family on the natural history of tics such as waxing/waning, exacerbating factors and tendency for a natural reduction in the frequency and severity of tics as the child grows older. Teachers and classmates may also need to be told that the tics are not voluntary or purposeful.

Treatment of tics with a combination of cognitive–behavioural therapy and medications is often the most effective. Before starting any medication for tics, it must first be established that the tics are adding to dysfunction by adequately assessing for tic duration, frequency, intensity, quantity, complexity and anatomical location. The Yale Global Tic Severity Scale is a useful tool for this.[112] Mild tics can often be left untreated, but when starting medications for more bothersome tics, the patient and family require proper education about the side-effects of medication, especially those that may result in impaired learning and concentration due to sedation or cognitive impairment. Trial and error of medications may be needed in order to find an effective agent without troublesome side-effects. Further, it must be made clear that the goal of treatment is to improve function and not eliminate all tics.[113,114]

The two classes of medications most useful in reducing tic severity are dopamine-blocking agents and alpha-2 adrenergic drugs. The most common alpha-2 adrenergic agents are clonidine and guanfacine. Both of these have the potential to cause sedation, lightheadedness, headache and even irritability. These agents can sometimes also be useful for ADHD, if present; thus the choice of treatment may also depend on concurrent co-morbid issues.[111]

Dopamine-blocking agents with D2 properties are often most effective in reducing tics, but have an increased risk of side-effects such as sedation, cognitive impairment, weight gain, cardiac arrhythmia and tardive syndromes.[111,115] These medications are also effective in treating concurrent OCD symptoms.[116] The most common ones used due to their effectiveness at low doses are pimozide, haloperidol and fluphenazine. The newer dopamine-blocking neuroleptic medications such as risperidone, olanzapine, ziprasidone, and aripiprazole are also effective in reducing tics, but not clozapine and quetiapine.[111,113]

Other drugs that may be helpful for the treatment of tics include clonazepam. There is increasing evidence of the benefits of tetrabenazine in cases with persistent bothersome tics.[117,118] It was thought that gamma aminobutyric acid agents may have less potential side-effects, but there has not been any strong evidence to support the use of agents such as levetiracetam.[119–120] Dystonic tics, some vocal tics and some focal simple tics have been found to respond to a local injection of botulinum toxin.[121–124]

There is an increasing body of evidence supporting the effectiveness of deep brain stimulation therapy in reducing severe, disabling medication-refractory tics. Such therapy may be targeted at the thalamic nuclei (ventralis oralis complex and the centromedian parafascicular nuclei), globus pallidus internus, and nucleus accumbens/anterior limb of the internal capsule.[125–127]

One of the most effective therapies in the area of behavioural therapy is habit reversal training (HRT), which is repeated a few times a week over several months. This modality of treatment incorporates self-monitoring, awareness training, competing response training, motivation enhancement, generalization training, contingency management and relaxation training.[128] Behavioural treatment modalities include a number of psychosocial interventions, including massed negative practice, contingency management, exposure and response prevention, and cognitive–behavioural therapy.[129]

Conclusion

It is now recognized that tics represent a spectrum of disorders with neurological and psychological manifestations that usually begin in childhood, but can also affect adults. Though primarily a genetic disorder, there are increasing case reports of secondary causes of tic disorders, some of which have helped in identifying the pathological processes in tic generation. Irrespective of the aetiology of the tic disorder, it is important to establish that the goal of treatment is to improve overall function through a multidisciplinary approach. Treatment modalities include medication, behavioural therapy and surgical intervention. Early recognition of the disease may allow for a reduction in disability and improve the quality of life of those affected by tic disorders.

References

1. American Psychiatric Association. Task force on nomenclature and statistics. *Diagnostic and statistical manual of mental disorders.* 4th edition (DSM-IV). Washington DC: APA; 1994.
2. The Tourette Syndrome Classification Study Group. Definitions and classification of tic disorders. *Arch Neurol* 1993;**50**:1013–16.

3. Leckman JF, Peterson BS, King RA, *et al.* Phenomenology of tics and natural history of tic disorders. *Adv Neurol* 2001;**85**:1–14.

4. Erenberg G, Cruse RP, Rothner AD. Tourette syndrome: An analysis of 200 pediatric and adolescent cases. *Cleve Clin Q* 1986;**53**:127–31.

5. Leckman JF, Walker DE, Cohen DJ. Premonitory urges in Tourette's syndrome. *Am J Psychiatry* 1993; **150**:98–102.

6. Woods DW, Piacentini J, Himle MB, *et al.* Premonitory Urge for Tics Scale (PUTS): Initial psychometric results and examination of the premonitory urge phenomenon in youths with Tic disorders. *J Dev Behav Pediatr* 2005;**26**:397–403.

7. Himle MB, Woods DW, Conelea CA, *et al.* Investigating the effects of tic suppression on premonitory urge ratings in children and adolescents with Tourette's syndrome. *Behav Res Ther* 2007;**45**:2964–76.

8. Jankovic J. Tourette's syndrome. *N Engl J Med* 2001; **345**:1184–92. Comment in: *N Engl J Med* 2002;**346**: 710.

9. Jankovic J. Tics and Tourette's syndrome. In: Jankovic J, Tolosa E (eds). *Parkinson's disease and movement disorders*. 5th ed. Philadelphia: Lippincott Williams and Wilkins; 2007:356–75.

10. Gilles de la Tourette G. Etude sur une affection nerveuse caractérisée par de l'incoordination motrice accompagnée d'écolalie et de coprolalie. *Arch Neurol (Paris)* 1885;**9**:19–42,158–200.

11. Ward CD. Transient feelings of compulsion caused by hemispheric lesions: Three cases. *J Neurol Neurosurg Psychiatry* 1988;**51**:266–8.

12. Pulst SM, Walshe TM, Romero JA. Carbon monoxide poisoning with features of Gilles de la Tourette's syndrome. *Arch Neurol* 1983;**40**:443–4.

13. Kwak CH, Jankovic J. Tourettism and dystonia after subcortical stroke. *Mov Disord* 2002;**17**:821–5.

14. Gomis M, Puente V, Pont-Sunyer C, *et al.* Adult onset simple phonic tic after caudate stroke. *Mov Disord* 2008;**23**:765–6.

15. Sacks OW. Acquired tourettism in adult life. *Adv Neurol* 1982;**32**:89–92.

16. Singer C, Sanchez-Ramos J, Weiner WJ. A case of post-traumatic tic disorder. *Mov Disord* 1989;**4**:342–4.

17. Majumdar A, Appleton RE. Delayed and severe but transient Tourette syndrome after head injury. *Pediatr Neurol* 2002;**27**:314–17.

18. Wolfhart G, Ingvar DH, Hellberg AM. Compulsory shouting (Benedek's 'klazomania') associated with oculogyric spasms in chronic epidemic encephalitis. *Acta Psychiatr Scand* 1961;**36**:369–77.

19. Howard RS, Lees AJ. Encephalitis lethargica: A report of four recent cases. *Brain* 1987;**110**:19–33.

20. Dale RC, Church AJ, Heyman I. Striatal encephalitis after varicella zoster infection complicated by tourettism. *Mov Disord* 2003;**18**:1554–6.

21. Jankovic J, Kwak C. Tics in other neurological disorders. In: Kurlan R. *Handbook of Tourette's syndrome and related tic and behavioral disorders.* New York, NY: Marcel Dekker; 2004.

22. Riedel M, Straube A, Schwarz MJ, *et al.* Lyme disease presenting as Tourette's syndrome. *Lancet* 1998;**351**: 418–19.

23. Schrag A, Gilbert R, Giovannoni G, *et al.* Streptococcal infection, Tourette syndrome, and OCD: Is there a connection? *Neurology* 2009;**73**: 1256–63.

24. Mell LK, Davis RL, Owens D. Association between streptococcal infection and obsessive–compulsive disorder, Tourette's syndrome, and tic disorder. *Pediatrics* 2005;**116**:56–60.

25. Martino D, Dale RC, Gilbert DL, *et al.* Immuno-pathogenic mechanisms in Tourette syndrome: A critical review. *Mov Disord* 2009;**24**:1267–79.

26. Martino D, Chew NK, Mir P, *et al.* Atypical movement disorders in antiphospholipid syndrome. *Mov Disord* 2006;**21**:944–9.

27. Edwards MJ, Dale RC, Church AJ, *et al.* Onset tic disorder, motor stereotypies, and behavioural disturbance associated with antibasal ganglia antibodies. *Mov Disord* 2004;**19**:1190–6.

28. Jankovic J, Ashizawa T. Tourettism associated with Huntington's disease. *Mov Disord* 1995;**10**:103–5.

29. Scarano V, Pellecchia MT, Filla A, *et al.* Hallervorden–Spatz syndrome resembling a typical Tourette syndrome. *Mov Disord* 2002;**17**:618–20.

30. Pellecchia MT, Valente EM, Cif L, *et al.* The diverse phenotype and genotype of pantothenate kinase-associated neurodegeneration. *Neurology* 2005;**64**: 1810–12.

31. Nardocci N, Rumi V, Combi ML, *et al.* Complex tics, stereotypes, and compulsive behavior as clinical presentation of a juvenile progressive dystonia suggestive of Hallervorden–Spatz disease. *Mov Disord* 1994;**9**:369–71.

32. Hardie RJ, Pullon HW, Harding AE, *et al.* Neuroacanthocytosis. *Brain* 1990;**114**:13–49.

33. Kumar R, Lang AE. Tourette syndrome. Secondary tic disorders. *Neurol Clin* 1997;**15**:309–31.

34. Bharucha KJ, Sethi KD. Tardive tourettism after

exposure to neuroleptic therapy. *Mov Disord* 1995; **10:**791–3.

35. Polizos P, Engelhardt DM, Hoffman SP, *et al.* Neurological consequences of psychotropic drug withdrawal in schizophrenic children. *J Autism Child Schizophr* 1973;**3:**247–53.

36. Sotero de Menezes MA, Rho JM, Murphy P, *et al.* Lamotrigine-induced tic disorder: Report of five pediatric cases. *Epilepsia* 2000;**41:**862–7.

37. Kurlan R, Kersun J, Behr J, *et al.* Carbamazepine-induced tics. *Clin Neuropharmacol* 1989;**12:**298–302.

38. Cardoso FE, Jankovic J. Cocaine-related movement disorders. *Mov Disord* 1993;**8:**175–8.

39. Daniels J, Baker DG, Norman AB. Cocaine-induced tics in untreated Tourette's syndrome. *Am J Psychiatry* 1996;**153:**965.

40. Davis RE, Osorio I. Childhood caffeine tic syndrome. *Pediatrics* 1998;**101:**E4.

41. Denckla MB, Bemporad JR, MacKay MC. Tics following methylphenidate administration. A report of 20 cases. *JAMA* 1976;**235:**1349–51.

42. Lowe TL, Cohen DJ, Detlor J, *et al.* Stimulant medications precipitate Tourette's syndrome. *JAMA* 1982;**247:**1729–31.

43. Leckman JF, Zhang H, Vitale A, *et al.* Course of tic severity in Tourette syndrome: The first two decades. *Pediatrics* 1998;**102:**14–19.

44. Robertson MM. The prevalence and epidemiology of Gilles de la Tourette syndrome: Part 1. The epidemiological and prevalence studies. *J Psychosom Res* 2008;**65:**461–72.

45. Robertson MM. The prevalence and epidemiology of Gilles de la Tourette syndrome: Part 2. Tentative explanations for differing prevalence figures in GTS, including the possible effects of psychopathology, aetiology, cultural differences, and differing phenotypes. *J Psychosom Res* 2008;**65:**473–86.

46. Shapiro AK, Shapiro ES, Braun RD, *et al. Gilles De la Tourette syndrome.* New York: Raven; 1978.

47. Bloch MH, Leckman JF. Clinical course of Tourette syndrome. *J Psychosomatic Res* 2009;**67:**497–501.

48. Scahill L, Sukhodolsky DG, Williams SK, *et al.* Public health significance of tic disorders in children and adolescents. *Adv Neurol* 2005;**96:**240–8.

49. Robertson MM. Annotation: Gilles de la Tourette syndrome—an update. *J Child Psychol Psychiatry* 1994;**35:**597–611.

50. Khalifa N, von Knorring AL. Prevalence of tic disorders and Tourette syndrome in a Swedish school population. *Dev Med Child Neurol* 2003;**45:**315–19.

51. Kadesjo B, Gillberg C. Tourette's disorder: Epidemiology and comorbidity in primary school children. *J Am Acad Child Adolesc Psychiatry* 2000; **39:**548.

52. Peterson BS, Leckman JF. The temporal dynamics of tics in Gilles de la Tourette syndrome. *Biol Psychiatry* 1998;**44:**1337–48.

53. Kurlan R, McDermott MP, Deely C, *et al.* Prevalence of tics in schoolchildren and association with placement in special education. *Neurology* 2001;**57:** 1383–8.

54. Rickards H. Tourette's syndrome and other tic disorders. *Pract Neurol* 2010:**10:**252–9.

55. Sukhodolsky DG, Scahill L, Zhang H, *et al.* Disruptive behavior in children with Tourette's syndrome: Association with ADHD comorbidity, tic severity, and functional impairment. *J Am Acad Child Adolesc Psychiatry* 2003;**42:**98–105.

56. Diniz JB, Rosario-Campos MC, Hounie AG, *et al.* Chronic tics and Tourette syndrome in patients with obsessive-compulsive disorder. *J Psychiatr Res* 2006; **40:**487–93.

57. Saccomani L, Fabiana V, Manuela B, *et al.* Tourette syndrome and chronic tics in a sample of children and adolescents. *Brain Development* 2005;**27:**349–52.

58. Kurlan R, Como PG, Miller B, *et al.* The behavioral spectrum of tic disorders: A community-based study. *Neurology* 2002;**59:**414–20.

59. Khalifa N, von Knorring AL. Psychopathology in a Swedish population of school children with tic disorders. *J Am Acad Child Adolesc Psychiatry* 2006; **45:**1346–53.

60. Shady GA, Fulton WA, Champion LM. Tourette syndrome and educational problems in Canada. *Neurosci Behav Rev* 1988;**12:**263–5.

61. Elstner K, Selai CE, Trimble MR, *et al.* Quality of life (QOL) of patients with Gilles de la Tourette's syndrome. *Acta Psychiatr Scand* 2001;**103:**52–9.

62. Bernard BA, Stebbins GT, Siegel S, *et al.* Determinants of quality of life in children with Gilles de la Tourette syndrome. *Mov Disord* 2009;**24:**1070–3.

63. Bloch MH, Peterson BS, Scahill L, *et al.* Adulthood outcome of tic and obsessive–compulsive symptom severity in children with Tourette syndrome. *Arch Pediatr Adolesc Med* 2006;**160:**65–9.

64. March JS, Franklin ME, Leonard H, *et al.* Tics moderate treatment outcome with sertraline but not cognitive-behavior therapy in pediatric obsessive–compulsive disorder. *Biol Psychiatry* 2007;**61:**344–7.

65. Bloch MH, Landeros-Weisenberger A, Kelmendi B,

et al. A systematic review: Antipsychotic augmentation with treatment refractory obsessive–compulsive disorder. *Mol Psychiatry* 2006;**11**:622–32.

66. Bloch MH, Panza KE, Landeros-Weisenberger A, *et al.* Metaanalysis: Treatment of attention-deficit hyperactivity disorder in children with comorbid tic disorders. *JAACAP* 2009;**48**:884–93.

67. Tourette's Syndrome Study Group. Treatment of ADHD in children with tics: A randomized control trial. *Neurology* 2002;**58**:527–36.

68. Kurlan R, Fett K, Parry K, *et al.* School problems in Tourette's syndrome. *Ann Neurol* 1991;**30**:275–6.

69. Kurlan R. Tourette's syndrome: Current concepts. *Neurology* 1989;**39**:1625–30.

70. Hagin RA, Beecher R, Pagano G, *et al.* Effect of Tourette syndrome on learning. *Adv Neurol* 1982;**35**:323–8.

71. Bornstein RA. Neuropsychological performance in children with Tourette syndrome. *Psychiatr Res* 1990;**33**:73–81.

72. Schuerholz LJ, Baumgardner TL, Singer HS, *et al.* Neuropsychological status of children with Tourette's syndrome with and without attention deficit hyperactivity disorder. *Neurology* 1996;**46**:958–65.

73. Aronowitz BR, Hollander E, DeCaria C, *et al.* Neuropsychology of obsessive–compulsive disorder: Preliminary findings. *Neuropsychiatry Neuropsychol Behav Psychol* 1994;**7**:81–6.

74. Savage CR, Keuthen NJ, Jenike MA, *et al.* Recall and recognition memory in obsessive–compulsive disorder. *J Neuropsychiatry Clin Neurosci* 1996;**8**:99–103.

75. Factor SA, Molho ES. Adult-onset tics associated with peripheral injury. *Mov Disord* 1997;**12**:1052–55.

76. Chouinard S, Ford B. Adult onset tic disorders. *J Neurol Neurosurg Psychiatry* 2000;**68**:738–43.

77. Tiffen J. *Purdue Pegboard test.* Chicago: Scientific Research Associates; 1968.

78. Tanner CM, Goldman SM. Epidemiology of Tourette syndrome. *Neurol Clin* 1997;**15**:395–402.

79. Goetz CG, Tanner CM, Stebbins GT, *et al.* Adult tics in Gilles de la Tourette's syndrome: Description and risk factors. *Neurol* 1992;**42**:784–8.

80. Eapen V, Pauls DL, Robertson MM. Evidence for autosomal dominant transmission in Tourette syndrome: United Kingdom cohort study. *Br J Psychiatry* 1993;**162**:593–6.

81. Walkup JT, LaBuda MC, Singer HS, *et al.* Family study of segregation analysis of Tourette syndrome. *Am J Hum Genet* 1996;**59**:684–93.

82. Pauls DL, van de Wetering BJM. The genetics of tics and related behaviours. In: Robertson MM, Eapen V (eds). *Movement and allied disorders in childhood.* Chichester, UK: John Wiley; 1996.

83. Pauls DL, Cohen DJ, Heimbuch R, *et al.* Familial pattern and transmission of Gilles de la Tourette syndrome and multiple tics. *Arch Gen Psychiatry* 1981;**38**:1091–3.

84. Tourette Syndrome Association International Consortium for Genetics: Genome scan for Tourette disorder in affected-siblingpair and multigenerational families. *Am J Hum Genet* 2007;**80**:265–72.

85. Abelson JF, Kwan KY, O'Roak BJ, *et al.* Sequence variants in SLITRK1 are associated with Tourette's syndrome. *Science* 2005;**310**:317–20.

86. Simonic I, Nyholt DR, Gericke GS, *et al.* Further evidence for linkage of Gilles de la Tourette syndrome (GTS) susceptibility loci on chromosome 2p11, 8q22 and 11q23-24 in South African Afrikaners. *Am J Med Genet* 2001;**105**:163–7.

87. Merette C, Brassard A, Potvin A, *et al.* Significant linkage for Tourette syndrome in a large French Canadian family. *Am J Hum Genet* 2000;**67**:1008–13.

88. Diaz-Anzaldua A, Riviere J-B, Dube M-P, *et al.* Chromosome 11-q24 region in Tourette syndrome: Association and linkage disequilibrium study in the French Canadian population. *Am J Med Genet Part A* 2005;**138A**:225–8.

89. Curtis D, Brett P, Dearlove AM, *et al.* Genome scan of Tourette syndrome in a single large pedigree shows some support for linkage to regions of chromosomes 5, 10 and 13. *Psychiatr Genet* 2004;**14**:83–7.

90. Kalanithi PS, Zheng W, Kataoka Y, *et al.* Altered parvalbumin-positive neuron distribution in basal ganglia of individuals with Tourette syndrome. *Proc Natl Acad Sci USA* 2005;**102**:13307–12.

91. Stern E, Silbersweig DA, Chee KY, *et al.* A functional neuroanatomy of tics in Tourette syndrome. *Arch Gen Psychiatry* 2000;**57**:741–8.

92. Singer HS, Minzer K. Neurobiology of Tourette syndrome: Concepts of neuroanatomical localization and neurochemical abnormalities. *Brain Dev* 2003;**25**(Suppl):S70–S84.

93. Tekin S, Cummings JL. Frontal-subcortical neuronal circuits and clinical neuropsychiatry: An update. *J Psychosom Res* 2002;**53**:647–54.

94. Alexander GE, Crutcher MD, DeLong MR. Basal ganglia-thalamocortical circuits: Parallel substrate for motor, oculomotor, prefrontal, and limbic function. *Prog Brain Res* 1990;**85**:119–46.

95. Kimber TE. An update on Tourette syndrome. *Curr*

Neurol Neurosci Rep 2001;**10**:286–91.

96. Rickard H. Functional neuroimaging in Tourette syndrome. *J Psychosomatic Res* 2009;**67**:575–84.

97. Mink JW. Neurobiology of basal ganglia and Tourette syndrome: Basal ganglia circuits and thalamocortical outputs. *Adv Neurol* 2006;**99**:89–8.

98. Peterson BS, Thomas P, Kane MJ, *et al.* Basal ganglia volumes in patients with Gilles de la Tourette syndrome. *Arch Gen Psychiatry* 2003;**60**:415–24.

99. Bloch M, Michael H, Leckman JF, *et al.* Caudate volumes in childhood predict symptom severity in adults with Tourette syndrome. *Neurology* 2005;**65**:1253–8.

100. Peterson BS, Staib L, Scahill L, *et al.* Regional brain and ventricular volumes in Tourette syndrome. *Arch Gen Psychiatry* 2001;**58**:427–40.

101. Sowell ER, Kan E, Yoshii J, *et al.* Thinning of sensorimotor cortices in children with Tourette syndrome. *Nat Neurosci* 2008;**11**:6–8.

102. Fahim C, Yoon U, Das S, *et al.* Somatosensory-motor bodily representation cortical thinning in Tourette: Effects of tic severity, age and gender. *Cortex* 2010;**46**:750–60.

103. Neuner I, Kupriyanova Y, Stocker T, *et al.* White-matter abnormalities in Tourette syndrome extend beyond motor pathways. *Neuroimage* 2010;**51**:1184–93.

104. Plessen KJ, Wentzel-Larsen T, Hugdahl K, *et al.* Altered interhemispheric connectivity in individuals with Tourette's disorder. *Am J Psychiatry* 2004;**161**:2028–37.

105. Thomalla G, Siebner HR, Jonas M, *et al.* Structural changes in the somatosensory system correlate with tic severity in Gilles de la Tourette syndrome. *Brain* 2009;**132**:765–77.

106. Bohlhalter S, Goldfine A, Matteson S, *et al.* Neural correlates of tic generation in Tourette syndrome: An event-related functional MRI study. *Brain* 2006;**129**:2029–37.

107. Peterson BS, Skudlarski P, Anderson AW, *et al.* A functional magnetic resonance imaging study of tic suppression in Tourette syndrome. *Arch Gen Psychiatry* 1998;**55**:326–33.

108. Stern E, Silbersweig DA, Chee KY, *et al.* A functional neuroanatomy of tics in Tourette syndrome. *Arch Gen Psychiatry* 2000;**57**:741–8.

109. Moll GH, Wischer S, Heinrich H, *et al.* Deficient motor control in children with tic disorder: Evidence from transcranial magnetic stimulation. *Neurosci Lett* 1999;**272**:37–40.

110. Ziemann U, Paulus W, Rothenberger A. Decreased motor inhibition in Tourette's disorder: Evidence from transcranial magnetic stimulation. *Am J Psychiatry* 1997;**154**:1277–84.

111. Shprecher D, Kurlan R. The management of tics. *Mov Disord* 2008;**24**:15–24.

112. Leckman JF, Riddle MA, Hardin MT, *et al.* The Yale Global Tic Severity Scale (YGTSS): Initial testing of a clinician-rated scale of tic severity. *J Am Acad Child Adolesc Psychiatry* 1989;**28**:566–73.

113. Bloch MH. Emerging treatments for Tourette's disorder. *Current Psychiatry Reports* 2008;**10**:323–30.

114. Peterson AL, Azrin NH. Behavioral and pharmacological treatments for Tourette syndrome: A review. *Applied and Preventive Psychology* 1993;**2**:231–42.

115. Kurlan R. Treatment of tics. *Neurol Clin North Am* 1997;**15**:403–9.

116. Leckman JF. A systematic review: Antipsychotic augmentation with treatment refractory obsessive–compulsive disorder. *Mol Psychiatry* 2006;**11**:622–32.

117. Jankovic J, Orman J. Tetrabenazine therapy of dystonia, chorea, tics, and other dyskinesias. *Neurology* 1988;**38**:391–4.

118. Gonce M, Barbeau A. Seven cases of Gilles de la tourette's syndrome: Partial relief with clonazepam: A pilot study. *Can J Neurol Sci* 1977;**4**:279–83.

119. Hedderick EF, Morris CM, Singer HS. Double-blind, crossover study of clonidine and levetiracetam in Tourette syndrome. *Pediatr Neurol* 2009;**40**:420–5.

120. Smith-Hicks CL, Bridges DD, Paynter NP, *et al.* A double blind randomized placebo control trial of levetiracetam in Tourette syndrome. *Mov Disord* 2007;**22**:1764–70.

121. Jankovic J. Botulinum toxin in the treatment of dystonic tics. *Mov Disord* 1994;**9**:347–9.

122. Salloway S, Stewart CF, Israeli L, *et al.* Botulinum toxin for refractory vocal tics. *Mov Disord* 1996;**11**:746–8.

123. Scott BL, Jankovic J, Donovan DT. Botulinum toxin injection into vocal cord in the treatment of malignant coprolalia associated with Tourette's syndrome. *Mov Disord* 1996;**11**:431–3.

124. Marras C, Andrews D, Sime E, *et al.* Botulinum toxin for simple motor tics: A randomized, double-blind, controlled clinical trial. *Neurology* 2001;**56**:605–10.

125. Servello D, Porta M, Sassi M, *et al.* Deep brain stimulation in 18 patients with severe Gilles de la Tourette syndrome refractory to treatment: The surgery and stimulation. *J Neurol Neurosurg Psychiatry* 2008;**79**:136–42.

126. Welter M-L, Mallet L, Houeto J-L, *et al.* Internal pallidal and thalamic stimulation in patients with Tourette syndrome. *Arch Neurol* 2008;**65:**952–7.

127. Houeto JL, Karachi C, Mallet L, *et al.* Tourette's syndrome and deep brain stimulation. *J Neurol Neurosurg Psychiatry* 2005;**76:**992–5.

128. Azrin NH, Nunn RG. Habit-reversal: A method of eliminating nervous habits and tics. *Behaviour Research and Therapy* 1973;**11:**619–28.

129. Cook CR, Blache J. Evidence-based psychosocial treatments for tic disorders. *Clinical Psychology: Science and Practice* 2007;**14:**252–67.

20

Acute endovascular stroke treatment

SANJEEV DEVESHWAR, PRAMOD SETHI

Stroke is the third leading cause of death, after heart attacks and cancer, in adults in the United States of America.[1] Approximately 700,000 people suffer a stroke each year, 180,000 of which are recurrent strokes.[2] The majority of these are ischaemic strokes caused by blockage of blood supply to the brain, resulting in irreversible injury or infarction. A large majority of patients lose functional independence and have deficits, which impact their work and home life.

Acute stroke care has evolved considerably in last few decades with the approval in 1996 of intravenous tissue plasminogen activator, which as of now remains the only approved therapy for acute stroke by the United States Food and Drug Administration (FDA). Unfortunately, this therapy is available only to a minority of acute stroke patients and is not effective in patients with large-vessel occlusions. Several promising endovascular treatment options are being developed to enhance recanalization rates and improve outcomes in patients with large-vessel occlusions. These include newer thrombolytic agents as well as mechanical thrombolysis or sonolysis, or a combination of several of these approaches.

Intravenous thrombolysis

A variety of 'clot busters' have been used, including streptokinase, urokinase (UK), recombinant tissue plasminogen activator (rt-PA), recombinant prourokinase (r-proUK), and reteplase. These medications differ only slightly in their half-life, fibrin selectivity, stability, and mechanism of action.

Eight large, multicentre randomized trials of intravenous thrombolysis were conducted in the last 30 years. The first three trials—Multicentre Acute Stroke Trial (Europe), Australian Stroke Trial, and Multicentre Acute Stroke Trial (Italy) —were terminated early because of increased haemorrhage rates and failure to demonstrate benefit within 4–6 hours of acute stroke. However, later the European Cooperative Acute Stroke Study (ECASS) I and the ECASS II, and ATLANTIS (Alteplase Thrombolysis for Acute Non-interventional Therapy in Ischemic Stroke), which also looked at intravenous thrombolysis between 4–6 hours, failed to show significant benefit in primary outcome of neurological improvement at 90 days; but they did show that under certain conditions the medications might be beneficial. These two trials were pivotal in identifying patients who would benefit the most and established the correct rt-PA dosing range. They also provided the rationale for doing the National Institutes of Neurologic Disorders and Stroke (NINDS) trial. The NINDS trial was positive and results led to FDA approval in 1996 of first therapy to treat patients with acute stroke (Table 1).[3] Patients who received rt-PA were 30% more likely to have minimal or no disability at 90 days compared with those who received placebo. Despite the symptomatic haemorrhage risk (6.4% versus 0.6%), this did not translate into higher mortality.

Only 5% of acute stroke patients actually receive intravenous rt-PA, despite its approval by the FDA. The low treatment rates are mainly because of a delay in patient presentation. Several studies looked at patients who might benefit from intravenous thrombolysis beyond the 3-hour window; in 2009, ECASS III ½ hours from symptom onset. The ECASS III protocol has been accepted now by most stroke societies, even though it is not FDA-approved in the USA. The use of intravenous rt-PA in the 3–4.5 hours time window is considered off-label use.[4]

Intra-arterial thrombolysis

Intravenous thrombolysis results are encouraging as they can be achieved with minimal infrastructure and equipment. However, intravenous thrombolysis does not work well in patients with large-vessel occlusion. Intra-arterial delivery allows for a greater concentration of the thrombolytic agent at the site of arterial occlusion and a lower systemic concentration of the thrombolytic agent, leading to a decreased risk of haemorrhage, as well as the potential for mechanical clot disruption (Table 2). Prolyse in Acute Thromboembolism Clinical Trials I (PROACT I) and Prolyse in Acute Thrombo-embolism Clinical Trials II (PROACT II) studied a homogenous population of stroke patients with middle cerebral artery (MCA) occlusion and established the safety and efficacy of r-proUK.[5] Recanalization rates of up to 70% were achieved with significant improvement in neurological outcome. Haemorrhage rates were higher but did not lead to a higher mortality rate. Intra-arterial rt-PA is used off-label, either as an adjunct to intravenous rt-PA or alone. However, randomized studies showing definite benefit are lacking.

Combination of intravenous and intra-arterial therapy

The Emergency Management of Stroke (EMS) Bridging Trial in 1999 showed that combining intravenous and intra-arterial thrombolysis resulted in more complete MCA recanalization (55% *versus* 10%) but failed to show a significant difference in clinical outcome. In 2001, Keris *et al.* studied combined intra-arterial and intravenous thrombolysis *versus* intra-arterial therapy alone in a randomized fashion. They noted an

Table 1. rt-PA benefit in NINDS trial[3]
(624 patients with ischaemic stroke treated within 3 hours)

	Intravenous alteplase (0.9 mg/kg) (%)	Placebo (%)
Improvement at 24 hours	47	39
Favourable outcome at 3 months	43	27
Intracerebral haemorrhage	6.4	0.6

Table 2. Results of PROACT II Trial[5]
(188 patients with occlusion of middle cerebral artery treated within 6 hours of onset)

	Intra-arterial r-prourokinase (9 mg) (%)	Placebo (%)
Recanalization	66	18
Symptomatic intracerebral haemorrhage	25	10
Favourable outcome	40	25

increased rate of haemorrhage in the combination group without a difference in significant incidence of symptomatic haemorrhage, mortality or functional outcome.[6]

International Management of Stroke (IMS) I Trial compared patients with combined intravenous and intra-arterial thrombolysis with NINDS trial patients who had received only intravenous rt-PA.[7] Eighty patients who had a National Institutes of Health Stroke Scale score (NIHSS) of ≥18 received intravenous rt-PA followed by a 2-hour infusion of intra-arterial rt-PA. Three-month mortality was only 16%, although there was a 64% rate of symptomatic intracerebral haemorrhage. Nevertheless, outcomes at 3 months for all outcome measures performed were better than the NINDS intravenous rt-PA group. Regression analysis of haemorrhage rates identified atrial fibrillation and arterial obstruction of proximal large vessels as independent risk factors for haemorrhage.

IMS II is ongoing; comparisons are being made between intravenous rt-PA and various forms of intra-arterial intervention, such as mechanical embolus removal in cerebral ischaemia (MERCI), EKOS ultrasound micro-infusion catheter, or intra-arterial rt-PA.

Other interventional therapies under development

In addition to intra-arterial rt-PA and FDA-approved MERCI and Penumbra [(Penumbra Inc., Alameda, CA, USA) devices for mechanical thrombectomy, several other modalities are being currently investigated, including angioplasty, with/without stenting, for acute occlusion/severe stenosis, snares and sonothrombolysis. Recent developments in endovascular technology for the treatment of ischaemic stroke, such as angioplasty, stenting, mechanical thrombectomy or clot disruption are providing evidence that safe and effective revascularization can be achieved.[8] Endovascular mechanical intervention can be combined with little or no amounts of intra-arterial or intravenous thrombolytics. With the rapid advancement in technology and introduction of easier systems, more effective and safer endovascular treatments will be available for routine use.

Mechanical revascularization

Endovascular mechanical revascularization techniques have several advantages over endovascular delivery of pharmacological fibrinolytics. Mechanical devices have the following advantages:

- A potentially more rapid, efficacious and safer method of clot removal
- Alternative treatment when fibrinolytics are contraindicated
- Combine with fibrinolytic agents to accelerate clot lysis
- A quick reduction in clot burden in large, proximal cerebral vessels, followed by pharmacological thrombolysis of distal fragments of clot in smaller vessels.

A recent introduction is the concept of augmenting cerebral blood flow and perfusion by partial and transitory obstruction of the abdominal aorta using a double balloon system in order to potentially open collateral blood supply.[9] Endovascular-induced, local and moderate hypothermia may be promising. Disadvantages of mechanical revascularization are as follows:

- Possibility of occlusion/damage to perforators
- Vessel dissection/endothelial injury
- Intracranial haemorrhage
- Vessel occlusion
- Clot fragmentation with distal emboli, which can occur with intravenous and/or intra-arterial thrombolysis.

Intra-arterial mechanical interventions in acute stroke can be classified into endovascular thrombectomy, mechanical clot disruptions or fragmentation, and augmented fibrinolysis devices (Table 3).

Table 3. Endovascular treatment strategies

Mechanical disruption	Mechanical retrieval	Augmented fibrinolysis
Balloon catheters	MERCI	Clot busters
Snares	Penumbra device	Laser
EKOS catheter	Alligator retrieval device	Ultrasound
Angioget	Amplatz gooseneck	
	Microsnare	
Neuroget	In-time snare retreiver	
	Neuronet	

MERCI mechanical embolus removal in cerebral ischaemia

Thrombectomy

Endovascular thrombectomy devices are designed to extract occlusive thrombi from target vessels via a transcatheter approach. There are two general types: (i) Devices that retrieve cerebral emboli by grasping and pulling; and (ii) suction thrombectomy devices that aspirate.

Clot retrieval devices

These devices can ensnare a thrombus and withdraw from the body through a guide catheter. Examples of clot retrieval devices available are the MERCI retrieval device, the Amplatz gooseneck microsnare, neuronet, in-time retrieval device, the alligator retrieval device, and the penumbra retrieval device.

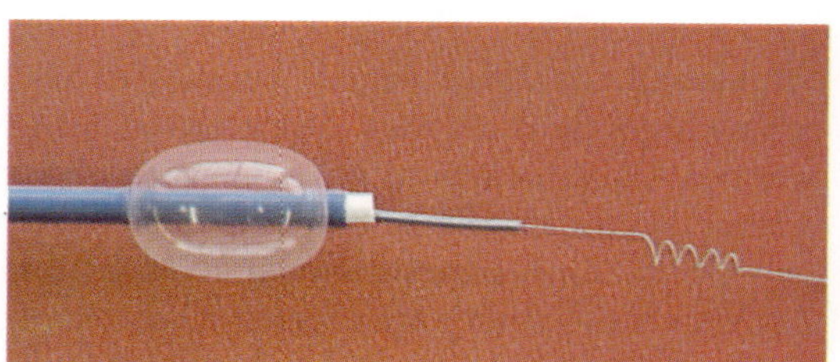

Fig. 1. Merci Retrieval Device with balloon

MERCI retriever X5/X6/LS (Concentric Medical)

This was the first approved by the FDA for mechanical thrombectomy in acute ischaemic stroke. X5/X6 devices consist of platinum-tipped nitinol wire—a moderately stiff, gradually enlarging helix that is displayed through the microcatheter. An 8F/9F/5F balloon-tipped guide catheter is used for flow arrest or reversal within the internal carotid artery (ICA) or vertebral artery during retrieval.

The MERCI retriever X5 and X6 devices were used in the MERCI trial.[10] The trial evaluated the safety and efficacy of these devices to restore patency of occluded blood vessels within the first 8 hours of acute ischaemic stroke.

The MERCI trial was conducted in two parts. Part I enrolled 55 patients and Part II enrolled 96 patients, making a total of 151 patients. Recanalization was achieved in 46% of patients with markedly improved clinical outcomes (90 day modified rankin score 0–2 in 46% of recanalizers *versus* in 10% of non-recanalizers). Symptomatic intracranial haemorrhage occurred in 7.8% of patients treated with the device alone.

The LX type version of the MERCI retriever, consisting of concentric helical loops with polymer filaments attached that increase clot traction, has achieved higher recanalization rates in preclinical studies than the X5/X6 versions.

Recent data from the multi MERCI trial using the modified clot retriever L5 were more promising.[11] Overall recanalization rates in the

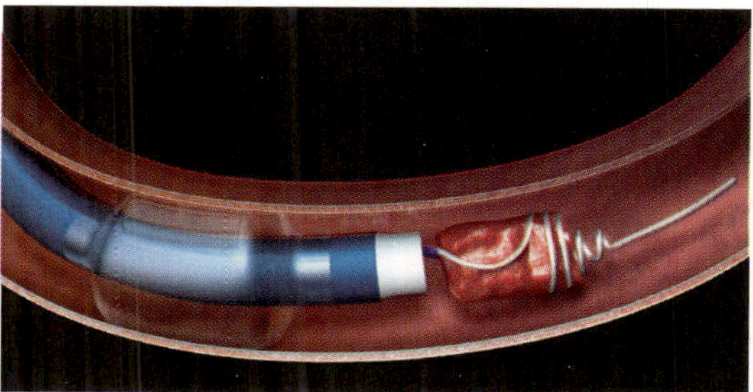

Fig. 2. Merci snares a clot

164 patients enrolled was 54.9% with the device alone, and 68.3% with use of adjuvant therapy (prior use of intravenous rt-PA and intra-arterial rt-PA). Patients entered the study with severe ischaemic stroke and baseline NIHSS of 19.3±6.4. The site of occlusion was ICA/ICA-T in 52 patients, MCA in 60 patients, and vertebrobasilar in 14 patients. Favourable outcome at 90 days was seen in 36% (mRS ≤2); mortality at 90 days was 34%.

Amplatz gooseneck microsnare

The Amplatz gooseneck microsnare is a wire loop snare that exits the microcatheter at a 90° angle, which is designed to improve its ability to capture foreign bodies. The device is delivered through a microcatheter positioned just proximal to the occlusion. A retrieval snare with the same diameter as the occluded vessel is then introduced with the loop pushed just distal to the microcatheter. The microcatheter is then pushed with the snare into the embolus. The snare is pulled back slightly into the microcatheter. Following this, the two are pulled out a few centimeters. If the embolus is caught in the snare, the whole assembly, including the guide catheter, is pulled as a unit.

Alligator retrieval device (Chestnut Medical)

This device has three micro prongs on the end of a micro wire that can be pushed through the microcatheter to open the jaws. It can then be pulled back inside the microcatheter to close the jaws; it seems to grasp the foreign body more securely.

Suction thrombectomy devices

These devices use vacuum aspiration to remove an occlusive clot in acute ischaemic stroke. Compared with the mechanical thrombectomy devices, suction thrombectomy has a reduced risk of causing uncontrolled thrombus fragmentation and embolization. Simple syringe suction applied to an endovascular catheter may be successful in treating large, ICA thrombi. More sophisticated vortex aspiration devices have been developed for extracranial circulation using high-pressure streams to generate Venturi forces that physically fragment, draw in and aspirate thrombi.

Angiojet

An angiojet is an endovascular thrombectomy device that combines local vortex suction with mechanical disruption to draw in, trap and fragment the adjacent thrombus. The debris is then simultaneously removed through the recovery lumen. The system lacks flexibility, making navigation into the intracranial circulation difficult.

Neurojet

This suction device is a single-channel device that uses the same physics as the angiojet but is designed for intracranial navigation. Although dramatic success has been reported in some cases, its failure is still related to its inability to navigate through tortuous intracranial circulation.

Clot disruption/fragmentation

Mechanical clot disruption can be accomplished simply by using guide wire manipulation or in a complex fashion, such as with laser shockwave devices. As the thrombus is disrupted and flow re-established, small emboli are created and carried into the distal circulation. In case of larger clot fragments, a further reperfusion may require endogenous or exogenous enzymatic thrombolysis.

Simple micro-guide wire

The simple micro-guide wire is the most basic device and easy to use. In intra-arterial thrombolysis, a microcatheter is navigated over a micro-guide wire up to the thrombus. The micro-guide wire, which has a soft and flexible tip, can be advanced through the thrombus. The micro-guide wire tip can be shaped variously to avoid vessel perforation. Multiple passes through the clot with the micro-guide wire and the microcatheter is one form of mechanical disruption that may fragment the thrombus. In combination with fibrinolytic agents, this disruption aids in the process by exposing more of the thrombus to the thrombolytic agent.

Penumbra system[12–13]

A wire with an olive-shaped tip is navigated into the clot through a larger braided microcatheter. Simultaneously, suction is applied to the microcatheter allowing aspiration of the fragmented clot. FDA approval for clot retrieval was based on the results from a single-arm, multicentre trial conducted in the United States of America and Europe.[14]

In the study, 125 patients were treated at 24 international centres. The average time from symptom onset to arterial puncture was 4.1 hours. Baseline NIHSS was 17.6, with angiographically confirmed T1M1 0 flow in 96% of

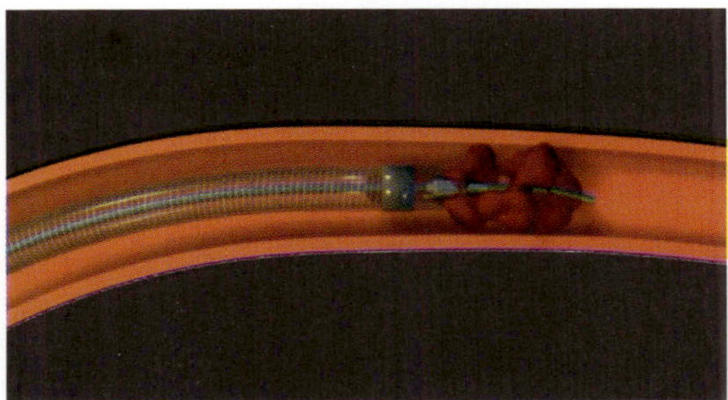

Fig. 3. Penumbra system (Penumbra Inc., Alameda, CA). Used with permission from Penumbra, Inc. © 2009 Penumbra, Inc. All rights reserved.

patients. ICA and vertebrobasilar occlusion was seen in 18% and 9% of patients, respectively. In 81.6% of the patients, T1M1 2 or 3 revascularization was achieved using the Penumbra system. Procedural related, serious adverse events were encountered in 4 (3.2%) of cases. mRS ≤2 was achieved in 25% of patients and 46% of the patients had a 4-point improvement in NIHSS at discharge. Good clinical outcome after 30 days, defined as a ≥4-point NIHSS improvement or mRS ≤2, was recorded in 46% of patients in whom recanalization was achieved, versus only 22% of patients in whom the occluded vessel was not recanalized (p<0.05).

Microsnares and net devices

Microsnares and net devices can also be used to fragment a thrombus more aggressively. However, one needs to avoid dissections and perforations when using these as a mechanical disruption device. As an adjunctive technique, the use of snares should result in more fragmentation and, theoretically, more rapid recanalization than micro-guide wires.

Laser thrombolysis

At least two devices are being tested presently, viz. the endovascular photoacoustic recanalization (Endovasix, Inc.) and the LATIS laser device (Latis, Inc.). These devices use laser energy to assist clot fragmentation for cerebrovascular occlusion in an ischaemic stroke. The laser is designed to disrupt effectively or dissolve the clot without damaging the endothelium.[15] Technical challenges remain and further improvements will allow their safe use clinically.

Augmented fibrinolysis

Several mechanical techniques, as described, may enhance pharmacological fibrinolysis. An increase in recanalization rates after combined aggressive mechanical clot disruption and thrombolytic agents has been described without significant increase in haemorrhage rates (Table 4 and Table 5).[16]

Ultrasonification

Ultrasonification is used in conjunction with thrombolytic therapy. Non-thermal effects of low frequency ultrasound energy have been found to accentuate enzymatic fibrinolysis *in vitro*. Externally applied low frequency pulse nerve ultrasonography has suggested that, in combination with rt-PA, there is shortening of time to vessel recanalization compared with rt-PA alone. The exact mechanism is unclear, although there could be contributing factors, such as rectified diffusion, which facilitates drug transport into the thrombus, reformation and opening of the fibrin matrix of the clot, cleavage of fibrin polymers and surface expansion, and improved binding of alteplase to fibrin.

Currently, only one ultrasound thrombolytic infusion catheter is available (EKOS Corporation), which combines an ultrasound transducer at the microcatheter tip with simultaneous infusion of a thrombolytic agent through the microcatheter. The EKOS device was evaluated for safety and feasibility in combination with intravenous and intra-arterial treatment of acute ischaemic stroke IMS II study and is presently being used in the IMS III trial.

Angioplasty and stenting for acute stroke intervention

Intracranial percutaneous transluminal angioplasty (PTA) in acute stroke can be used primarily to mechanically fragment the clot, or for combined intravenous or intra-arterial thrombolysis. It can also be helpful for treatment of an acute ischaemic stroke associated with an occlusion of a haemodynamically significant intracranial atherosclerotic lesion, when chemical thrombolysis is ineffective, or only partially so.

Stenting of an occluded ICA or an occluded intracranial artery in selected patients presenting with an acute stroke has gained more attention.

Revascularization of acute carotid occlusion

Patients with an acute ICA occlusion and poor collateral blood flow are considered to have a poor prognosis. Often this results in a 'T' occlusion with a massive clot burden; 16%–55% of these patients will die of complications from infarction, 40%–69% will be left with severe disability, and only 2%–12% will make a good recovery. This, therefore, represents a challenging problem.

Two important factors correlating with poor prognosis have been identified—the presence of an associated MCA occlusion and lack of collateral flow. Several studies strongly suggest that an early revascularization with local intra-

Table 4. Comparison of recanalization rates between different strategies

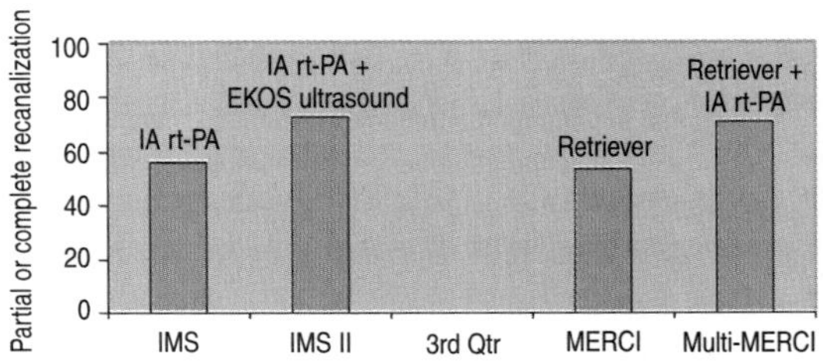

IA intra-arterial; rt-PA recombinant tissue plasminogen

Table 5. Comparison of symptomatic intracranial haemorrhages (ICH) between different strategies

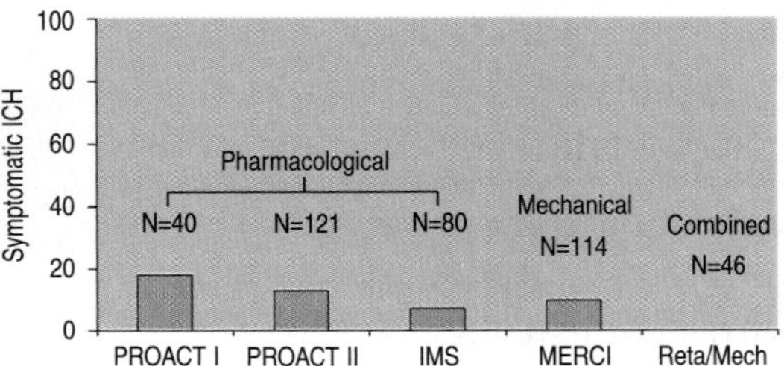

arterial thrombolytic or mechanical devices is vital for a clinical improvement in patients with an ICA occlusion. To gain access to the intracranial circulation through the ipsilateral occluded ICA, it is necessary to either recanalize the ICA or navigate directly through the occluded segment. Several recent studies have shown that neither intravenous nor intra-arterial thrombolysis is effective in recanalizing an occluded ICA. Higher doses of thrombolytics do not seem to correlate with success. Mechanical thrombectomy has been described to be technically feasible, requiring small expenditures of time.

During the first hours and days after a stroke, the risk of re-occlusion or recurrent anterio-arterial embolism remains. To reduce this risk, some investigators have developed protocols for endovascular treatment that include stent implantation in the proximal ICA with or without intra-arterial thrombolysis. The patient has to be placed on dual antiplatelet therapy after stenting. Nedeltchev and colleagues combined invasive activity test and stent placement of the proximal ICA segment in 25 patients within 6 hours of symptom onset.[17] ICA recanalization of MCA was achieved in 11 patients. In 9 of these, recanalization of the MCA was achieved by using mechanical revascularization only. Symptomatic intracerebral haemorrhage occurred in 2 patients. When investigators compared their endovascular group with the medical group ($n=31$) at 3 months, 56% of the endovascular group and 26% of the medical group had a favourable outcome. Mortality was 20% in the endovascular group and 16% in the medical group. Major risks include thrombus fragmentation and distal emboli, vessel perforation and dissection.

Revascularization of symptomatic middle cerebral artery occlusion

MCA occlusion syndromes are the most recognized because of the blood supply to the lateral two-thirds hemisphere and deep basal ganglia. Although thromboembolism is the predominant mechanism affecting the MCA territory, primary atherosclerosis at this site occurs in a subset of patients. A higher prevalence of MCA atherosclerosis is noted in African-Americans and Asians compared with Caucasians. Many patients with intracranial atherosclerosis have recurrent cerebral ischaemic events despite standard medical therapy with antiplatelets or oral anticoagulants.

As seen in the Extracranial/Intracranial Bypass Trial, two-thirds of the patients present with an initial infarction without a warning transient ischaemic attack. In these patients the stenosis progresses from atherosclerotic disease rather than a thromboembolic process. Anticoagulants would, therefore, appear to aid in preventing only an acute final occlusion caused by a thrombus and not the progression of the disease to an inevitable occlusion.

The high recurrent stroke rates in these patients indicate the need for more aggressive treatment methods for patients with symptomatic MCA atherosclerotic occlusive disease. PTA has recently been proposed as a promising treatment for such patients.[18] However, it may be complicated by symptomatic recurrent stenosis, which may require retreatment. Stent-assisted angioplasty has the advantage of coverage of the plaque, reduced risk of dissection, and prevention of vessel recoil and rupture. Therefore, the availability of recently introduced flexible self-expanding stents, the development of potent antiplatelet inhibitors, and increasing evidence from experimental and clinical studies of intracranial stents have encouraged the use of stents in the management of ischaemic intracranial cerebrovascular disease.

Current management of acute ischaemic stroke patients at Moses Cone Stroke Center, Greensboro, NC, USA

Patients with suspected acute stroke are rapidly evaluated by emergency medical system personnel. They are specially trained to use standardized tools to triage patients to the nearest acute care hospital. The stroke team at Moses Cone Stroke Center is available to the emergency department and outlying hospitals for referrals of stroke patients. In the absence of contraindications and if the patient qualifies for treatment, intravenous rt-PA is administered. From outlying facilities, patients are then transported to Moses Cone via our 'drip and ship' protocol. Work up is tailored to the patient's presenting symptoms and history to decide whether acute endovascular treatment is beneficial. Candidates with clinical or radiological evidence of large vessel occlusion are brought to the neuroangiography suite for possible intervention, which may include intra-arterial thrombolysis and/or mechanical embolectomy (Table 6).

Conclusion

Aggressive and prompt management of acute stroke has been shown to improve clinical outcomes. Intravenous rt-PA remains the only FDA-approved treatment for acute stroke. Unfortunately, it is available to only a minority of patients. Newer endovascular technologies have greatly enhanced the treatment options for stroke physicians with a combination of intravenous and intra-arterial thrombolysis, mechanical embolectomy, and angioplasty with or without stent placement. Several of these approaches have shown improved recanalization rates without a significant increase in haemorrhage, but have not yet been shown to improve clinical outcomes in controlled clinical trials. The currently ongoing IMS-II and MR RESCUE (MR and recanalization of stroke clots using embolectomy), and future trials will hopefully offer new opportunities for patients with large-vessel occlusion and acute stroke.

Several important strategies are prevalent that will impact the future of acute ischaemic stroke treatment. First is that the high rate of recanalization can be achieved using the third generation thrombolytics, glycoprotein 2B/3A receptor antagonist, and mechanical thrombolysis. Second, the ability to recanalize occluded vessels will continue to improve with newer agents and devices. Third, recanalization is important but it is not the only factor that determines clinical outcome. And finally, expedited transfers, ready availability, and appropriate selection of patients are the ultimate determinates of the future of acute stroke treatment.

Illustrative Case #1

A 65-year-old right-handed woman who collapsed while shopping with aphasia and right-sided hemiplegia with right gaze deviation. Patient was brought to the ER within 40 minutes

Table 6. Algorithm for acute ischaemic stroke treatment

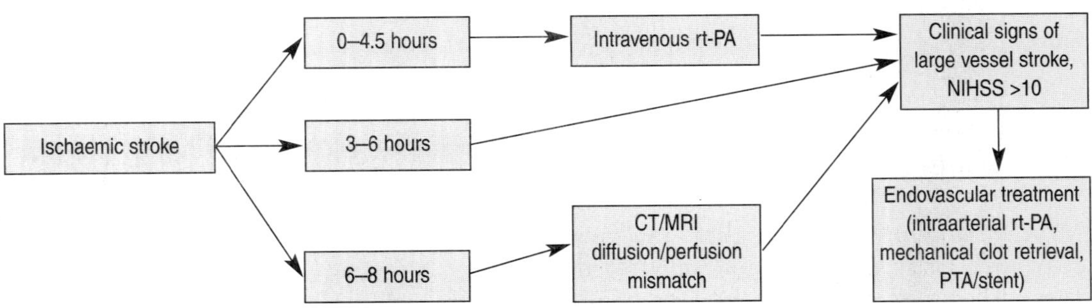

with NIH stroke scale of 18 and CT scan of the brain demonstrated hyperdense left middle cerebral sign without other overt signs of infarction (Image 1). Patient received two-thirds intravenous t-PA. Initial angiogram revealed a left middle cerebral artery proximal occlusion without significant collaterals (Image 2).

A 054 penumbra reperfusion microcatheter with 032 penumbra reperfusion catheter were advanced over a 0.014 inch microguidewire into the distal clot; 4 mg of intra-arterial t-PA was infused into the clot and aspiration performed without recanalization (Image 3). Through the 054 system additional 4 mg of intra-arterial t-PA was infused followed by aspiration with complete recanalization (Image 4).

Illustrative Case #2

62-year-old right-handed male who collapsed at work with aphasia, right gaze deviation, and right

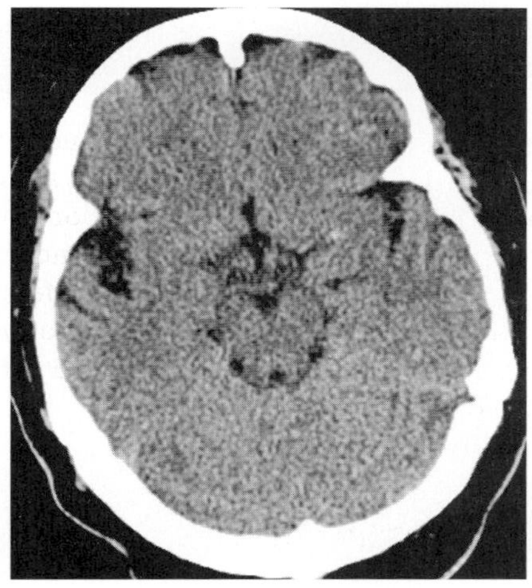

Image 1

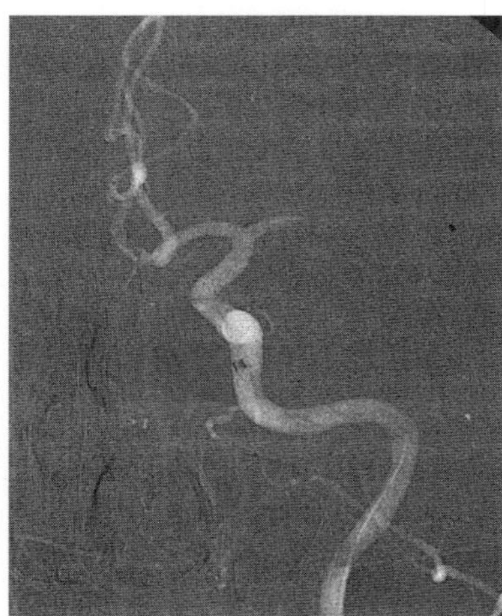

Image 2

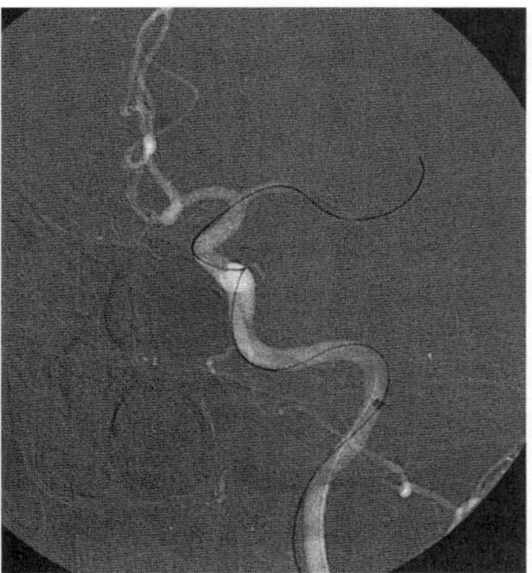

Image 3

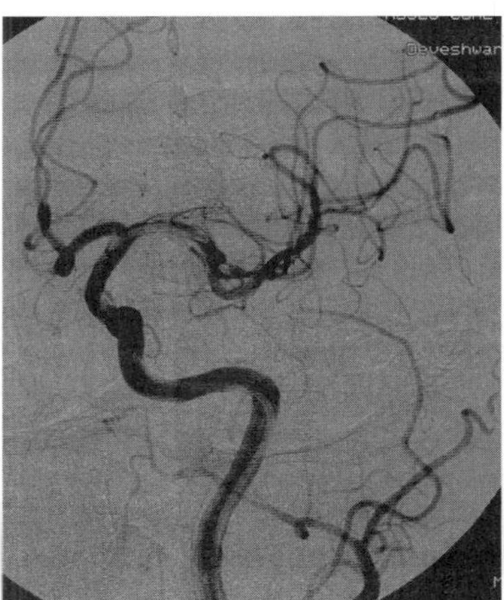

Image 4

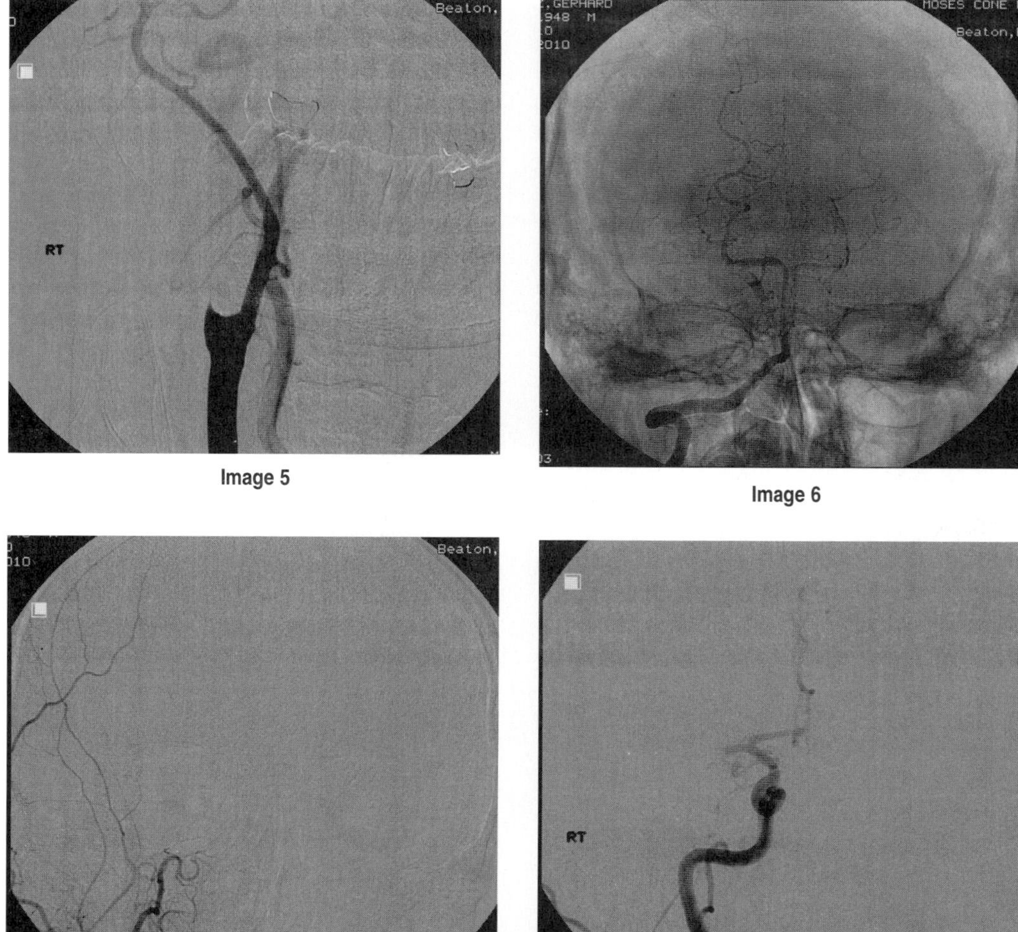

Image 5

Image 6

Image 7

Image 8

hemiplegia. NIH stroke scale 17 on admission. Initial CT scan of the brain performed within 1 hour of symptom onset was negative for haemorrhage catheter angiography reveals complete ICA occlusion (Image 5) without distal reconstitution or collateral flow (Image 6 and Image 7).

MERCI 18 L microcatheter was advanced to the right middle cerebral artery through the ICA and 10 mg of intra-arterial t-PA was infused. An L5 MERCI retrieval device was advanced through the microcatheter and deployed into the clot. With proximal flow arrest in the right ICA rigorous aspiration was performed as the combination of the microcatheter and the retrieval device was performed. Huge chunks of clot were aspirated (Image 8). Controlled angiogram showed revascularization of the ICA and proximal middle right cerebral artery and of the right anterior cerebral artery (Image 9). 7 mg of intra-arterial t-PA was then infused into the main trifurcation branch with complete recanalization (Image 10).

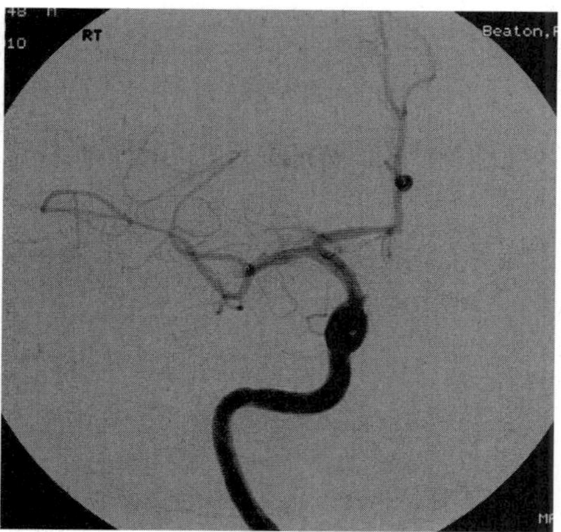

Image 9

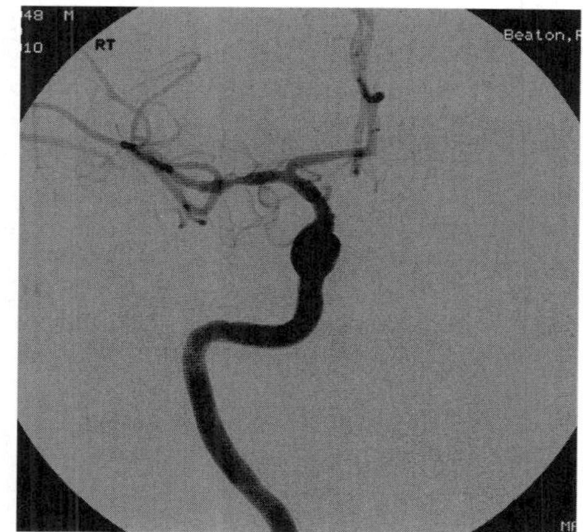

Image 10

References

1. Xu J, Kochanek KD, Tejada-Vera B. Deaths: Preliminary data for 2007. National Vital Statistics Reports 2009;**58**:5.
2. Rosamond W, Flegal K, Friday G, *et al.* American Heart Association Statistics Committee and Stroke Statistics Subcommittee. Heart disease and stroke statistics-2007 update: A report from the American Heart Association Statistics Committee and Stroke Statistics subcommittee. *Circulation* 2007;**115**:e172.
3. The National Institute of Neurological Disorders and Stroke rt-PA Stroke Study Group. Tissue plasminogen activator fir acute ischemic stroke. *N Engl J Med* 1995;**333**:1581–87.
4. Del Zoppo GJ, Saver JL, Jauch EC, Adams HP; on behalf of the American Heast Association Stroke Council. Expansion of the time window for treatment of acute ischemic stroke with intravenous tissue plasminogen activator: A science advisory from the American Heart Association/American Stroke Association. *Stroke* 2009;**40**:2945–48.
5. Furlan A, Higashida R, Wechsler L, *et al.* Intra-arterial prourokinase for actue ischemic stroke: The PROACT II study: A randomized controlled trial. Prolyse in Acute Cerebral Thromboembolism. *JAMA* 1999;**282**:2003–11.
6. Keris V, Rudnicka S, Vorona V, *et al.* Combined intraarterial/intravenous thrombolysis for acute ischemic stroke. *Am J Neuroradiol* 2001;**22**:352–8.
7. The IMS Study Investigators. Combined intravenous and intra-arterial recanalization for acute ischemic stroke: The Interventional Management of Stroke Study. *Stroke* 2004;**35**:904–11.
8. Nesbit GM, Luh G, Tien R, *et al.* New and future endovascular treatment strategies for acute ischemic stroke. *J Vasc Interv Radiol* 2004;**15**:S103–S110.
9. Lylyk P, Vila JF, Miranda C, *et al.* Partial aortic obstruction improves cerebral perfusion and clinical symptoms in patients with symptomatic vasospasm. *Neurol Res* 2005;**27** (Suppl 1):S129–S135.
10. Smith WS, Sung G, Starkman S, *et al.* MERCI Trial Investigators. Safety and efficacy of mechanical embolectomy in acute ischemic stroke: Results of the MERCI trial. *Stroke* 2005:**36**:1432–38.
11. Smith W, Sung G, Sever J, *et al.* Mechanical thrombectomy for acute ischemic stroke: Final results of Multi MERCI trial. *Stroke* 2008;**39**:1205–12.
12. Bose A, Henkes H, Alfke K, *et al.* Sit SP for the Penumbra Phase 1 Stroke Trial Investigators. The penumbra system: A mechanical device for the treatment of acute stroke due to thromboembolism. *Am J Neuroradiol* 2008;**29**:1409–13.
13. Kulcsár Z, Bonvin C, Pereira VM, *et al.* Penumbra system: A novel mechanical thrombectomy device for large-vessel occlusions in acute stroke. *Am J Neuroradiol* 2010;**31**:628–33.
14. McDougall C, Clark W, Mayer T, *et al.* The penumbra stroke trial: Safety and effectiveness of a new generation of mechanical devices for clot removal in acute ischemic stroke. Late-Breaking Science Abstracts presented at the International Stroke Conference, New Orleans, LA; 20–22

February 2008.

15. Berlis A, Lutsep H, Barnwell S, *et al.* Mechanical thrombolysis in acute ischemic stroke with endovascular photoacoustic recanalization. *Stroke* 2004; **35**:1112–16.

16. Qureshi AI. Endovascular treatment of cerebrovascular diseases and intracranial neoplasms. *Lancet* 2004;**363**:804–13.

17. Nedeltchev K, Brekenfeld C, Remonda L, *et al.* Internal carotid artery stent implantation in 25 patients with acute stroke: Preliminary results. *Radiology* 2005; **237**:1029–37.

18. Ueda T, Hatakeyama T, Kohno K, *et al.* Endovascular treatment for acute thrombotic occlusion of the middle cerebral artery: Local intra-arterial thrombolysis combined with percutaneous transluminal angioplasty. *Neuroradiology* 1997;**39**: 99–104.

21

Thunderclap headache

ATUL AGARWAL

Thunderclap headache (TCH), so named because it is like a 'clap of thunder', is an acute, explosive and severe headache with a maximum intensity at onset.[1] The term was first used in 1986 to describe the presenting symptom of an unruptured cerebral aneurysm.[2] Since then, several other causes have been ascribed to a TCH (Table 1). Diagnosis for primary TCH is positive when diagnostic testing fails to identify other potential underlying causes.

Subarachnoid haemorrhage

Subarachnoid haemorrhage (SAH) is the most common cause of secondary TCH and should be the focus of the initial assessment, given the significant associated morbidity and mortality. Initial misdiagnosis and subsequent re-bleeding corresponds to a worsening prognosis. SAH is most commonly (85%) caused by rupture of an intracranial aneurysm but can also have uncommon causes (Table 2).[3]

Headache, which may occur in isolation or in association with other signs and symptoms, is the most common symptom in SAH. The percentage of patients presenting with TCH who may have

Table 1. Symptomatic causes of TCH

Subarachnoid haemorrhage
Sentinel headache
Cerebral venous sinus thrombosis
Cervical artery dissection
Spontaneous intracranial hypotension
Pituitary apoplexy
Retroclival haematoma
Intraparenchymal, subdural, extradural haemorrhage
Ischaemic stroke
Acute hypertensive crisis
Reversible cerebral vasoconstriction syndrome
Third ventricle colloid cyst
Intracranial infection
Primary cough, sexual and exertional headache

SAH was shown to vary from 11% (in a community-based study) to 25% (hospital-based study).[4,5] In the community-based, prospective study, 70% of patients with SAH presented with headache alone, without loss of consciousness or focal symptoms.[4] By contrast, in the hospital-based study, <50% of patients with SAH presented with isolated headache.[5] Headaches

Table 2. Causes of SAH

Rupture of an intracranial aneurysm
Non-aneurysmal perimesencephalic haemorrhage
Transmural arterial dissection
Cerebral arteriovenous malformation
Dural arteriovenous fistula
Mycotic aneurysm
Cocaine abuse

can be of maximum intensity at onset or develop rapidly, reaching their maximum within a few minutes. Typically, a SAH headache lasts a few days; it is atypical for the headache to resolve in <2 hours. Although physical exertion or sexual intercourse may precede SAH, it can occur without physical stress; such stressors are also commonly associated with benign attacks of acute, severe headache.

Loss of consciousness occurs in one-third of patients with SAH. Other associated symptoms and signs include seizures (6%–9%), delirium (16%), stroke (caused by intracerebral haematoma), visual disturbances (due to intraocular haemorrhage), nausea, vomiting, dizziness, photophobia, neck stiffness and fundal haemorrhages.[3]

How to investigate a patient with SAH

Non-contrast CT (computed tomography) of the brain is the first diagnostic test in the assessment of suspected SAH. CT scan should be done as soon as possible after the onset of symptoms as its sensitivity approximates 100% within the first 12 hours of SAH; after 1 week it falls to ~50%.[3] If CT results are unrevealing, lumbar puncture must be done for cerebrospinal fluid (CSF) examination for RBCs and visual inspection for xanthochromia. Its analysis by spectrophotometry should also be done if this facility is available as it has been shown to be 100% sensitive for detecting SAH when analyzed between 12 hours and 2 weeks from the time of ictus.[6]

Magnetic resonance angiography (MRA) and CT angiography (CTA)

As MRA and CTA are non-invasive investigations, they are often used to identify unruptured aneurysms. The yield of these tests is 85%–95% if the aneurysm is >6 mm in size.[7] CTA has disadvantages over MRA in that it requires an injection of iodine-based contrast, exposes patients to radiation, and carries a small risk of an allergic reaction or deterioration in renal function.[8]

Need for conventional angiography

It is a difficult to decide if a catheter angiography is required to exclude definitively a symptomatic but unruptured intracranial aneurysm in a patient presenting with TCH. The literature dealing with this question has yielded conflicting results. An initial retrospective study of unselected patients presenting with TCH concluded that angiography is indicated in all patients with sudden severe head pain and normal clinical, CT and CSF.[4] Similar views have been expressed by Moussouttas and Mayer.[9] But later a retrospective study of 71 patients with TCH and normal CT and lumbar puncture found no patients with SAH during an average follow up of 3.3 years.[10] Many prospective studies involving 225 patients with primary TCH found no patients with SAH or sudden death during at least the next one year after onset of headache.[11–14] These data, which are of higher quality than isolated case reports, suggest that patients with TCH do not require angiography if head CT and CSF are normal.[15]

What causes headache in cases of unruptured aneurysm?

As already stated, the term 'thunderclap headache' was originally coined to describe what was believed to be the presenting symptom of an unruptured cerebral aneurysm, and suggested a possible mechanism of headache to morphological expansion of the aneurysm, luminal thrombosis, or intramural haemorrhage.

Sentinel headache

A distinctive and unusually severe headache in the days or weeks preceding a presenting haemorrhage is reported by 20%–50% of patients with SAH.[16] This headache is often referred to as a warning or sentinel headache. It has often been thought to represent a 'warning leak' or small SAH. Sentinel headaches are clinically similar to headaches that occur with SAH; they develop rapidly, reach maximum intensity within minutes, and can last for hours to days. However, unlike SAH, patients with sentinel headaches generally do not have meningismus, altered consciousness, or focal neurological symptoms and signs. A recent study demonstrated a frequency of severe headache in only 11% of patients in 1 month preceding a SAH.[5] The authors of this study suggested that in the context of serious brain disease, the severity of a prior headache episode may be over interpreted (recall bias) and this may account for the higher frequency (40%–50%) of sentinel headaches reported in many studies.[17]

Crash migraine

The term 'crash migraine' was earlier used to describe an unusual, sudden, severe headache that was self-limited and accompanied by nausea and vomiting in patients with a history of migraine.[18] In view of the fact that this term may suggest that it is a legitimate presentation of migraine, its usage has been abandoned.[19]

Cerebral venous sinus thrombosis (CVST)

TCH is the predominant symptom in 2%–10% of patients with CVST. Although headache is the most common symptom, occurring in 75%–95% of patients, its onset tends to be more gradual and sub-acute. The headaches associated with CVST could be localized or diffuse, are persistent, and exacerbated by the transient increases in intracranial pressure that occur during coughing, sneezing, or other valsalva maneuvers. Headaches can also worsen when in the recumbent position and upon awakening. Although headaches are most commonly accompanied by other symptoms and signs of CVST, including seizures, papilloedema, altered level of consciousness, and focal neurological symptoms or signs, 15%–30% of patients present with an isolated headache.[19,20]

CVST is more common during puerperium and these patients typically have an acute presentation that may include TCH. Headache in CVST can be caused directly by distention of veins or sinuses, increased intracranial pressure, or associated ischaemic or haemorrhagic stroke. CT scan may be normal in 25% patients who have no abnormality on physical examination, but abnormal in up to 90% of patients with focal neurological deficits. CT abnormalities include venous infarcts, evidence of oedema, or hyperdensity within the occluded sinus. MRI with venography is usually needed for the diagnosis of CVST; it should be considered as the investigation of first choice whenever CVST is suspected.[21]

Cervical artery dissection

Headache is the most common symptom in patients presenting with cervical artery dissection. It is reported in 60%–95% of patients with carotid artery dissections and in ~70% of patients with vertebral artery dissections.[22] Although the headaches most commonly have a gradual onset, 20% of patients present with TCH. According to the International Headache Society's (IHS) diagnostic criteria, headaches secondary to cervical artery dissection must be ipsilateral to the dissected artery.[1] Headaches from carotid artery dissection are invariably ipsilateral to the dissection and most commonly involve the jaw, face, ears, periorbital, and frontal or temporal regions. Headaches caused by vertebral artery dissection are commonly located in the occipital-nuchal region; however, with dissection of any of these arteries, headaches may less commonly be diffuse and bilateral. Neck pain accompanies head pain in 50% of patients with vertebral artery dissection and in 25% of patients with carotid artery dissection. Associated neurological symptoms and signs include amaurosis fugax, Horner syndrome, pulsatile tinnitus, dysgeusia, diplopia, or other stroke manifestations.

Diagnostic tests include doppler study, CTA, MRA, conventional angiography, or MRI of the neck with a fat saturation protocol. Unless accompanied by ischaemic stroke, CT and lumbar puncture are not helpful.

Spontaneous intracranial hypotension

Spontaneous intracranial hypotension (SIH) usually appears as a positional headache that worsens when upright and improves after lying down. SIH is typically preceded by minor trauma, such as trivial falls, lifting, coughing, and sports activities. Most headaches are bilateral, in the frontal, fronto-occipital, holocranial, or occipital regions, and can be associated with throbbing. However, ~15% of patients with SIH present with TCH.[23]

Lumbar puncture is done to exclude other processes, such as SAH. Opening pressure is typically low and can even be undetectable. CSF is generally clear and colourless, protein concentration is normal or slightly high (<100 mg/dl), erythrocyte count can be normal or high, a lymphocytic pleocytosis of ≤50 cells per cubic mm is common, and glucose, cytological and microbiological tests are normal. Brain MRI with gadolinium typically reveals features of SIH, including diffuse pachymeningeal enhancement and evidence of 'brain sag' or cerebellar tonsillar descent. Crowding of the posterior fossa,

reduction in the prepontine space, descent of the optic chiasm, and subdural collections may also be present. MRI of the spine might show extra-arachnoid CSF collection. Nuclear cisternography, CT myelography, or magnetic resonance myelography may be required to confirm the presence and location of the CSF leak.

Pituitary apoplexy

Pituitary apoplexy is haemorrhage or infarction of the pituitary gland, usually in the setting of a pituitary adenoma. Patients with pituitary apoplexy most commonly present with a combination of acute headache, nausea, decreased visual acuity, ophthalmoplegia, and reduction in visual fields.[20] Cases have been reported of pituitary apoplexy in patients presenting with TCH and normal physical examinations, CT scans, and CSF.[24,25]

Reversible cerebral vasoconstriction syndrome (RCVS)

Some patients with TCH show evidence of vasospasm on angiography. In these patients, angiography shows alternating segments of vasoconstriction and dilation in the proximal and distal branches of the circle of Willis. It has been reported in various clinical settings (Table 3), a disturbance of vascular tone being the likely pathogenesis in all cases.

RCVS is a group of disorders characterized by reversible segmental cerebral vasoconstriction, and includes TCH with vasoconstriction, benign angiopathy of the CNS, Call-Fleming syndrome, postpartum angiopathy, migrainous vasospasm, and drug-induced vasospasm. Medications that have been associated with RCVS include SSRIs, cannabis, ecstasy and vasoactive drugs such as exercise stimulants, nasal decongestants, amphetamines, and cocaine. Other associated substances are red blood cell products, intravenous immune globulin, erythropoietin,

Table 3. The following conditions are associated with cerebral vasoconstriction syndromes[21]

---

1. **Pregnancy and puerperium**

   Early puerperium

   Late pregnancy

   Eclampsia, pre-eclampsia and delayed postpartum eclampsia

2. **Drugs and blood products**

   Phenylpropanolamine

   Pseudoephedrine

   Ergotamine tartrate

   Methergine

   Bromocriptine

   Lisuride

   SSRIs

   Sumatriptan

   Amphetamine derivatives

   Marijuana, LSD

   Cyclophosphamide

   Erythropoietin, i.v. IgG, red blood cell transfusion

3. **Miscellaneous**

   Acute hypertension

   Hypercalcaemia

   Porphyria

   Pheochromocytoma

   Bronchial carcinoid tumour

   Head trauma

   Spinal subdural haematoma

   Carotid endarterectomy

   Neurosurgical procedures

4. **Spontaneous, physical exertion and sexual intercourse**

---

tacrolimus, and interferon.

Diagnostic criteria for RCVS include the following:

- Documentation by transfemoral angiography, CTA, or MRA of multifocal segmental cerebral artery vasoconstriction
- No evidence of aneurysmal SAH
- Normal or near normal findings on CSF analysis (protein level <80 mg/dl; white blood cells <10/μl; normal glucose level)
- Severe, acute headaches, with or without additional neurological signs or symptoms
- Reversibility of angiographic abnormalities within 12 weeks after onset.[26]

Primary cough, exertional and sexual headache

Patients who present with acute onset of severe headache occurring only after precipitation by cough, physical exertion, or sexual activity, and with a normal comprehensive assessment for causes of secondary headache, can be classified as having primary cough, exertional, or sexual headache. Similar to primary TCH, these diagnoses require a normal diagnostic assessment, as headaches precipitated by such maneuvers might be secondary to many of the previously discussed causes of TCH as well as other structural abnormalities, such as Chiari malformation type I.

The IHS's diagnostic criteria stipulate that primary cough headache be precipitated by coughing, straining, or valsalva, has a sudden onset and a duration of 1 second to 30 minutes.[1] Primary exertional headache can be brought on by any form of exercise, must be pulsating, and lasts from 5 minutes to 48 hours. The primary sexual headaches are divided into those occurring preorgasmically and those occurring with orgasm. The orgasmic headaches are of the thunderclap variety whereas most preorgasmic headaches present as a dull ache in the head and neck that increases with sexual excitement. There have been case reports of sexual headache being caused by RCVS.[27]

Primary TCH

Patients with TCH in whom an underlying cause is not found are diagnosed with primary TCH. Primary TCH is both the diagnosis of exclusion, which can be made only after exhaustive assessment for all possible underlying causes, and the diagnosis of inclusion, as certain features must be present. The concept that TCH can be a primary headache disorder has only been considered recently, and diagnostic criteria for this have been proposed by the IHS (Table 4).[1] In developing these criteria, the second edition of International classification of headache disorders acknowledged that the evidence supporting this entity is inadequate.

The prevalence of primary TCH is not known but it is a rare entity. This predominantly affects individuals between 20–50 years of age and has a female predominance.[28] Primary TCH has a relatively benign prognosis. The clinical picture of primary TCH is characteristic. Headache appears suddenly and reaches a maximum within 30 seconds and lasts for several hours but may persist for weeks. Headache can be diffuse but is often occipital in location and can be accompanied by symptoms of migraine, such as photophobia, phonophobia, nausea and vomiting. In approximately two-thirds of patients, headache repeats over a period of 2 weeks, whereas the remaining one-third patients experience headache attacks for up to several years. Headache may appear spontaneously or may be triggered by exertion, vigorous exercise, bathing in hot water, hyperventilation, or by sexual intercourse. Valsalva-related maneuvers appear to be provoking factors in up to one-third of patients.

The pathophysiology of primary TCH is unclear, but hypersensitivity of the cranial autonomic system has been proposed. An excessive sympathethic activity, an abnormal vascular response to circulating cathecolamines, or an aberrant central sympathetic neurogenic reflex could explain the occurrence of TCH in patients who have pheochromocytoma, with acute hypertensive crisis in patients on amphetamine or cocaine, or who consume foods containing tyramine, while concurrently taking monoaminoxidase inhibitors.[2]

Diagnostic evaluation

TCH must be managed as a medical emergency in order to avoid potentially fatal consequences that can occur with secondary TCH. The initial diagnostic assessment must be focused on ruling out SAH. Non-contrast CT of the brain is the first test in this assessment followed by CSF examination. CT scan can be normal in many conditions of symptomatic TCH (Table 5). MRI will be necessary to diagnose many of the other possible causes of TCH and the diagnosis of primary TCH should be made only after a normal MRI.

Treatment of TCH depends on the cause. If initial investigations are negative, treatment is symptomatic. A short course of steroids can be justified to cover for cerebral vasculitis while awaiting the results of angiography. Primary TCH is usually a self-limiting disorder with no treatment recommendations. Nimodipine and verapemil have been demonstrated to prevent further attacks of TCHs in most patients and may be recommended for 2–3 months.

Conclusion

TCH is a clinical emergency that requires an urgent evaluation with investigations aimed at excluding a subarachnoid haemorrhage. Early CT has high sensitivity and specificity for detecting subarachnoid blood. However, when negative, lumbar puncture is required. In those patients with normal neurological, CT and CSF examinations, further imaging to detect an unruptured

Table 4. Primary TCH diagnostic criteria[1]

A. Severe head pain fulfilling criteria B and C
B. Both of the following characteristics:
Sudden onset, reaching maximum intensity in <1 minute
Lasting from 1 hour to 10 days
C. Does not recur regularly over subsequent weeks or months
D. Not attributed to another disorder (normal CSF and normal brain imaging a prerequisite)

Table 5. Conditions that can present with thunderclap headache and a normal CT scan[9]

Dural sinus thrombosis
Expansion or thrombosis of an unruptured intracranial aneurysm
Pituitary apoplexy
Dissection of the cerebral or cervical arteries
Hypertensive crisis
Posterior reversible leukoencephalopathy syndrome
Sympathomimetic-induced vasospasm
Cerebral vasculitis
Vasoconstrictive angiopathies (postpartum, exertional, coital)
Spontaneous intracranial hypotension
Viral or bacterial meningoencephalitis
Sphenoid sinusitis

intracranial aneurysm is not indicated. Acute neurological emergencies, such as cervical arterial dissection and CVST, may present with TCH as the only symptom in a minority of patients. Brain CT is often negative in these cases, and lumbar puncture is either negative, as in the case of arterial dissection, or may only demonstrate increased opening pressure in patients with cerebral venous thrombosis. In these cases, MRI with angio-venography is the imaging procedure of choice. When appropriate investigations have excluded all potential secondary causes, a diagnosis of primary TCH is appropriate.

References

1. Headache Classification Subcommittee of the International Headache Society. International classification of headache disorders. 2nd ed. *Cephalalgia* 2004;**24**(suppl 1):9–160.
2. Day JW, Raskin NH. Thunderclap headache: Symptom of unruptured cerebral aneurysm. *Lancet* 1986;**2**:1247–8.
3. van Gijn J, Rinkel GJ. Subarachnoid haemorrhage: Diagnosis, causes and management. *Brain* 2001;**124**:249–78.
4. Raps EC, Rogers JD, Galetta SL, *et al.* The clinical spectrum of unruptured intracranial aneurysms. *Arch Neurol* 1993;**50**:265–8.
5. Linn FHH, Rinkel GJE, Algra A, *et al.* The notion of 'warning leaks' insubarachnoid hemorrhage: Are such patients in fact admitted with a rebleed? *J Neurol Neurosurg Psychiatry* 2000;**68**:332–6.
6. Sean IS, Emily BL, Robert W, *et al.* Pooled analysis of patients with thunderclap headache evaluated by CT and LP. *J Neurol Sci* 2009;**276**:123–5.
7. Wardlaw JM, White PM. The detection and management of unruptured intracranial aneurysms. *Brain* 2000;**123**:205–21.
8. Hope JK, Wilson JL, Thomson FJ. Three-dimensional CT angiography in the detection and characterization of intracranial berry aneurysms. *Am J Neuroradiol* 1996;**17**:439–45.
9. Moussouttas M, Mayer SA. Thunderclap headache with normal CT and lumbar puncture: Further investigations are unnecessary: Against. *Stroke* 2008;**39**:1394–5.
10. Wijdicks EFM, Kerkhoff H, Van Gijn J. Long-term follow-up of 71 patients with thunderclap headache mimicking subarachnoid haemorrhage. *Lancet* 1988;**2**:68–70.
11. Linn FHH, Rinkel GJE, Algra A, *et al.* Follow-up of idiopathic thunderclap headache in general practice. *J Neurol* 1999;**246**:946–48.
12. Harling DW, Peatfield RC, Van Hille PT, *et al.* Thunderclap headache: Is it migraine? *Cephalalgia* 1989;**9**:87–90.
13. Landtblom AM, Boivie J, Fridriksson S, *et al.* Thunderclap headache: Final results from a prospective study of consecutive cases. *Acta Neurol Scand* 1996;**167** (suppl 94):23–24.
14. Markus HS. A prospective follow up of thunderclap headache mimicking subarachnoid hemorrhage. *J Neurol Neurosurg Psychiatry* 1991;**54**:1117–18.
15. Sean I. Savitz, Jonathan Edlow. Thunderclap headache with normal CT and lumbar puncture: Further investigations are unnecessary. *Stroke* 2008;**39**:1392–3.
16. Polmear A. Sentinel headaches in aneurysmal subarachnoid hemorrhage: What is the true incidence? A systematic review. *Cephalalgia* 2003;**23**:935–41.
17. Dodick DW, Wijdicks EFM. Pituitary apoplexy presenting as thunderclap headache. *Neurology* 1998;**50**:1510–11.
18. Miller Fisher C. Honored guest presentation: Painful states: A neurological commentary. *Clin Neurosurg* 1984;**31**:32–53.
19. Dodick DW. Thunderclap headache. *J Neurol*

Neurosurg Psychiatry 2002;**72:**6–11.

20. Schwedt TJ, Matharu MS, Dodick DW. Thunderclap headache. *Lancet Neurol* 2006;**5:**621–31.

21. Leys D, Cordonnier C. Cerebral venous thrombosis: Update on clinical manifestations, diagnosis and management. *Ann Indian Acad Neurol* 2008;**11:** S79–S87.

22. Silbert PL, Mokri B, Schievink WI. Headache and neck pain in spontaneous internal carotid and vertebral artery dissections. *Neurology* 1995;**45:** 1517–22.

23. Ferrante E, Savino A. Thunderclap headache caused by spontaneous intracranial hypotension. *Neurol Sci* 2005;**26:**S155–S157.

24. Dodick DW, Wijdicks EFM. Pituitary apoplexy presenting as thunderclap headache. *Neurology* 1998; **50:**1510–11.

25. Embil JM, Matthias K, Kinnear R. A blinding headache. *Lancet* 1997;**350:**182.

26. Zarkou S, Dilli E, Dodick DW. 55-year-old man with thunderclap headache. *Mayo Clin Proc* 2010;**85:** e44–e47.

27. Hu CM, Lin YJ, Fan YK, *et al.* Isolated thunderclap headache during sex: Orgasmic headache or reversible cerebral vasoconstriction syndrome? *J Clin Neurosci* 2010;**17:**1349–51.

28. Linn FH. Primary thunderclap headache. *Handb Clin Neurol* 2010;**97:**473–81.

22

Isolated neurosarcoidosis: Diagnostic and therapeutic dilemmas

JOY DESAI

Introduction

Sarcoidosis is a multisystem, autoimmune, inflammatory disorder of unknown cause that produces dysfunction within almost all the organ systems. Involvement of the nervous system occurs in approximately 10%–15% of cases. Diagnosis is not difficult when symptoms related to the nervous system arise in an individual who has already been diagnosed to suffer from sarcoidosis. However, when the patient's initial symptoms are restricted to the nervous system, diagnostic evaluation and treatment pose unique challenges. In this review, a few patients with variable clinical presentations in whom a final diagnosis of neurosarcoidosis was established are discussed and the relevant literature reviewed.

Clinical cases

Case 1

A 23-year-old man developed new onset of headaches associated with episodic hallucinations of vividly formed and coloured shapes appearing within his visual fields. These headaches were associated with nausea and vomiting and would last for a few hours. He was treated by a physician for new-onset migraine

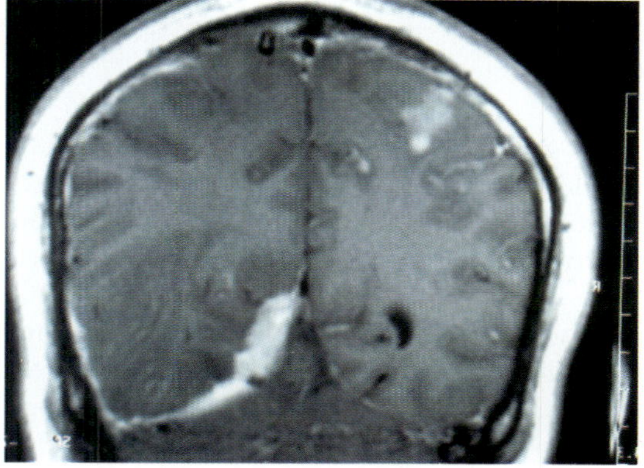

Fig. 1. Segmental occipital pachymeningeal enhancement on T₁-weighted image

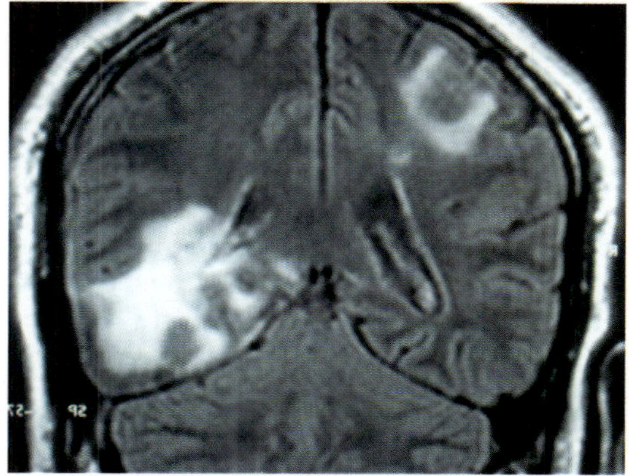

Fig. 2. Occipital and frontal white matter hyperintensities on T₂-weighted image

with standard therapy but the clinical response was poor. Neurological examination including fundus assessment was normal. The haemogram was normal, albeit with a high ESR of 67 mm/hour. Hepatorenal biochemistry, X-ray of the chest, urinary sediment, and thyroid function tests were all normal. MRI of the brain revealed localized T_2-weighted hyperintensities in the occipital white matter and an intense enhancement of the underlying pachymeninges in a segmentally localized distribution (Figs 1 and 2). CSF examination revealed euglycorachhia with raised proteins and a lymphocytic pleocytosis of 36 cells/cmm. A biopsy was taken from the lesion, which revealed typical non-caseating granulomas suggestive of sarcoidosis.

Case 2

A 64-year-old, well-controlled diabetic man developed subacute, progressive weakness without wasting in the lower limbs, which spread to involve the upper limbs within three weeks. This was associated with distal acral paraesthesiae without any sphincter dysfunction. Clinical examination revealed generalized areflexia. A single cervical lymph node was palpable on clinical examination. CSF examination revealed 10 cells/cmm with a lymphocytic predominance, normal sugar level but raised proteins. Nerve conduction velocity (NCV) study confirmed a demyelinating neuropathy. The serum angiotensin-converting enzyme (SACE) level was 47 mg/dl. FDG-PET study revealed multiple high-uptake areas in the cervical and mediastinal lymph nodes. An excision biopsy and histopathological examination of the cervical lymph node confirmed the changes of sarcoidosis (Fig. 3). On administration of intravenous steroids, the patient's diabetes worsened markedly, requiring increasing amounts of insulin. Finally, steroids were withdrawn and intravenous pulse cyclophosphamide therapy was initiated. After 10 pulses of cyclophosphamide at 3–4-weekly intervals, the patient went into

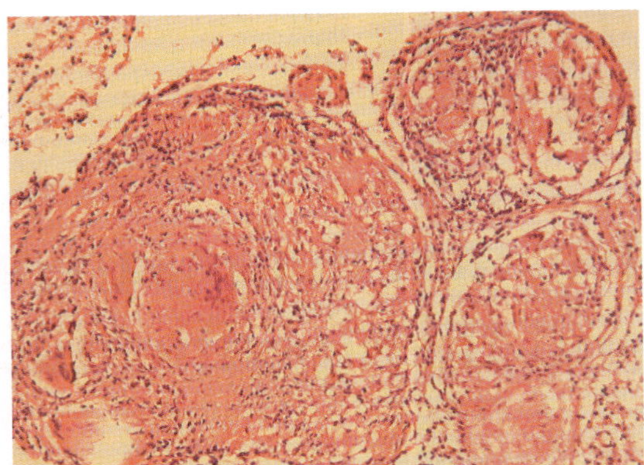

Fig. 3. Histopathological features of non-caseating granuloma consistent with sarcoidosis

total clinical remission with complete resolution of all his neurological symptoms and a remarkable improvement in the NCV findings.

Case 3

A 16-year-old adolescent girl from Gujarat presented at the local medical college with low-grade fever, bilateral parotid gland swelling and recurrent episodes of left-sided hemiparesis lasting for a few minutes, associated with slurring of speech and complete recovery within minutes. Physical examination revealed an anaemic individual with tachycardia, bilateral firm, mildly tender, parotid swelling and a normal CNS examination. Digital subtraction angiography (DSA) revealed a pseudoaneurysm of the right internal carotid artery (ICA) (Fig. 4). She was referred to Mumbai for stent insertion.

While awaiting evaluation, the patient had a cardiac arrest and had to be resuscitated. There was recurrent hypokalaemia while the patient was on replacement of potassium and this led to the unmasking of potassium-losing nephropathy. A renal biopsy revealed membranous glomerulonephritis with granulomatous interstitial nephritis. On examination, the renal granulomas were consistent with the features of sarcoidosis. The SACE level was normal. A diagnosis of systemic sarcoidosis was made and the patient

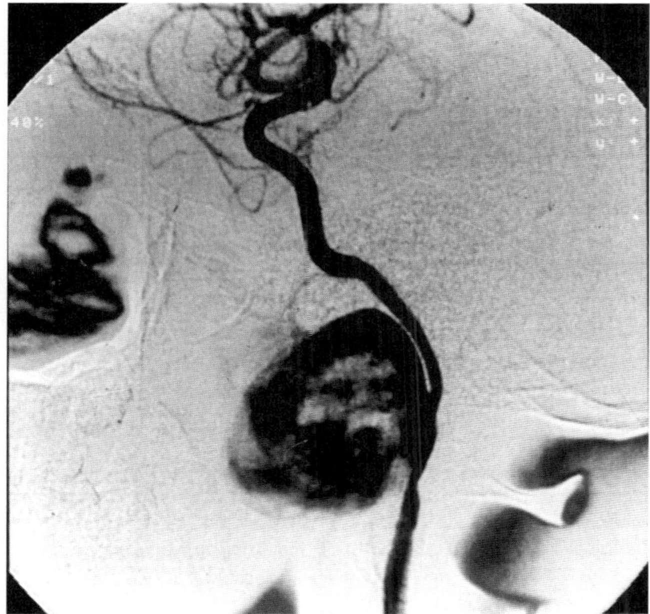

Fig. 4. Right internal carotid artery pseudoaneurysm adjacent to the parotid gland

was given pulsed methylprednisolone for 5 days followed by a course of oral steroids. The hypokalaemia remitted. DSA was repeated after 6 weeks and showed a dramatic regression in the size of the right ICA pseudoaneurysm. Ultimately, the proposed stenting for the pseudoaneurysm was deferred.

Case 4

An 18-year-old girl developed retro-orbital pain, pain on moving the eye, and sudden loss of vision in the left eye. This was followed within four days by a similar loss of vision in the opposite eye. Haemogram, serum biochemistry, auto-antibody panel for systemic vasculitides, and CSF examination were all normal. MRI of the brain was unremarkable. A clinical diagnosis of bilateral optic neuritis was made and she was treated with intravenous pulsed methylprednisolone therapy for 5 days with a good clinical response and near-complete visual recovery.

Twenty-four months later, she developed sudden onset of bilateral hearing loss without any accompanying neurological features. She was treated with oral steroids this time at a rural centre but there was no meaningful improvement in her hearing loss. Three years later, she presented with sudden onset of diplopia, slurring of speech and ataxia. Clinical examination revealed previous hearing loss, chaotic eye movements, and visible limb ataxia with normal reflexes and no other signs of CNS dysfunction. Haematological investigations including a systemic vasculitides panel were unrewarding except for a moderately high ESR. FDG-PET scan revealed multiple areas of high uptake in the mediastinal lymph nodes, and MRI of the brain revealed an irregular granulomatous enhancement pattern in the cerebellar folia with FLAIR hyperintensities in the subjacent cerebellar white matter (Figs 5 and 6). CSF examination showed lymphocytic pleocytosis with euglycorachhia. On the basis of these findings, a tentative diagnosis of possible neurosarcoidosis was made and the

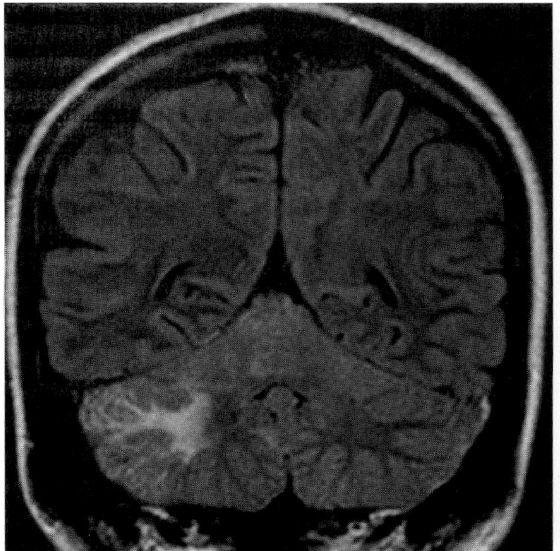

Fig. 5. Cerebellar white matter hyperintensities on FLAIR imaging

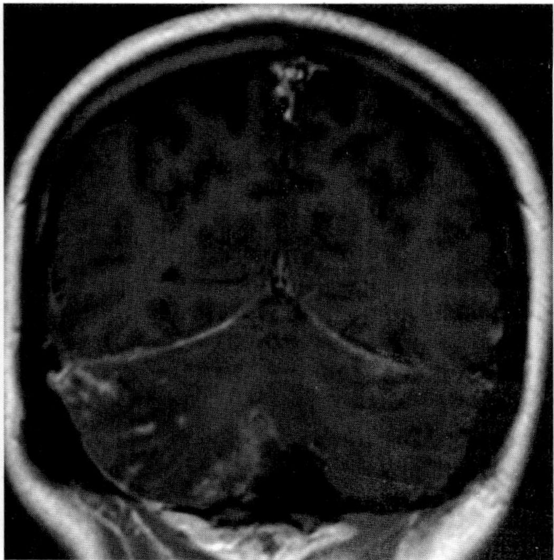

Fig. 6. Granulomatous enhancement in the cerebellar folia on T₁-weighted images

patient was treated with steroids followed by rewarding results of a near-complete resolution in 3 weeks.

Case 5

A 45-year-old man developed right-sided sharp, lancinating pain in the distribution of the V2 and V3 divisions of the trigeminal nerve. Despite multiple consultations and therapy with a variety of anticonvulsants, there was no clinical relief. CNS examination was normal. MRI of the brain revealed a homogeneously enhancing, well-demarcated lesion in the right trigeminal ganglion extending into the base of the skull. The radiological appearance appeared to be that of a meningioma. Clinical examination revealed an apparently incidental left cervical lymph node. A biopsy of the lymph node revealed a granulomatous lesion and the patient was treated with antituberculous therapy with no change in the lymph node size after 3 months. Steroids were empirically administered at an alternative centre, with full resolution of the lymph node and a bonus relief in the trigeminal symptoms. Follow-

up MRI showed a marked regression in the previous lesion thought to be a meningioma.

Discussion

The above cases illustrate the myriad ways in which neurosarcoidosis can present within the central and peripheral nervous system, at times mimicking other disorders. This can pose a diagnostic challenge. Recognizing the pattern of neurological symptomatology in the given clinical setting may aid in arriving at a diagnosis of neurosarcoidosis. Virtually any part of the central and peripheral neuraxis may be affected by sarcoidosis. The disease may involve the meninges in a segmental fashion producing aseptic meningitis and a striking appearance on contrast-enhanced MRI. Cerebral lesions may mimic tumours or space-occupying lesions (SOLs) and may be mistaken for meningiomas due to the homogeneous enhancement of gadolinium with the lesion. There is a predilection for involvement of the base of the brain and the lesion may even involve the hypothalamus. The optic, facial, trigeminal and

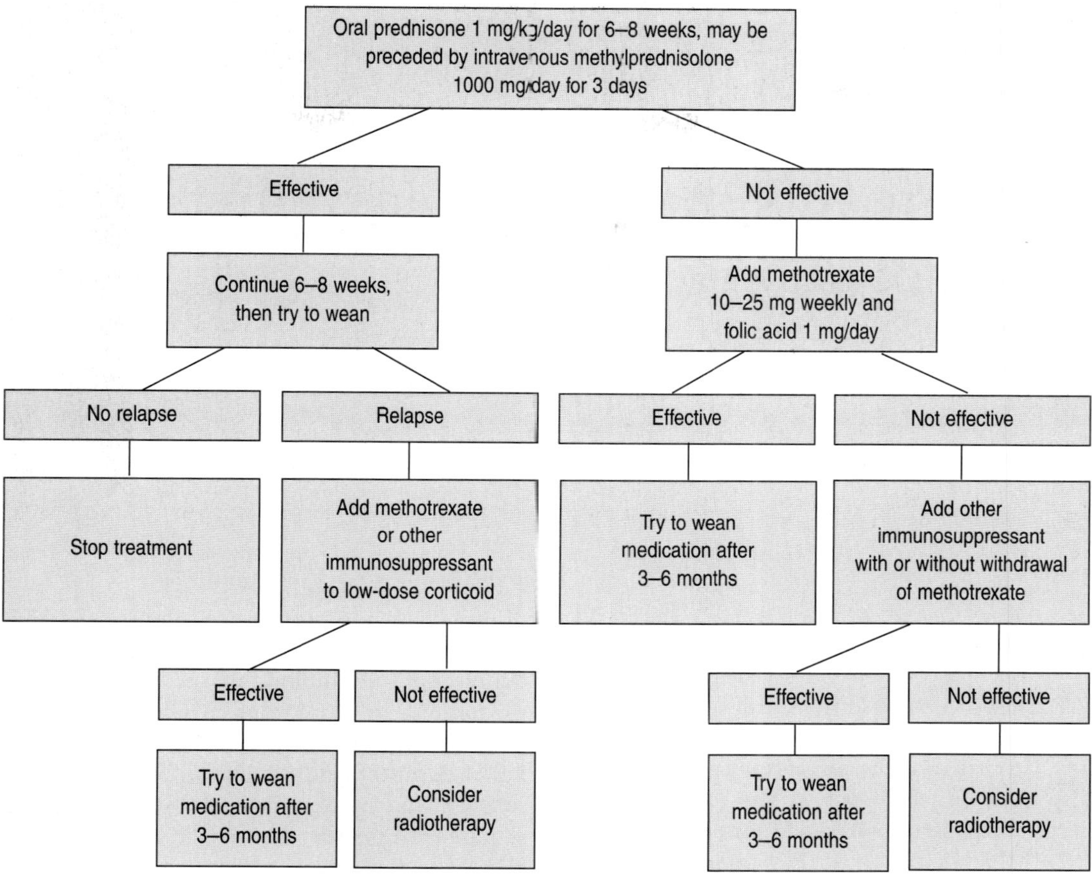

Fig. 7. Algorithm for the treatment of neurosarcoidosis

acoustic nerves are commonly involved in neurosarcoidosis. Spinal radiculomyelitis may make the distinction from tuberculosis difficult. Involve-ment of the peripheral nervous system often produces a demyelinating neuropathy or a myopathy. Gallium 67 scanning or FDG-PET scanning may aid in the diagnosis by revealing asymptomatic parotid uptake or asymptomatic uptake in the mediastinal lymph nodes producing a 'lambda' pattern. Asymptomatic uptake in the lacrimal and parotid glands bilaterally may sometimes produce the 'face of the Panda sign' on these functional imaging techniques. The therapy of neurosarcoidosis is not different from that of systemic sarcoidosis and can be summarized in the algorithm of Fig. 7.

References

1. Hoitsma E, Faber C, Drent M, *et al.* Neurosarcoidosis: A clinical dilemma. *Lancet Neurol* 2004;3:397–407.
2. Lower E, Weiss K. Neurosarcoidosis. *Clin Chest Med* 2008;29:473–92.
3. Yu J, Zhuang H, Mavi A, *et al.* Evaluating the role of flurodeoxyglucose PET imaging in the management of patients with sarcoidosis. *PET Clin* 2006;1:132–41.
4. Berliner A, Haas M, Choi M. Sarcoidosis: The nephrologist's perspective. *Am J Kid Dis* 2006;48:856–70.

23

Chronic inflammatory demyelinating polyradiculoneuropathy: Indian perspective and update

COL S.P. GORTHI

Introduction

Peripheral neuropathy, with its diverse aetiologies and a *de novo* presentation without any known association, presents a difficult diagnostic problem. We at the Armed Forces Medical College (AFMC) and Command Hospital (Southern Command), Pune, systematically studied 35 such cases of peripheral neuropathy between 2006 and 2008, and in the final analysis, chronic inflammatory demyelinating neuropathy emerged as a single large group (20 of 35 patients).

This chapter focuses on various clinical features of this important neuropathy, and where applicable, comparisons will be made between our group's studies and those cited in the literature.

Chronic inflammatory demyelinating polyradiculoneuropathy (CIDP) is an acquired multifocal neuropathy that commonly has symmetric, proximal and distal limb weakness, and distal sensory loss that progresses over 2 months.[1] Clinical and immunopathological studies suggest an aberrant immune mechanism. Treatment of this condition is with immunomodulatory medications. Whether CIDP is a disease or a syndrome remains controversial. The following neuropathies all have chronicity, demyelination, inflammation, or immune-mediation in common: Multifocal motor neuropathy with conduction block (MMNCB), Lewis–Sumner syndrome (multifocal acquired sensory and motor neuropathy) and distal acquired symmetric demyelinating neuropathy (DADS), and many others associated with various diseases.

Epidemiology

The reported prevalence is 1–1.9 per 100,000 population and incidence is 0.15 per 100,000. The mean age of onset in most studies is 47.6 years. A relapsing–remitting course is encountered in ~51% of patients. The ALS phenotype may have up to 1.6% cases of MMNCB. In the study conducted at the AFMC, Pune, the predominant age group was between 20–30 years (11/35) and 51–60 years (11/35) (Table 1). Eighty per cent of our cases were male (Figs 1a and 1b).

CIDP is usually idiopathic but it may be associated with other diseases. Most common associations are with diabetes mellitus, parapro-

Table 1. Diagnostic criteria of CIDP; European Federation of Neurological Societies (2006)

Mandatory clinical features

Weakness	**Typical:** Symmetric proximal and distal
	Atypical: DADS MADSAM pure motor and pure sensory
Reflexes	Arelexia or hyporeflexia
Time course	At least 2 months
Exclusion features	Clinical features of hereditary neuropathy, diphtheria, multifocal motor neuropathy, sphincteric disturbances, myelin-associated glycoprotein abnormalities

Laboratory features

Electrodiagnostic studies	One of the following must be met for definite diagnosis:
	
	Conduction block: CB of at least 50% if distal CMAP is at least 20% of LLN in two nerves or in one nerve plus one other nerve with feature of demyelination
	
	Temporal dispersion: >30% increase in duration in two nerves
	
	Distal CMAP dispersion: Distal CMAP duration >9 ms plus one of the following other feature of demyelination must be met:
	
	    Conduction velocity: At least 30% slowing of CV below LLN in two nerves
	
	    Distal latency: At least 50% prolongation of DL above ULN in two nerves
	
	    F latency: At least 20% increase in F wave above ULN (at least 50% increase if distal CMAP amplitude is <80 LLN); Absent F wave if distal CMAP amplitude is >20% of the LLN

Cerebrospinal fluid	Elevated CSF protein and cell count <10/mm³
Nerve biopsy features	Evidence of demyelination/remyelination on nerve biopsy with >5 fibres on EM or 6/60 teased fibres
Definitive diagnosis of CIDP	Clinical plus definite EDX criteria or probable EDX criteria plus one laboratory supportive criterion (CSF, nerve biopsy, MRI of roots, plexus or nerves showing thickening or enhancement, or clinical improvement with immunotherapy) **Or** possible EDX criteria plus two laboratory supportive criteria
Probable	Clinical and NCS showing CB <50% but >30% if distal CMAP is at least 20% of LLN in two nerves (excluding the posterior tibial) or in one nerve plus one other nerve with feature of demyelination
Possible	Clinical plus any one of the above EDX criteria found in only one nerve

teinaemias and monoclonal gammopathy of unknown origin (MUGS). Other notable associations are HIV infection, hepatitis C infection, Sjogren syndrome, lymphoma and melanoma.

CIDP occurs with both types 1 and 2 diabetes mellitus (DM) and may be more common than the idiopathic variety. When CIDP occurs in the setting of DM the disease is more severe with fewer relapses and a better response to intravenous immunoglobulin (IG).

CIDP associated with haematological malignancies characteristically involves plasma cells, such as plasmacytoma or osteosclerotic myeloma.[2]

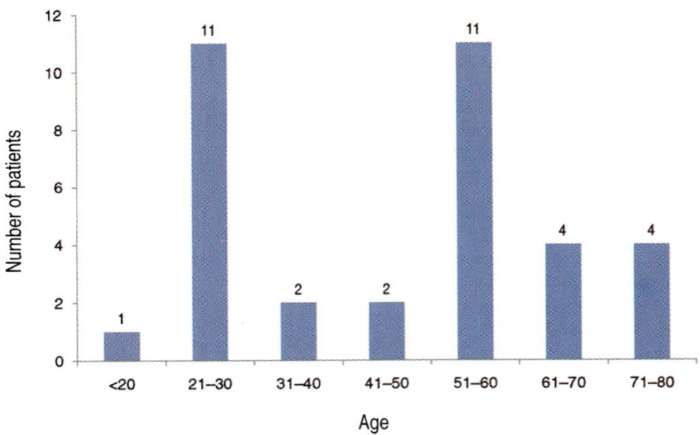

Fig. 1a. Age-wise distribution: 35 cases of peripheral neuropathy (AFMC study)

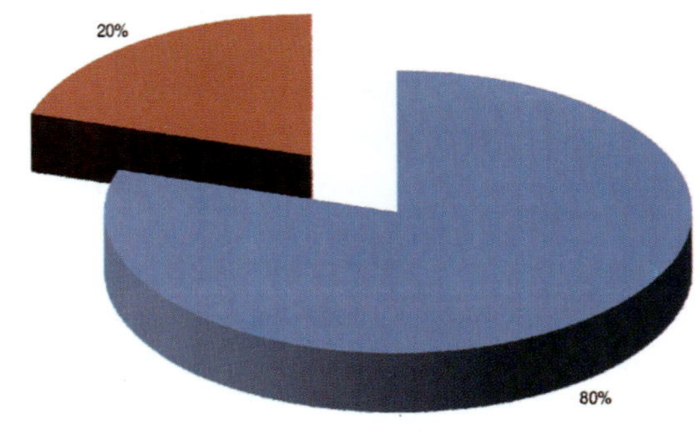

Fig. 1b. Sex distribution: 35 cases of peripheral neuropathy (AFMC study)

Pathogenesis

Both cell-mediated and humoral immunity-related abnormalities are implicated in the pathogenesis of CIDP. Involvement with cellular immunity is supported by evidence of T-cell activation, crossing of the blood–nerve barrier by activated T-cells, and by expression of cytokines, tumour necrosis factor, interferons, and interleukins. Humoral immunity is implicated by the demonstration of IG and complement deposition on myelinated nerve fibres.

Pathophysiology

The characteristic pathological features of CIDP include segmental demyelination and remyelination, and onion bulb formation. Some degree of axonal degeneration is usually present. Varying degrees of interstitial oedema and endoneurial inflammatory cell infiltrates, including lymphocytes and macrophages, are additional pathological features of CIDP.

Electrophysiology

Peripheral nerve demyelination underlies the characteristic electrophysiological features of CIDP, which are as follows: Partial conduction block, slowing of conduction velocity, prolonged distal motor latencies, delay or disappearance of F-waves, and dispersion and distance-dependent reduction of compound motor action potential (CMAP) amplitude.

Clinical features

Acute inflammatory demyelinating polyneuropathy (AIDP), the demyelinating form of Guillain–Barré syndrome, and CIDP show a temporal continuum. AIDP is a monophasic subacute illness that reaches its nadir within 3–4 weeks. CIDP continues to progress or has relapses for >8 weeks. Sub-acute inflammatory demyelinating polyneuropathy (SIDP) is the term used by some authors for disease that reaches its nadir between 4 and 8 weeks.[3]

In the classic form of CIDP, motor involvement is greater than sensory involvement, and neurological deficits are fairly symmetrical. Weakness is present in both proximal and distal muscles. Most patients have globally diminished or absent reflexes.

Sensory impairment in CIDP is usually greater for vibration and position sense than for pain and temperature sense, reflecting the involvement of larger myelinated fibres. Unlike the motor involvement, the sensory involvement tends to follow a distal to proximal gradient, although finger involvement is frequently seen as early as toe and foot involvement. Painful dysesthesias can occur in some patients. Cranial nerve and bulbar involvement occur in a minority of patients. The clinical course of CIDP is slowly progressive in a majority of patients, but a relapsing-remitting course is noted in at least one-third.

In the AFMC study, peripheral neuropathy, in which CIDP formed a major group, consisted of limb weakness and numbness in 71%, pain and numbness in 11%, numbness in 9%, pain alone in 6%, and weakness by itself in 3% of cases (Fig. 2).[4]

Progressive weakness in proximal muscles and sensory symptoms distally over 2 months is the most frequent presentation. This contrasts with the distal weakness seen in axonal neuropathies. Distal predominance of motor and sensory features is seen in 17% of cases (DADS variant) and pure motor features in 10% of cases (MMNCB). Subclinical cranial nerve dysfunction may occur in 6%–30% cases and presents as facial numbeness, facial weakness, papilloedema and hypoglossal neuropathies.

Diagnosis

The diagnosis of CIDP should be considered in patients with symmetric or asymmetric polyneuropathy who have a progressive or relapsing–remitting clinical course for >2 months, particularly if the clinical features include positive sensory symptoms, proximal weakness, areflexia without wasting, or selective loss of vibration or joint position sense. In our study of 35 cases of peripheral neuropathy, the clinical syndromes included symmetric distal motor

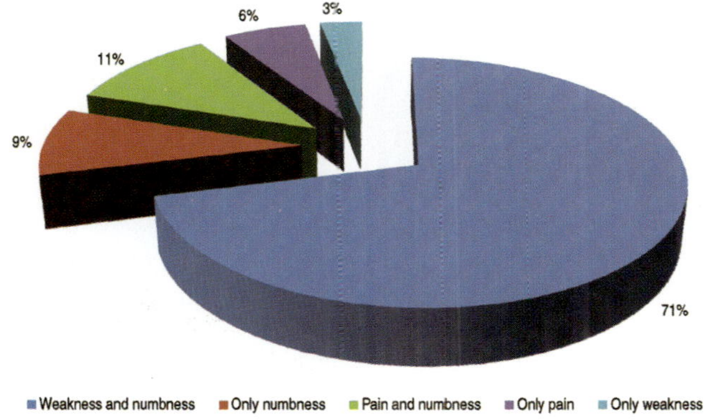

Fig. 2. Clinical symptomatology: 35 cases of peripheral neuropathy (AFMC study)

254 COL S.P. GORTHI

sensory peripheral neuropathy (SDMSPN; 74%), symmetric distal sensory polyneuropathy (SDSPN; 11%), asymmetric sensory neuropathy (9%), asymmetric motor peripheral neuropathy (3%), and mononeuritis multiplex (3%) (Fig. 3).[4] Both SDMSPN and SDSPN accounted for all cases of CIDP and unknown aetiology in this study. Our population may present more commonly with atypical features of CIDP or its variants.

Whereas the initial diagnosis of CIDP is clinical, the final diagnosis is confirmed by evidence from electrodiagnostic studies, and in some cases by cerebrospinal fluid (CSF) analysis, nerve biopsy findings, and other laboratory investigations. Peripheral nerve demyelination must be demonstrated by either electrodiagnostic findings or by nerve biopsy. The clinical features that distinguish CIDP from chronic length-dependent (i.e. axonal) peripheral neuropathies are the prominence of muscle weakness and the involvement of upper extremity and proximal muscles, as well as distal muscles. In contrast, axonal polyneuropathies are characterized by predominantly distal weakness. Furthermore, deep tendon reflexes are globally reduced or absent in CIDP, whereas only the ankle reflexes are diminished in typical axonal poly-neuropathies. The features of CIDP point to the multifocal or generalized nature of the disease even at early stages of the illness. Diagnostic criteria include the following:

- Progression over at least 2 months.
- At presentation, weakness felt more often than sensory symptoms and in that symmetric involvement of arms and legs with proximal muscle involvement more than distal muscle groups.
- Reduced deep tendon reflexes throughout
- Increased CSF protein without pleocytosis (the classic albuminocytological dissociation is present in >90% of patients with CIDP)
- Nerve conduction evidence of a demyelinating neuropathy, nerve biopsy evidence of segmental demyelination with or without inflammation. The diagnostic utility of nerve biopsy (typically of the sural nerve) for suspected CIDP is controversial. Nerve biopsy can provide solid evidence of demyelination. In addition, biopsy occasionally reveals other neuropathies that mimic CIDP, such as those caused by amyloidosis, sarcoidosis, and vasculitis. Supportive features for CIDP on nerve biopsy include the following: Endoneurial oedema, macrophage-associated demyelination, demyelinated and remyelinated nerve fibres, onion bulb formation, and endoneurial mono-nuclear cell infiltration variation between fascicles
- MRI with gadolinium of the spinal roots, cauda equina, brachial plexus, lumbosacral plexus, and other nerve regions can be used to look for enlarged or enhancing nerves. MRI abnormalities are useful as supportive criteria

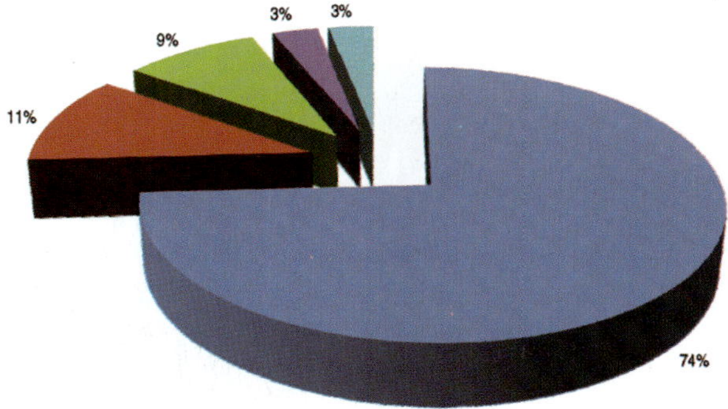

Fig. 3. Clinical syndromic pattern: 35 cases of peripheral neuropathy (AFMC study)

for CIDP in the European Federation of Neurological Societies and the Peripheral Nerve Society (EFNS/PNS) guidelines.

- Other laboratory studies: There are no blood tests that specifically point to CIDP. However, a number of studies are useful to identify disorders that are either associated with or mimic CIDP. These include the following: Fasting serum glucose and/or oral glucose tolerance test, glycated haemoglobin, thyroid function studies, hepatitis profiles, HIV antibody, serum and urine immunofixation electrophoresis (to detect paraprotein) complete blood count, renal function tests liver function tests, C reactive protein, antinuclear antibodies, extractable nuclear antigen antibodies, angiotensin converting enzyme, chest radiograph, and skeletal survey (if a paraprotein is found).

There is still no gold standard set of diagnostic criteria for the electrophysiological identification of demyelination or for the clinical diagnosis of CIDP and its variants, even though at least 8 sets of diagnostic criteria have been published since 1989. The current CIDP guideline from the EFNS/PNS (Table 1) is the most useful for clinical diagnosis.[5]

The EFNS/PNS guideline defines CIDP as typical (i.e. classic) or atypical. Atypical CIDP encompasses variants of CIDP with predominantly distal weakness, such as DADS, and variants with pure motor or pure sensory presentations. For definite CIDP, it is mandatory to have a typical or atypical clinical picture with clear demyelinating electrodiagnostic changes in 2 nerves, or probable demyelinating features in 2 nerves, plus at least one supportive feature (from CSF analysis, nerve biopsy, MRI, or treatment response to immunotherapy). The EFNS/PNS guidelines relegate CIDP with concomitant disease to a 'possible' category. IgM paraprotein-related neuropathies with anti-MAG antibodies are considered as distinct from CIDP, but IgM disorders without anti-MAG are considered to be a CIDP variant.[6] Our study showed features of both axonal and demyelinating features more commonly than pure demyelination features. Only 7 of 23 cases had pure features of demyelination, and 16 cases showed electrophysiological findings of both axonopathy and demyelination (Fig. 4).[4]

Evidence-based medicine (EBM) point: Which electrophysiological criteria should be used for the diagnosis of CIDP?

After studying and analyzing eight different studies, the following criteria are recommended for the diagnosis of CIDP:[6]

In two or more nerves

- *Distal latency:* >150% of upper limit of normal
- *Conduction velocity:* >70% of lower limit of

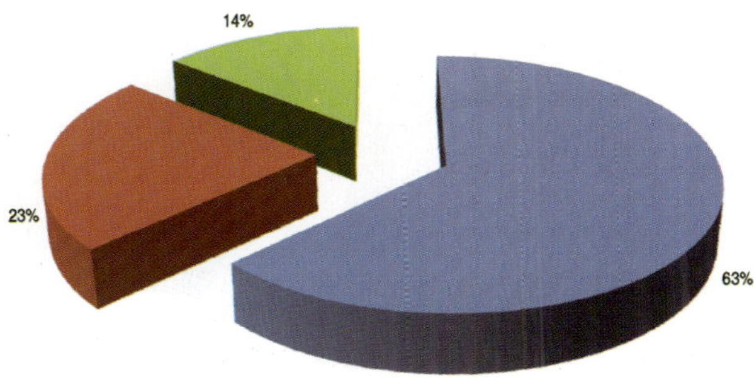

Fig. 4a. Electrophysiological patterns: 35 cases of peripheral neuropathy (AFMC study)

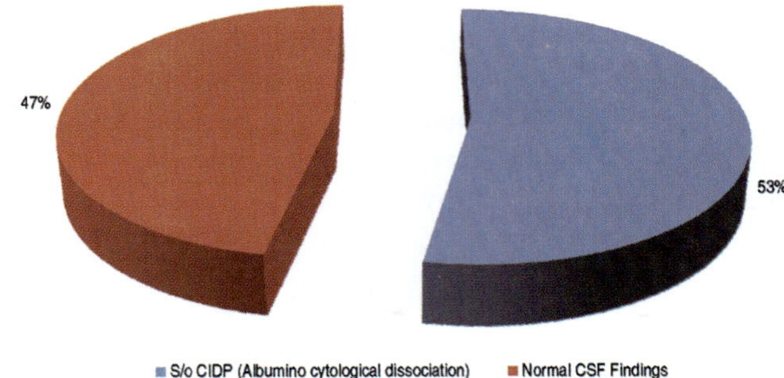

Fig. 4b. CSF Analysis: 35 cases of peripheral neuropathy (AFMC study)

normal
- *Conduction block:* 30%–50% loss of amplitude
- *F-response:* >120% or absent F-wave with CMAP >20% of normal amplitude

Any single criterion is sufficient for the diagnosis of CIDP. If conduction block is demonstrated in one nerve, any other one nerve should show one other abnormality. The sensitivity is 75% and specificity is 100%.

The CSF examination was done in 20 of 23 cases of CIDP; typical albumin–cytological dissociation was found in 18 cases (90%). Two cases with normal CSF were diagnosed by sural nerve biopsy (Fig. 5).[4]

EBM point: What is the utility of nerve biopsy in the diagnosis of CIDP?

The issue is controversial. Elevated CSF protein, neurophysiological evidence for demyelination, and the absence of an alternative aetiology for the neuropathy were the 3 factors that most strongly predicted CIDP. The results of sural nerve biopsy were found to have no significant additional predictive value.[7] The future advances consisting of a teased fibre preparation and studies under electron microscope should give a positive diagnosis.

In the AFMC study, sural nerve biopsy was

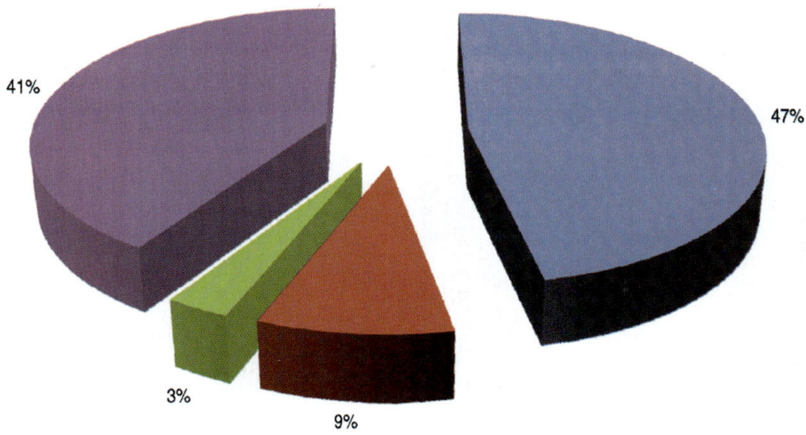

Fig. 5. Sural nerve biopsy findings: 35 cases of peripheral neuropathy (AFMC study)

performed in 32 of 35 cases. The histopathology report showed changes suggestive of CIDP (segmental demyelination) in 15 patients, vasculitis in 1 patient, and focal axonolysis in 3 patients. Thirteen patients showed normal histopathological findings (Figs 6–9). Sural nerve biopsy was carried out in 17 of 20 cases of CIDP; it proved to be confirmatory in 15 of 17 cases (88%).

Treatment[8–12]

Plasma exchange, intravenous IG, and glucocorticoids are the main treatment modalities for CIDP; all three appear to be equally effective. Intravenous IG and plasma exchange may lead to a more rapid improvement in CIDP than glucocorticoid therapy, but are less likely to

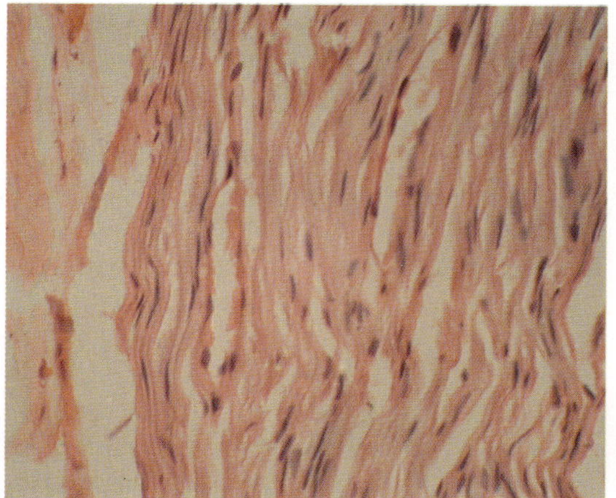

Fig. 6. Sural nerve biopsy: Peripheral nerve showing vacuoles in myelin fibres, segmental demyelination (B/241/06 dt 11 feb 06, H&E X600)

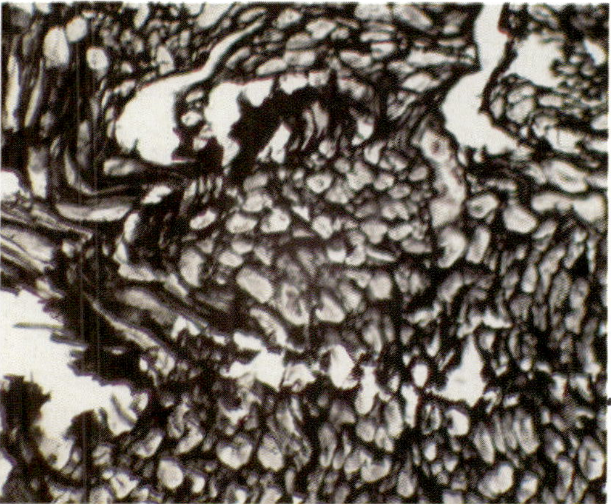

Fig. 7. Sural nerve biopsy: Peripheral nerve showing vacuoles in myelin fibres, segmental demyelination as well as severe axonal degeneration (B/711/06 dt 19 april 06, Solochrome cynanine X600)

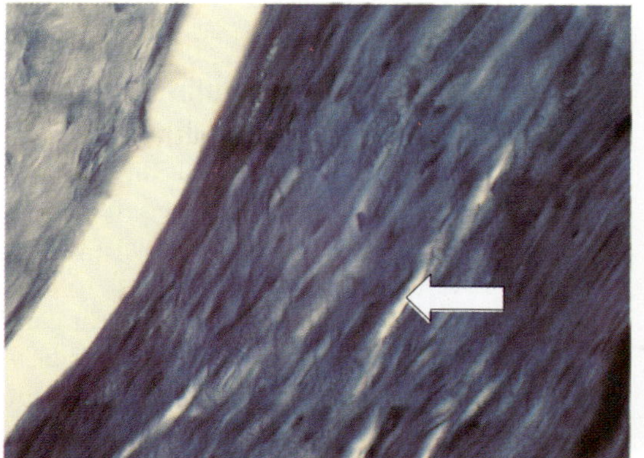

Fig. 8. Sural nerve biopsy: Peripheral nerve showing vacuolar degeneration of myelin (B/241/06 dt 11 Feb 06, Solchrome cynanine X600)

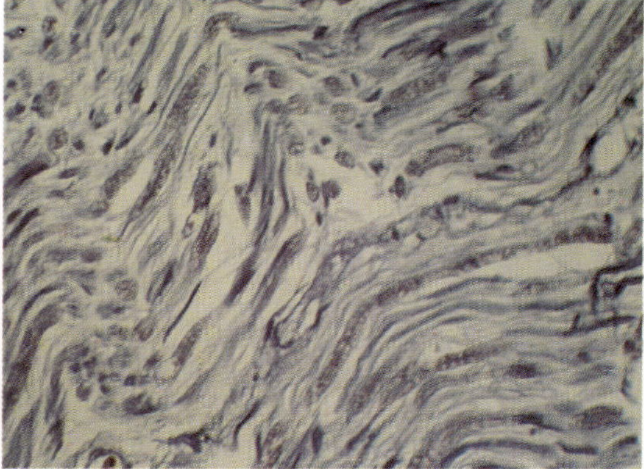

Fig. 9. Sural nerve biopsy. Peripheral nerve showing complete degeneration of axonal fibres (B/178/06 dated 3 February 2006, Solchrome cynanin X600)

produce a remission than glucocorticoids. Intravenous IG is expensive and its supply is sometimes limited. Glucocorticoids are inexpensive, but chronic use is limited by common and clinically important side-effects. Plasma exchange is expensive, invasive and available only at specialized centres. The rate of disability improvement within 1 month of treatment was significantly higher with intravenous IG than with placebo (RR [relative risk] 2.4, 95% CI 1.72–3.36).[10] To obtain improvement in 1 patient, the number needed to treat was 3. Overall, intravenous IG improved disability for 2–6 weeks. The benefit of intravenous IG was similar to that of plasma exchange and oral prednisolone. The ICE study confirmed evidence from earlier trials that intravenous IG is effective for the treatment of CIDP.[11] In addition, the ICE results suggested that the benefit of intravenous IG extends for as long as 48 weeks with a maintenance dose of 1 g/kg every 3 weeks. Whereas intravenous IG therapy can usually control CIDP, most patients require repeated expensive treatments every 2–6 weeks for many years, as intravenous IG monotherapy does not usually lead to remission. The initial dose of intravenous IG is 2 g/kg infused over 2–5 days (e.g. 0.4 g/kg per day for 5 days). Many patients with CIDP require repeat intravenous IG maintenance dosing every 2–6 weeks. For patients who respond well to initial treatment and remain clinically stable, the maintenance dose can be tapered to 1.0 g/kg, or as low as 0.4 g/kg, given over 1–2 days.

Substantial data from retrospective series suggest that oral glucocorticoids are beneficial for CIDP. The maximum benefit of glucocorticoid therapy in these studies was seen for 1–6 months of treatment. However, relapses were common, particularly when tapering the dose.[10] Clinical experience suggests that glucocorticoid therapy is more likely to produce a clinical remission than either intravenous IG or plasma exchange. Although less well studied, retrospective evidence

suggests that weekly pulse methylprednisolone (500 mg once a week) is also an effective option for long-term treatment of CIDP.[11] For patients with severe CIDP who are refractory to treatment with intravenous IG, glucocorticoids and plasma exchange, and are also refractory to glucocorticoids combined with intravenous IG or plasma exchange, alternative immunosuppressant treatment options include methotrexate, cyclosporine, azathioprine, mycophenolate, and cyclophosphamide. Whereas the long-term prognosis of CIDP is generally favourable, data are limited, and up to 15% of patients are severely disabled despite treatment.

EBM point: What is the evidence that steroids are of benefit to patients with CIDP?

Based on the results of a single randomized study (28 patients) as well as the data from the uncontrolled case series, the conclusion seems to be that prednisolone leads to a small but significant improvement in disability in previously untreated patients of CIDP.[10] The latency from the start of treatment to the onset of improvement is unclear, with the available data suggesting that the norm is 4–8 weeks, but that it may take as long as 5 months.[10,12]

Is intravenous immunoglobulin effective in the treatment of patients with CIDP?[8,9]

Available data suggest that intravenous IG is effective in the treatment of patients with CIDP, although fewer than one-half of patients treated with intravenous IG will show a significant improvement in their level of disability. Furthermore, the effect of intravenous IG is often not lasting in patients with relapsing–remitting disease, and these patients may require regular infusions in order to maintain a clinical response.

Prognosis

At present, 70%–75% of patients with CIDP will have only slight or no residual disability following appropriate therapy. Probable good prognostic factors include: (i) Female gender, (ii) younger age, (iii) relapsing-remitting pattern, and (iv) electrophysiological studies suggesting pure demyelination without axonal loss.

Conclusion

On the basis of a thorough clinical examination, electrophysiological studies, relevant biochemical tests, including CSF analysis, and histopathological evidence of the sural nerve biopsy. In this large sural nerve biopsy-based study of peripheral neuropathy the various aetiological factors can be summarized as follows (after exclusion of common secondary causes): CIDP=20 (includes variants, such as MUGS-1, CML-1), vitamin B_{12} deficiency=1, vasculitis=1, neuroacanthocytosis=1, and anterior horn cell disorder=1. The most common neuropathy in this study is CIDP (58%). In 11 cases (34%), a proper aetiology could not be established despite a thorough evaluation.

References

1. European Federation of Neurological Societies/Peripheral Nerve Society Guideline on management of chronic inflammatory demyelinating polyradiculoneuropathy. Report of a joint task force of the European Federation of Neurological Societies and the Peripheral Nerve Society. *J Peripher Nerv Syst* 2005;**10**:220–8.

2. Kelly JJ Jr, Kyle RA, Miles JM, *et al.* Osteosclerotic myeloma and peripheral neuropathy. *Neurology* 1983;**33**:202–10.

3. Oh SJ, Kurokawa K, De Almeida DF, *et al.* Subacute inflammatory demyelinating polyneuropathy. *Neurology* 2003;**61**:1507–12.

4. Gorthi SP, Mehata A, Bewal N, *et al.* A sural nerve biopsy based study of peripheral neuropathy. Free paper presentation. 56th annual conference of Neurology Society of India (NSI) Dec 2007, Agra.

5. Hughes RA, Bouche P, Cornblath DR, *et al.* European Federation of Neurological Societies/Peripheral Nerve Society guideline on management of chronic inflammatory demyelinating polyradiculoneuropathy: Report of a joint task force of the European Federation of Neurological Societies and the Peripheral Nerve Society. *Eur J Neurol* 2006;**13**:326.

6. Van den Bergh PY, Pieret F. Electrodiagnostic criteria for acute and chronic inflammatory demyelinating polyradiculoneuropathy. *Muscle Nerve* 2004;**29**:565–74.

7. Molenaar DS, Vermuelen M, de Haan R. Diagnostic value of sural nerve biopsy in chronic inflammatory demyelinating polyneuropathy. *J Neurol Neurosurg Psychiatry* 1998;**64**:84–9.

8. Eftimov, F, Winer, JB, Vermeulen, M, *et al.* Intravenous immunoglobulin for chronic inflammatory demyelinating polyradiculoneuropathy. *Cochrane Database Syst Rev* 2009;**1**:CD001797.

9. Hughes, RA, Donofrio, P, Bril, V, *et al.* Intravenous immune globulin (10% caprylate-chromatography purified) for the treatment of chronic inflammatory demyelinating polyradiculoneuropathy (ICE study): A randomized placebo-controlled trial. *Lancet Neurol* 2008;**7**:136.

10. Benator M. Chronic inflammatory demyelinating polyradiculoneuropathy. In: *Neuromuscular diseases: Evidence and analysis in clinical neurology.* New Jersy, Totowa: Human Press; 2006:209–22.

11. Lopate G, Pestronk A, Al-Lozi M. Treatment of CIDP with high dose intermittent intravenous methyl prednisolone. *Arch Neurol* 2005;**62**:649.

12. Mehandiratta MM, Hughes RA. Corticosteroids for chronic inflammatory demyelinating Polyneuropathy. *Cochrane database Syst Rev* 2002;**1**:CD002062.

24

Unusual manifestations of neurocysticercosis (NCC)

MANVINDER SAPPAL, GAGANDEEP SINGH

Introduction

Taeniasis and cysticercosis, caused by *Taenia solium* and commonly referred to as pork tapeworm, is a classic zoonosis recognised since antiquity. The disorder has emerged as an increasingly important disease in the regions where it has long been endemic, e.g. South and Central America and India, as well as in the regions in which it has been imported or introduced as a result of a variety of demographical, technological and the political factors, e.g. the United States of America. The two-host life cycle of the tapeworm involves humans as definitive hosts and swine as intermediate hosts. The magnitude of transmission may be as high as 25% of humans infected at a given time in hyperendemic villages in Latin America, and may easily be >10% in many endemic zones.[1] Whereas seroprevalence rates are high, neurologically symptomatic individuals constitute only the tip of iceberg. The manifestations of neurocysticercosis are a puzzling concern to clinicians. No symptom or sign is specific to the disorder. Furthermore, a plethora of clinical presentations have been described, giving neurocysticercosis (NCC) the appropriate title of the modern day successor of syphilis, the master imitator of all the diseases. In non-endemic regions, which are experiencing a re-emergence of this disorder, the lack of awareness of NCC often leads to delay in diagnosis and resort to unnecessary invasive, potentially harmful and time consuming tests, such as stereotactic biopsy and so forth. Contrariwise, in endemic areas clinicians often pronounce diagnosis of NCC only to arrive at an alternative diagnosis much later.[2,3] Because of this, it is important to classify the disorder, put down diagnostic criteria and familiarize clinicians with salient clinical manifestations, which have been extensively described elsewhere.[4,5]

The lack of pathognomic clinical features was recognised very early by medical scientists, despite the large number of clinical presentations of human *T. solium* cysticercosis. This led to attempts at systematic classification of the disease. A major objective of classification is to guide the management approaches and obtain prognostic information. Several orderly classifications were given; that of Stepien and Chorobski is the most well known.[6] Classifying NCC according to the anatomical compartment of involvement is advantageous to clinicians,

Table 1. Anatomical classification of neurocysticercosis (NCC)

---

1. Parenchymal NCC
2. Extraparenchymal NCC
   Subarachnoid
   Intraventricular
3. Mixed

---

radiologists and the pathologists. However, the purely anatomically oriented classification does not take into account the evolutionary stage of NCC, which also influences clinical presentation (Table 1). In 1995, Sotelo *et al.* proposed to classify NCC into active and inactive disease.[7]

Meningeal cysticercosis

The meningeal form of NCC was first described by Virchow in 1860. He noticed membranous structures at the base of brain in a necropsy of an individual who died of a chronic neurological disorder. It has been common practice to describe cysticerci located in the brain parenchyma or within the cortical sulci between 2 cerebral convolutions as 'cysticercus cellulosae' and those cysticerci located within the basal cisterns as 'cysticercus racemosus'.

The clinical pleomorphism of meningeal cysticercosis is related to individual variations in number, size and location of the parasites, as well as the severity of subarachnoid inflammatory reaction.[8,9] A typical syndrome of meningeal cysticercus cannot be defined: focal neurological deficits, meningitis and intracranial hypertension in varying combinations are the most common presenting features.[8–10]

Focal neurological deficits

Arachnoiditis caused by cysticercus can cause entrapment of nerves exiting from the brainstem. The third nerve, which runs a long course along the base of brain, is very much susceptible to this kind of entrapment. It can manifest as diplopia

on account of extraocular muscle paralysis, and blurring of vision caused by pupillary abnormalities. Encasement of optic nerves or the optic chiasm can lead to visual field defects and decreased visual acuity.[11,12] Large cysts in the cerebellopontine angle can present with a syndrome of vertigo, facial palsy, sensorineural hearing loss, facial numbness and pain, which may be combined with the signs of long tract involvement, motor weakness and cerebellar ataxia. Contralateral motor weakness, sensory deficits and the language disturbances can be a manifestation of clumps of cyst in the sylvian fissure. Stroke-like presentation can be seen in 3% of patients with subarachnoid cysticercosis. Ischaemic cerebrovascular complications can be in the form of lacunar infarcts or the large cerebral infarcts (Fig. 1a). Lacunar infarcts may be located in the midbrain or the thalamus, when the thalamopeduncular branches of the mesencephalic artery are involved by the process of angiitis. They can then present as impaired vertical gaze, pupillary abnormalities, somnolence, paraparesis, and urinary incontinence.[13] Large cerebral infarcts are caused by occlusion of the

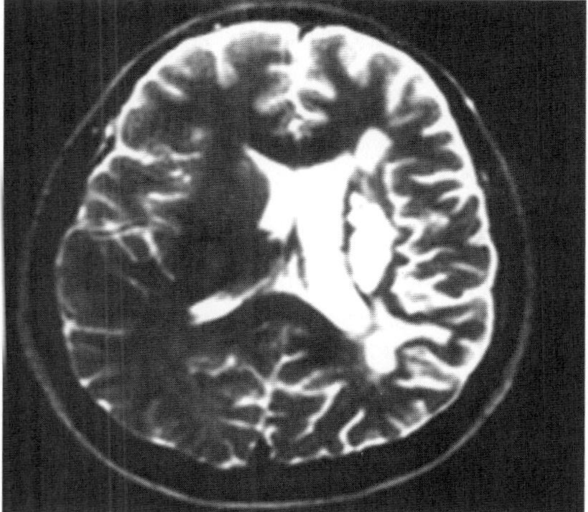

Fig. 1a. Axial T₂-weighted MRI scan reveals cerebral infarction in the left middle cerebral artery territory secondary to vasculitis associated with a suprachiasmatic cyst (Source: Fernando Barinagarrementeria, Carlos Cantu. In: G. Singh, S. Prabhakar (eds). *Taenia solium Cysticercosis: From basic to clinical sciences.* CABI Publishing, CAB International, Oxon UK).

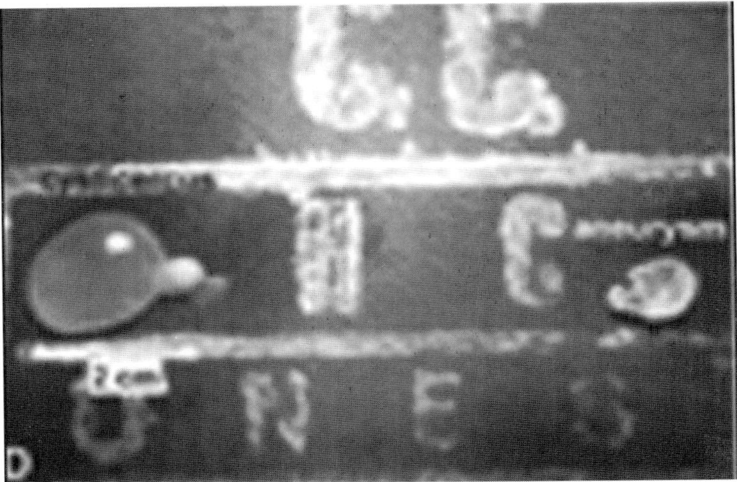

Fig. 1b. Mycotic aneurysm of the middle cerebral artery formed in relation to a degenerating cysticercus after surgical removal of both (Source: Svetlana Agapejev, Sao Paulo, Brazil In: G. Singh, S. Prabhakar (eds). *Taenia solium Cysticercosis: From basic to clinical sciences.* CABI Publishing, CAB International, Oxon UK).

internal carotid artery, middle cerebral artery or anterior cerebral artery.[8–10] Infarcts can occur in basal ganglia or the cerebral cortex. There are reports of patients presenting with subarachnoid haemorrhage due to rupture of mycotic aneurysm of the basilar artery, caused by large subarachnoid cysticerci (Fig. 1b).

Meningitis

Often, the meningitis is sub-acute to chronic.[9] Symptoms or signs of increased intracranial pressure or cranial nerve dysfunction can be presenting features. Meningeal cysticerci generally do not cause acute meningitis.[8] In a report by Bonametti *et al.*, fever was reported in 74% and neck stiffness in 44% of cases.[14]

Intracranial hypertension

Patients may present with signs of raised intracranial pressure, the cause of which is inflammatory occlusion of foramina of Lushcka and Magendie. They have headache, vomiting and papilloedema. It may be accompanied by signs and symptoms of cranial nerve dysfunction and cerebral infarcts. Cysts in the sylvian fissure and the anterior interhemispheric fissure may also present with intracranial hypertension. However, in these cases the focal neurological deficits will precede the signs of raised intracranial pressure by several weeks to months.

Seizures

Although seizures are characteristic symptoms of parenchymal NCC, these may also occur in meningeal cysticercosis. Irritation of subjacent cerebral cortex by overlying subarachnoid cysticerci may cause seizures. The seizures caused by these lesions are probably partial seizures with secondary generalization.[15]

Myelopathy and radiculopathy

Subarachnoid cysticerci of the spinal canal cause

a non-specific clinical picture of radicular pains and motor deficit of sub-acute onset and progressive course.[15–17] Cysts in the cervical region may cause signs of upper motor neuron damage in the lower limbs, and the lower motor neuron features of atrophy and fasciculations in upper limbs. Cauda equina cysts may present as flaccid paralysis and areflexia in the lower limb.

Heavy multi lesional cysticercotic syndromes

Among the various manifestations of human cysticercosis, a small subset of individuals harbour massive infections and develop clinical manifestations thereof.[18–20]

Cysticercotic encephalitis

Multiple parenchymal cysts causing a syndrome of raised intracranial pressure were first described by Stepien and Chorobsky.[6] The manifestations are due to severe inflammatory response around the dying cysts (Fig. 2a). As many parasites are degenerating simultaneously, it creates a booster

effect. The severity of clinical features depends upon the number of parasites and degree of inflammation and can be severe enough to be fatal.

Cysticercotic encephalitis occurs frequently in women and at a younger age group; a series of paediatric NCC has also been described.[21,22] Patients present with headache, that intensifies rapidly prior to diagnosis and seizures, although these symptoms may have been present earlier for about a period of 18 months (mean 6 months). Papilloedema, secondary optic atrophy, false localizing III and VI nerve palsy, deep tendon hyperreflexia and Babinski response are main presenting features.

Heavy non-encephalitic NCC

Heavy non-encephalitic NCC differs from cysticercotic encephalitis in a sense that no

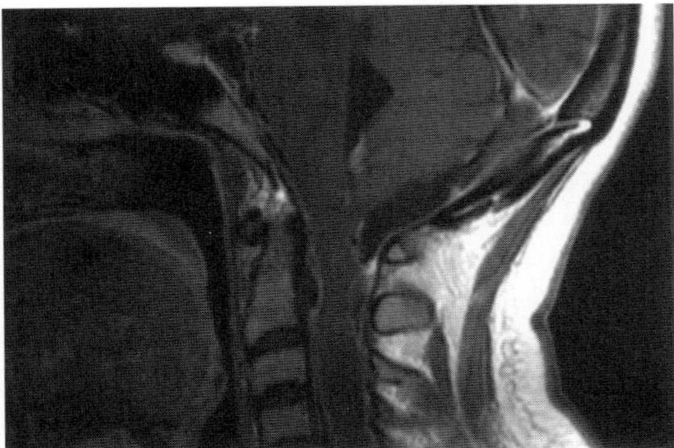

Fig. 2a. T₁ sagittal MRI section demonstrating that intradural extramedullary cysticercosis represents an extension of cranial subarachnoid cysticercosis into the spinal canal (Source: E. Citfci and A. Hayman, Baylor, Texas, USA. In: G. Singh, S. Prabhakar (eds). *Taenia solium Cysticercosis: From basic to clinical sciences.* CABI Publishing, CAB International, Oxon UK).

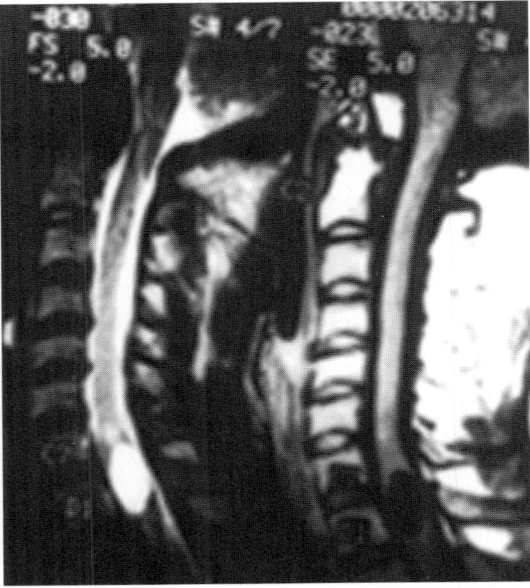

Fig. 2b. Intramedullary spinal cysticercosis. T₂ (left) and T₁ (right) sagittal MRI of the cervical cord revealing a cystic intramedullary lesion (Source: Prakash Singh, New Delhi, India. In: G. Singh, S. Prabhakar (eds). *Taenia solium Cysticercosis: From basic to clinical sciences.* CABI Publishing, CAB International, Oxon UK).

inflammatory reaction is seen around the cysts, and that all parasites are viable and do not enhance upon contrast in computed tomography (CT)/magnetic resonance imaging (MRI) (Fig. 2b). It has a few hundred live parasites in contrast to the disseminated form, which has a few thousand parasites. This variety of cysticercosis is more common during the third or fourth decades of life and has no gender predilection. It presents as a mild syndrome. Patients present with seizures and neuropsychological abnormalities. Intracranial hypertension is not seen. The involvement of other body parts is seen but it is not predominant. Intestinal tapeworms were detected in 90% of cases in one series.[23]

Disseminated cysticercosis

The term was first used by Priest in 1926.[24] The symptom complex of this is because of 2 main reasons—a large number of cysts and the absence of host inflammatory response in contrast to heavy non-encephalitic NCC. The disorder presents in the younger age group (mean age at presentation 22±10 years); males are affected twice as commonly as females. In reported cases, muscular pseudohypertrophy was the main presenting feature.[25,26] In other series, seizures, dementia, subcutaneous nodules and muscle pains were the main manifestations.[24,25,27] The muscle hypertrophy follows these initial features in a few weeks to 1 year. The onset is often marked by fever and skin rash. Due to associated cognitive impairment, muscle pain and tightness may not be presenting features. Muscular involvement is seen mainly in calves, thighs, arms, glutei, trapezius, nuchal muscles and the masseters. Muscles may be tender on palpation. Muscle weakness is mild and not profound. Deep tendon reflexes may be normal, absent or even brisk. The cerebral and ocular features are more noticeable, although the subcutaneous cysticerci can be easily identified during examination. Strangely, these are reported more often from Asia than Latin America. An ocular cyst may be noticed on careful examination. In 50% of cases, dementia and behavioural changes are noticed.[25,27] Focal neurological deficit and intracranial hypertension are rare.[27]

Intraventricular NCC

The cysticerci are present inside the cerebral ventricular system. Approximately 30% of patients with NCC have intraventricular cysts.[28,29] Intraventricular cysts have an aggressive behaviour in comparison to parenchymal cysts. The intraventricular cysts become symptomatic at the time of implantation due to obstruction of the cerebrospinal fluid (CSF) flow, with consequent hydrocephalus and signs and symptoms of raised intracranial pressure. As the involution occurs, inflammation around dead or dying cysts produces ependymitis, scarring, obstruction and ventriculitis. The patients with parenchymal cysts may incidentally be found to have intraventricular cysts.

CSF outflow obstruction

Intraventricular cysts may obstruct the CSF flow. It can be an abrupt or gradual obstruction. Abrupt obstruction leads to acute hydrocephalus with symptoms, such as headache, diplopia, dizziness, vomiting, restlessness, drowsiness, respiratory changes, bradycardia, elevation of arterial blood pressure, seizures and alteration of consciousness. Sudden changes in the position of the head may produce or alleviate headache caused by changes in the position of cysts. Sudden change in position of the head may produce loss of muscle strength and tone. Abrupt permanent obstruction leads to acute hydrocephalus with stupor, coma and death due to brain herniation. Any obstructing cyst leads to non-communicating hydrocephalus that requires prompt therapeutic intervention. In the fourth ventricle, direct compression of the brainstem and the midcerebellar structures may produce focal deficits on account of local mass lesions, such as gait ataxia, dysmetria and the diplopia. The superior aqueductal syndrome, caused by blockade of aqueduct of sylvius, may cause paralysis of vertical gaze and features of raised intracranial pressure.

Chronic obstruction

A large cyst in the fourth ventricle may obstruct CSF circulation. The patients may present with the features of headache, nausea, vomiting, somnolence, memory and behavioural changes, gait disturbances for several months before presentation. Impairment of frontal lobe functions may be a presenting feature because of the enlarging lateral ventricles. If untreated, these patients may decompensate and deteriorate rapidly.

Symptoms caused by obstruction of CSF flow and inflammation

When the cysticerci degenerate, the involution process and inflammation turn asymptomatic cysts into symptomatic ones. The antigenic substances liberated by cysts generate an inflammatory reaction throughout the ventricular system. This leads to adhesions and fibrosis in the ventricular system, producing irreversible blockade of CSF circulation. The fourth ventricle is frequently affected. The patient presents with features of increased intracranial pressure, focal neurological deficits and inflammatory reaction in the CSF. Cerebral and brainstem infarcts, caused by angiitis, hypothalamic dysfunction, repeated shunt failure, progression of disease with arachnoiditis, ependymitis, ventriculitis and irreversible tissue damage, are the main causes of clinical deterioration. This leads to enlargement of the fourth ventricle, which may persist despite a ventriculoperitoneal shunt for relief of hydrocephalus. At times no cysts can be seen on neuroimaging.

Cerebrovascular manifestations of NCC

Arteritis or vasculitis may involve blood vessels in close proximity to the cysts. All the three layers of the vessel may be involved, leading to panarteritis. Cysticercotic endarteritis is a small-vessel disease related to cysts in close relation to basal arteries. Small deep lacunar infarcts are commoner than the large vessel infarcts.

The frequency of stroke in NCC is 2%–15%.[7,9] Barinagarrementeria and Del Brutto reported an incidence of lacunar stroke at ~2%.[30] In another report from the same group, the lacunar syndrome caused by NCC was reported in 8% of cases.[31]

Lacunar syndromes

Patients may present with typical lacunar syndromes, including pure motor hemiparesis, ataxic hemiparesis and sensorimotor paralysis. Lacunar infarcts are located in the posterior limb of the internal capsule or the corona radiata. The cyst and surrounding meningeal inflammatory response, and the subsequent arachoidnitis, lead to occlusion of penetrating branches of the proximal segment of the middle cerebral artery.

Thalamomesencephalic syndrome

A thalamomesencephalic syndrome occurs because of severe perimesencephalic arachnoiditis and occlusion of thalamopeduncular branches of mesencephalic arteries. Patients present with impaired vertical gaze, pupillary abnormalities, somnolence, paraparesis and urinary incontinence.

Large territorial infarcts

Occlusion of large cerebral vessels, such as the internal carotid, middle cerebral and the anterior cerebral arteries, can occur in NCC. They are infrequent in comparison to small vessel infarcts. At times, large vessel arteritis and the infarcts may occur on account of inflammatory response precipitated by anticysticercal drugs; the latter should therefore be given with caution in patients with extensive cyst load, particularly in relation to a large vessel.

Haemorrhagic stroke

NCC may produce subarachnoid, parenchymal, or intracystic haemorrhage.[11,32,33] These are the rare complications of NCC. Subarachnoid haemorrhage may be the result of rupture of a mycotic aneurysm that develops in relation to racemose cyst adherent to an artery.

Spinal cysticercosis

The first description of the cervical spinal cyst was given by Walton in 1881.[34] The number of cases of spinal cysticercosis reported to date are few and far between. Its incidence is ~3%.[35] It is classified on the basis of the location of the cysts. The disease may be extradural, intradural, extramedullary, and intramedullary in location. Extradural cysticercosis is rare.[36–38]

Intradural extramedullary cysticercosis

According to Rocca, intradural extramedullary cysticercosis is most common in the cervical spinal canal.[38] However, the literature suggests that cysts can produce symptoms at any location, with lumbosacral and cervical cord involvement being more common (Fig. 3a). Zee et al. reported hydrocephalus as a presenting symptom.[39] In many cases the intracranial signs and symptoms precede myelopathy. Extramedullary spinal cysts are mostly asymptomatic by themselves and produce signs and symptoms of spinal involvement because of arachnoiditis when they

degenerate. Three varieties of spinal syndrome have been classified by Canelas et al. (i) Spinal cord compression syndrome (ii) Tabes dorsalis syndrome and, (iii) Meningomyelitis.[40] Rarely, a cauda equina-conus medullaris syndrome, amyotrophic lateral sclerosis and syringomyelia have also been reported.[40–42] In the amyotrophic lateral sclerosis-like presentation, pathologically speaking, degeneration of the anterior horn cells and the lateral funiculi and cysticercal arachnoiditis in cervical spinal cord have been noted.[42] Finally, occlusion of the fourth ventricle outlet by cysticercal arachnoiditis and meningeal fibrosis may lead to syringomyelia in association with syringobulbia.

Intramedullary spinal cysticercosis

This condition occurs mostly in young adults (Fig. 3b). Myelopathy develops over a few weeks

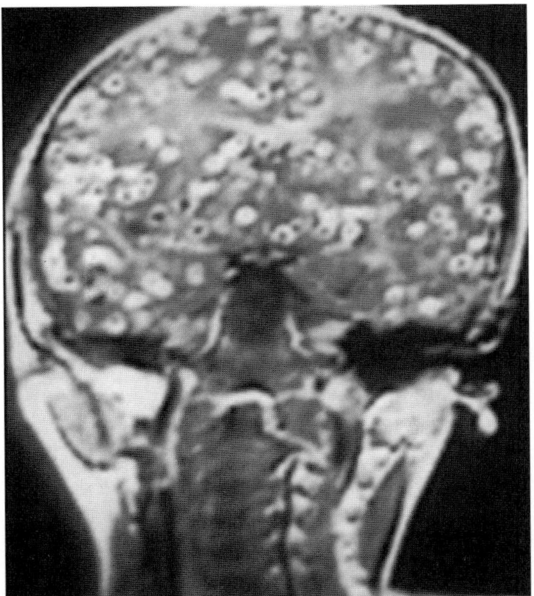

Fig. 3a. Post-gadolinum T_1 weighted coronal MRI manifesting cysticercotic encephalitis (Source: Oscar H. Del Brutto and Hector H. Garcia. In: G. Singh, S. Prabhakar (eds). *Taenia solium Cysticercosis: From basic to clinical sciences.* CABI Publishing, CAB International, Oxon UK).

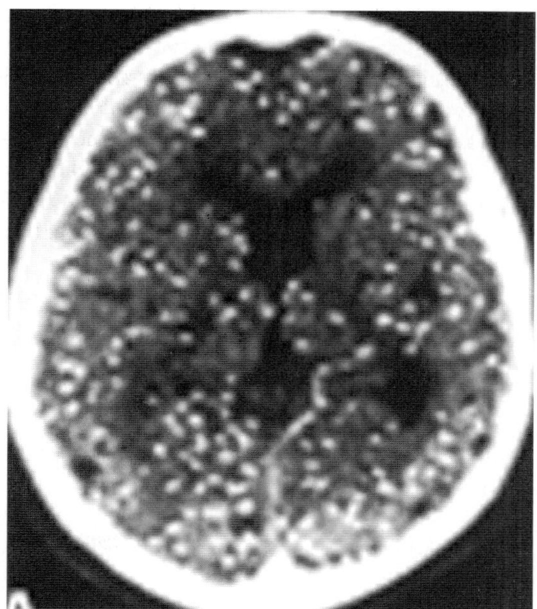

Fig. 3b. CT scan of the brain of patient with disseminated cysticercosis (Source: Noshir H. Wadia. In: G. Singh, S. Prabhakar (eds). *Taenia solium Cysticercosis: From basic to clinical sciences.* CABI Publishing, CAB International, Oxon UK).

to months. Acute spinal cord syndrome can be precipitated by anticysticercal drugs given for cerebral cysticercosis in a patient with symptomatic intramedullary cysticercosis.[43] The patients may present with sensorimotor paralysis below the level of the lesion, with or without bladder and bowel involvement. Local pain is a significant symptom. There may be signs of meningeal irritation. Intramedullary spinal cysticercosis is found mainly in the thoracic cord. It occasionally may also involve the cervical cord. Conus medullaris has also been reported to be affected. Usually one, but rarely multiple, cysts may be present.

Sellar cysticercosis

Pituitary fossa and the areas alongside are infrequent sites for cysticercosis. Eight pathologically verified cases have been reviewed

by Del Brutto.[44] Sellar cysticercosis may present as symptomatic sellar enlargement in skull radiographs. Incidental sellar cysts have been reported at necropsy.[45] Other symptoms are described below.

Visual loss

Chiasmal compression by sellar or suprasellar cysts or arachnoiditis may result in visual loss. Visual loss is usually bilateral with associated bitemporal field defects. In contradistinction to other pituitary tumours in which visual loss occurs in months to years, here it develops rapidly in 3–12 weeks.[44] Optic atrophy may be evident on opthalmoscopic examination; papilloedema is rare and signifies associated hydrocephlaus caused by associated meningeal cysticercosis or raised intracranial pressure due to involuting parenchymal cysticerci. Growth in the cavernous sinus may produce exopthalmos.

Endocrine disturbances

Panhypopituitarism, diabetes insipidus and galactorrhoea have been reported in 33%–50% of cases of reported series.[44,46] Seizures may be a manifestation of sellar cysticerci in 40% of patients.[44] The occurrence of seizures should invoke a search for parenchymal cysts; similarly, the presence of intracranial hypertension indicates an association with parenchymal cysticerci and the associated hydrocephlaus. Intrasellar cysticerci do not cause cerebrovascular involvement. However, a large cyst may occlude the blood vessels and lead to infarcts.

Psychiatric manifestations of NCC

Psychiatric disturbances typically present in the course of cerebral cysticercosis, both in association with the neurological syndrome and as a dominant feature. The several psychiatric syndromes that have so far been attributed to NCC include conditions similar to dementia praecox, paranoia, neurosyphilis, Korsakoff psychosis and dementia. Chronic delusions and hallucinations, as well as the variations of mood compatible with diagnosis of major depression and bipolar disorder, are additionally reported. Leukart, in 1886, suggested that the cysticerci located in the ventricles and the basal ganglia were more liable to induce mental abnormality than the cortical lesions.[47] In a number of such cases, neuropsychiatric findings were compatible with major cognitive impairment, delirium and dementia.[47] NCC can cause mental illness through association with intracranial hypertension, meningitis and epilepsy, in which case mood and perceptual disorders and acute and chronic psychosis have been described.

As a general rule, ventricular cysticerci and the subarachnoid cysticercosis, which are usually associated with meningitis and intracranial hypertension, may result in a greater amount of cognitive dysfunction, attention deficits, impaired consciousness and delirium. Patients with parenchymal cysticercosis are prone to experiencing neuropsychiatric complications of epilepsy, intracranial hypertension and the space occupying lesions. Ventriculosubarachnoid forms are likely to present with psychomotor agitation, sleep–wake cycle disturbances, and other behavioural symptoms suggestive of acute cognitive dysfunction. Massive and scattered infections of the brain and the sub-acute form of intraventricular cysticercosis have been associated with dementia. It is not possible to classify the disease according to the areas of brain involved because the parenchymal lesions may be located anywhere in the brain, although the gray–white matter transition tissue is the preferred site.[48]

Ophthalmic cysticercosis

Schott and Sommering in 1829 gave the earliest description of living cysticerci in the human eye.[49] In a South American study of 153,528 patients, only 111 cases were found to have ophthalmic cysticerci.[50] In another report from the same place, the frequency was 30 cases per 100,000.[51] Malik *et al.* reported that 68% of their patients were in the age group of 10–30 years.[52]

Ocular involvement was seen in 13%–46% in a large series of patients with cysticercosis.[53,54] Ocular involvement is typically unilateral, but can be bilateral in cases of disseminated cysticercosis. The left eye is affected more commonly than the right one, probably because of the direct origin of the left internal carotid from the aorta; this has, however, not been proven. The medial side of the eye is involved more frequently than the lateral side, on account of the anatomical course of the ophthalmic artery, which, after giving out lacrimal arteries,[52] runs along the medial side of the orbit before dividing into terminal branches. Cysticerci can lodge in any part of the eye or its adenexa; they have also been reported to migrate within the eyes.[55]

Lid and subconjuctival cysticercosis

This condition may present as a painless, subcutaneous mass that remains unchanged for long periods of time.[56] Conjunctival cysts and, rarely, abscesses have been reported. The cyst can be spontaneously extruded from the eye.

Extraocular myocysticercosis

Recurrent inflammation, proptosis, restricted ocular motility, and ptosis are the signs of extraocular cysticercosis. There can be restricted ocular motility in the direction of action of the involved muscle, in the direction opposite to the involved extraocular muscle, recurrent inflammation with conjuctival congestion, and acquired blepharoptosis. There can be restricted infraduction, acquired ptosis and proptosis due to involvement of the superior rectus muscle, levator palpebrae, and the orbital involvement.

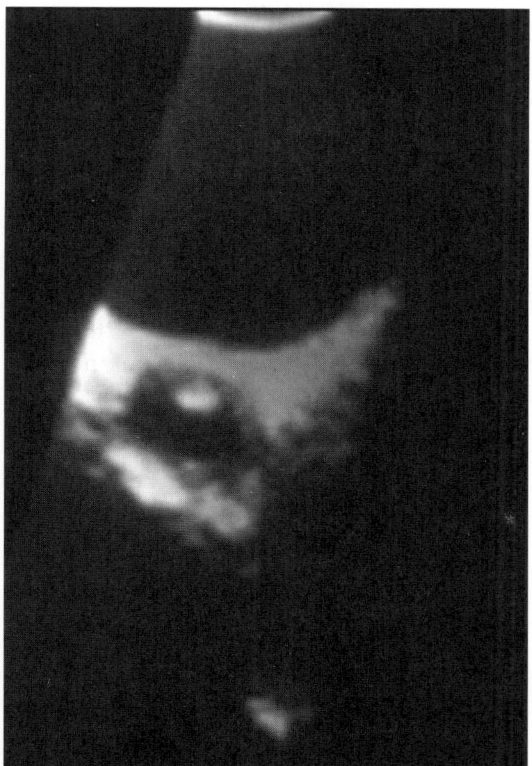

Fig. 4. Communicating cysticercosis, upon B-mode ultrasound scan. The posterior wall of the cyst was not distinguishable from the retinoscleral echo, raising suspicion that the cyst was communicating. (Source: Atul Kumar and Namrata Sharma. In: G. Singh, S. Prabhakar (eds). *Taenia solium Cysticercosis: From basic to clinical sciences.* CABI Publishing, CAB International, Oxon UK).

Vitreal, subretinal and anterior chamber cysticercosis

Intraocular cysticercosis can cause painless, gradual, progressive loss of vision (Fig. 4). The cyst is well tolerated as long as it is alive; however, when the parasite dies, toxic products released from the cysts cause an intense inflammation, and the patient presents with blind, painful eyes. Unilateral iritis may be a presentation of cysticercus larvae in the anterior chamber. Intarvitreal live cysticercosis can be recognized as a white cyst with a dense, white spot formed by the invaginated scolex. Subretinal cysticercosis can present as an acute central retinitis and subretinal exudates. The macular area is the preferred site because of its rich vascularization. The diagnosis of ocular cysts becomes difficult when the parasite dies and an intense inflammatory response develops. Marked circumcorneal congestion, keratin precipitates, flare in anterior chamber, and the opacification of the vitreous are similar to any other inflammatory ocular condition.

Conclusion

The principal manifestations of NCC depend on the site or location of the cysts. Cysts present in remote areas in the CNS produce uncommon manifestations. They often present as diagnostic and therapeutic challenges to the treating physician in both endemic and non-endemic areas.

Disclosures

None

References

1. Garcia HH, Martinez M, Gilman RH, *et al.* Diagnosis of cysticercosis in endemic regions. *Lancet* 1991;**33**:549–51.
2. Bandres JC, White AC Jr, Samo T, *et al.* Extra-parenchymal neurocysticercosis: A report of five cases and review of management. *Clin Infect Dis* 1992;**15**:799–811.
3. Keane JR. Neuroopthalmic signs and the symptoms of cysticercosis. *Arch Ophthalmol* 1982;**100**:1445–8.
4. Del Brutto OH, Dumas M, *et al.* Proposal of diagnostic criteria for human cysticercosis and NC. *J Neurol Sci* 1996;**142**:1–6.
5. Del Brutto OH, Rajshekhar V, White AC Jr, *et al.* Proposed diagnostic criteria for neurocysticercosis. *Neurology* 2001;**57**:177–83.
6. Stepien L, Chorobski J. Cysticercosis cerebri and its operative management. *Arch Neurol Psychiatr (Chicago)* 1949;**61**:499–527.

7. Sotelo J, Guerrero V, Rubio F. Neurocysticercosis new classification based on active and the inactive forms. A study of 753 cases. *Arch Intern Med* 1985;**145:**442–5.

8. Ter Penning B, Litchmann CD, Heier L. Bilateral middle cerebral artery occlusion due to neuro-cysicercosis. *Stroke* 1992;**28:**280–3.

9. McCormick GF, Giannotta S, Zee CS, *et al.* Carotid occlusion in cysticercosis. *Neurology* 1983;**33:**1078–80.

10. Levy AS, Lillehei KO, Rubinstein D, *et al.* Subarachnoid neurocysticercosis with occlusion of the major intracranial arteries: Case report. *Neurosurgery* 1995;**36:**183–8.

11. Soto-Hernandez JH, Gomez-Llata S, Rojas-Echeverri LA, *et al.* Subarachnoid haemorrhage secondary to a ruptured inflammatory aneurysm: A possible manifestation of the neurocysticercosis, case report. *Neurosurgery* 1996;**38:**197–200.

12. Bonametti AM, Baldy JLS, Bortoliero AL, *et al.* Neurocysticercose com quadro clinico inicial de meningite aguda. *Revists do Instituto de Medicina Tropical de Sau Paulo* 1994;**36:**27–32.

13. Cantu C, Barinagarrementeria F. Cerebrovascular complications of neurocystucercosis.Clinical and the neuroimaging spectrum. *Arch Neurol* 1985;**53:**233–9.

14. Bonametti AM, Baldy JLS, Bortoliero AL, *et al.* Neurocysticercose com quadro clinico inicial de meningite aguda. *Revists do Instituto de Medicina Tropical de Sau Paulo* 1994;**36:**27–32.

15. Keane JR. Death from cysticercus. Seven patients with unrecognised hydrocephlaus. *West J Med (San Franscisco)*1984;**140:**787–9.

16. Del Brutto OH, Santibanez R, Noboa CA, *et al.* Epilepsy due to neurocysticercosis: Analysis of 203 patients. *Neurology* 1992;**42:**389–92.

17. Bandres JC, White AC Jr, Samo T, *et al.* Extra-pyramidal Neurocysticercosis: Report of five cases and management. *Clin Infect Dis* 1992;**15:** 799–811.

18. Del Brutto OH, Sotelo J, Roman GC. *Neuro-cysticercosis: A clinical handbook.* The Netherlands: Swets and Zeiliger, Lisse; 1997:207.

19. Garcia HH, Martinez SM. *Taenia solium Taeniasis/cysticercosis.* 2nd ed. Lima, Peru: Editorial Universo; 1999:346.

20. Garcia HH, Del Brutto OH. T. Solium/cysticecosis. *Infect Dis Clin North Am* 2000;**14:**97–120.

21. Del Brutto OH, Garcia E, Talamas O, *et al.* Sex related severity of inflammation in peranchymal brain cysticercosis. *Arch Intern Med* 1988;**148:**544–7.

22. Lopez-Hernandez A, Garayzar C. Analysis of 89 cases of infantile cerebral Cysticercosis. In: Flissser A, Willms K, Laclete JP (eds). *Cysticercosis: Present state of knowledge and perspective.* New York: Academic Press; 1982:127–38.

23. Garcia HH, Del Brutto OH and the cysticercosis working group in Peru. Heavy non-encephalitic cerebral cysticercosis in tapeworm carriers. *Neurology* 1999;**53:**1582–4.

24. Priest R. A case of extensive somatic dissemination of Cysticercus cellulosae in man. *Br Med J* 1926;**ii:**471–2.

25. Jolly SS, Pallis C. Muscular pseudohypertrophy de to Cysticercosis. *Neurology* 1971;**18:**767–71.

26. Sawhney BB, Chopra JS, Banerji AK, *et al.* Pseudo-hypertrophic mopathy in cysticercosis. *Neurology* 1976;**26:**270–2.

27. Mc Gill RJ. Csticercosis resembling myopathy. *Lancet* 1948;**ii:**728–30.

28. Madrazo I, Garcia-Renteria JA, Sandowal M, *et al.* Intraventricular cysticercosis. *Neurosugery* 1983;**12:** 148–51.

29. Cuetter AC, Garcia-Bobadilla J, Guerra LG, *et al.* Neurocysticercosis: Focus on inyraventriculardisease. *Clin Infect Dis* 1997;**24:**157–64.

30. Barinagarrementeria F, Del Brutto OH. Lacunar syndromes due to neurocysticercosis. *Arch Neurol* 1989;**46:**415–17.

31. Barinagarrementeria F. Non-vascular etiology of lacunal syndromes. *J Neurol Neurosurg Psychiatr* 1990;**53:**1111.

32. Ferris EJ, Levine HL. Cerebral arteritis: Classification. *Radiology* 1973;**109:**327–41.

33. Del Brutto OH. Cysticercosis and the cerebrovascular disease: A review. *J Neurol Neurosurg Psychiatr* 1992;**55:**252–4.

34. Walton L. A case of cysticercosis in the substance of spinal cord. *Boston Med Surg J* 1881;**105:**511–12.

35. Briceno CE, Biagi F, Martinez BB. Cysticercosis: Observaciones sobre 97 casos de autopsia. *Presna Medicina Mexico* 1961;**26:**193–7.

36. Mohanty A, Das S, Kolluri S, *et al.* Spinal extradural ctsticecosis: A case report. *Spinal Cord* 1998;**36:**285–7.

37. Kurrien F, Vickers AA. Cysticercosis of spine. *Annal Trop Med Parasitol* 1977;**71:**213–17.

38. Rocca ED. Cisticercosis intramedular. *Revista Neuropsiquiatria (Lima)* 1959;**22:**166–73.

39. Zee CS, Segall HD, Boswell W, *et al.* MR Imaging of neurocysticercosis. *J Computer Assisted Tomography* 1988;**12:**927–34.

40. Canelas HM, Riccardi-Cruz O, Escalante OAD.

Cysticercosis of the narvous system: Less frequent clinical forms. III. Spinal cord forms. *Arquivos de Neuropsiquiatria* 1963;**21**:77–86.

41. Escobar A, Vega J. Syringomyelia and syringobulbia secondary to arachnoiditis and the fourth ventricle blockage due to cysticercosis. A case report. *Acta Neuropathologica (Berlin)* 1981;**7**:389–91.

42. Kahn P. Cysticercosis of the central nervous system with amyotrophic lateral sclerosis; case report and the review of literature. *J Neurol, Neurosurg Psychiatr* 1972;**35**:81–7.

43. Corral I, Quereda C, Moreno A, *et al.* Intramedullary cysticercosis cured with drug treatment. A case report. *Spine* 1996;**21**:2284–7.

44. Del Brutto OH, Guevara J, Sotelo J. Intrasellar cysticercosis. *J Neurosurg* 1988;**69**:58–60.

45. Briceno CE, Biagi F, Martinez B. Cysticercosis: Observaciones sobre 7 casos de autopsia. *Presna Medicina Mexico* 1961;**26**:193–7.

46. Dickenson CJ. Cysticercosis and panhypopituitarism. *Proc R Soc Med* 1955;**48**:892.

47. Leukart R. *The parasites of man, and the diseases which proceed from them.* A textbook for students and the practitioners. Young J (ed). Pentl and Edinburgh, UK; 1886:488–551.

48. Brown WJ, Voge M. Cysticercosis; A modern day plague. *Pediatr Clin North Am* 1985;**32**:953–69.

49. Junior L. Ocular cysticercosis. *Am J Ophthalmol* 1949;**32**:528–58.

50. Cano MR. Ocular cysticercosis. In: Ryan SJ (ed). *Retina*, vol. 2. St Louis, Missouri: CV Mosby; 1989: 583–7.

51. Santos R, Dalma A, Ortiz E, *et al.* Management of subretinal and vitreous cysticercosis: Role of photocoagulation and surgery. *Ophthalmology* 1979;**86**: 1501–7.

52. Malik SRK, Gupta AK, Chaudhary S. Ocular cysticercosis. *Am J Opthalmol* 1968;**66**:1168–71.

53. Reddy PS, Reddy DB. Ocular Cysticercosis. *Curr Med Pract* 1957;**1**:642.

54. Katz M, Despommier DD, Gwadz RW. *Parasitic diseases.* New York: Springer-Verlag; 1982.

55. Fishman M, Kerman B, Foxman S. Intraocular cysticercosis: Migratory. In: Ossoing KC (ed). *Ophthalmic Echography*. Proceedings of the 10th SIDOU Congress. Dordrecht: Martinus Nijhoff, 1987.

56. Jampol LM, Caldwell JBH, Albert DM. Cysticercus cellulosae in the eyelid. *Arch Opthalmol* 1973;**89**: 318–20.

25

Non-surgical (or medical) aspects of pituitary lesions

T.N. DUBEY, SANDEEP JULKA

Introduction

Case vignette 1

A 20-year-old woman with acne, hirsutism and oligomenorrhoea was treated by a dermatologist and was intermittently seen by a gynaecologist. The woman had received several sittings of laser therapy for her hirsutism but with no significant improvement. Her baseline tests were performed, which included thyroid-stimulating hormone (TSH), serum prolactin, serum dehydroepiandrosterone sulphate (DHEAS), serum total testosterone and a pelvic ultrasonogram (USG). The woman had marginally high prolactin and the USG showed polycystic ovaries. On this basis, the diagnosis of polycystic ovary syndrome (PCOS) was made and, over the years, she was advised oestogen and cyproterone acetate, metformin, etc. Then she was referred to an endocrinologist as the oligomenorrhoea did not respond. On examination, she was found to have expressive galactorrhoea and a fasting pooled prolactin level of >100 ng/dl. A dynamic MRI was done, which revealed a pituitary micro-adenoma. The woman was started on cabergoline

and with which she had regular cycles and her prolactin levels normalized.

Case vignette 2

A 33-year-old woman was diagnosed to have a growth hormone-secreting pituitary macro-adenoma. She underwent trans-sphenoidal resection of the tumour. Her postoperative post-glucose challenge growth hormone (GH) levels were >1 ng/ml and the insulin-like growth factor-1 (IGF-1) level was found to be high for her age. The reports meant that the acromegaly had not been biochemically cured, although the follow-up MRI showed almost complete removal of the adenoma. After 2 years of the surgery, the woman developed diabetes, which is one of the metabolic derangements known to occur with GH excess. Treatment options were discussed but the patient refused radiotherapy, so she was advised long-acting analogues of octreotide to bring the GH levels to normal.

Case vignette 3

A 72-year-old man with carcinoma prostrate,

now cured, was diagnosed to have adreno-corticotrophic hormone (ACTH)-dependent Cushing's syndrome. An MRI of the brain showed a possible 4 mm lesion in the pituitary. Rare cases of carcinoma prostrate are known to secrete corticotrophin-releasing hormone (CRH), which leads to Cushing's syndrome. Immuno-cytochemistry of the prostrate tissue was done, which was negative, and inferior petrosal sinus sampling (IPSS) was planned to localize the source of the excess ACTH. The patient refused IPSS. Subsequently, he was taken up for trans-sphenoidal resection of the tumour. Unfortunately, the procedure had to be abandoned due to heavy bleeding. Ultimately, a decision to perform bilateral adrenalectomy was taken. The patient was started on ketoconazole to block steroid production from the adrenals while he waited for surgery. After a month, the patient underwent successful bilateral adrenalectomy.

The three cases described above demonstrate that pituitary tumours or lesions can be encountered by a host of medical specialties and can be managed medically if required. They also demonstrate that all specialists should have a basic understanding of the types of pituitary lesions and their management, whether surgical or medical.

Classification of pituitary tumours

Tumours of the pituitary may be classified as given below (Tables 1 and 2).

Classified according to size, pituitary tumours can be divided into microadenomas (<1 cm diameter) and macroadenomas (>1 cm diameter). They can also be classified on the basis of staining characteristics, as chromophobic and chromophilic tumours. The latter can be further subdivided using haematoxylin and eosin stains (i.e. eosinophilic or basophilic).

However, this classification has proven to be of no clinical value and has been replaced by a more functional classification that involves electromicroscopy and immunohistochemistry.

Table 1. Classification of pituitary lesions

Developmental

Primary empty sella syndrome

Rathke's cyst

Traumatic

Surgical resection

Radiation injury

Head injury

Neoplastic

Adenoma

Pituitary metastasis from breast, colon, lung

Infiltrative/inflammatory

Lymphocytic infiltration

Haemochromatosis

Sarcoidosis

Histiocytosis X

Granulomatous lesions

Vascular

Pituitary apoplexy

Postpartum necrosis

Infections

Histoplasmocytosis

Toxoplasmosis

Tuberculosis

Frequency of pituitary tumours

Table. 2. Hormonal types of pituitary tumours

Type	Frequency (%)
Prolactin secreting	25–30
Non-functioning pituitary tumours	25–30
ACTH secreting	15
GH secreting	15
Pleurihormonal	12
TSH secreting	2

These techniques have identified hormonal production in many chromophobe adenomas, enabling pathologists to identify hormones that are produced by eosinophilic tumours. The coricotrophs, somatotrophs, lactotrophs and thyrotrophs hypersecrete while the gonadotrophs are silent tumours. These techniques have also demonstrated that many tumours produce more than one hormone. The mutated form of *p53*, a tumour suppressor gene, can also be determined histologically. The presence of this mutated gene suggests a tumour with rapid growth.

Clinical history

The presentation of a pituitary macroadenoma relates to its mass effect and pressure on the surrounding structures. About 50%–60% present with visual symptoms due to compression of the optic nerve structures. Non-specific headache may be present. Lateral extension can result in compression of the cavernous sinuses and may cause ophthalmoplegia. Talkad *et al.* recently reported an isolated, painful, postganglionic Horner syndrome as the initial sign of lateral extension of a large prolactinoma.[1] Extension into the sphenoid sinuses can cause spontaneous cerebrospinal fluid (CSF) rhinorrhoea. In addition to visual symptoms, endocrine dysfunction can result.

Clinical effects, morbidity and mortality

The endocrinological morbidity that is associated with pituitary tumours is dependent on the specific underproduction or overproduction of a hormone or hormones associated with the tumour. Macroadenomas can compress the optic nerve structures. The optic chiasm is the most frequently affected structure, and bitemporal field defects are the most common findings.

Hormonal deficiency

Can result from the pressure effect of the mass, pituitary apoplexy, Sheehan's syndrome or empty sella.

a. Growth hormone deficiency
- Adults—Increased rate of cardiovascular disease, obesity, reduced muscle strength and exercise capacity, and increased cholesterol
- Infants—Hypoglycaemia
- Children—Decreased height and growth velocity.

b. Gonadotrophin deficiency
- Men—Diminished libido and impotence; testes shrink in size, but spermatogenesis generally preserved
- Women—Diminished libido and dyspareunia; breast atrophy in chronic deficiency
- Children—Delayed or frank absence of puberty

c. Thyrotrophin deficiency or secondary hypothyroidism—Malaise, weight gain, lack of energy, cold intolerance and constipation

d. Corticotrophin deficiency—Unlike primary adrenal insufficiency, mineralocorticoid function (which is dependent on the angiotensin–renin axis) is not affected; the deficiency is limited to glucocorticoids and adrenal androgens. Initially, the symptoms are non-specific (e.g. weight loss, lack of energy, malaise); severe adrenal insufficiency may present as a medical emergency.

e. Panhypopituitarism—Refers to deficiency of several anterior pituitary hormones, and may occur in a slowly progressive fashion (e.g. pituitary adenomas)

Hormonal excess

a. Prolactin
- Hypogonadism, if hyperprolactinaemia sustained
- Women—Amenorrhoea, galactorrhoea, and infertility
- Men—Decreased libido, impotence, and rarely galactorrhoea

b. Growth hormone
- Children and adolescents—May result in pituitary gigantism
- Adults—Acromegaly

Changes are seen in the size of the hands and feet;

there is coarseness of the face, frontal bossing and prognathism. Further changes in the voice and hirsutism are pointers towards the diagnosis. Acromegaly frequently results in glucose intolerance, with 20% of patients progressing to diabetes mellitus. Respiratory difficulty and sleep apnoea are fairly common. Cardiac complications result from acromegalic cardiomyopathy. Although patients have a bulky appearance, they are generally weak as a result of associated myopathy. Carpal tunnel syndrome is frequently seen. Lumbar canal stenosis can present with a syndrome resembling amyotrophic lateral sclerosis. Acromegaly may be associated with colonic polyps, although an increased incidence of colon cancer has not been shown definitively.

c. Cushing's disease
- Weight gain, centripetal obesity, moon facies, violet striae, easy bruisability, proximal myopathy and psychiatric changes
- Other possible effects—Arterial hypertension, diabetes, cataracts, glaucoma and osteoporosis

Mortality/morbidity

Mortality due to pituitary tumours is low. Advances in the medical and surgical management of these lesions and the availability of hormonal replacement therapies have contributed to successful management. Pituitary apoplexy can be a lethal complication. Morbidity associated with macroadenomas may include permanent visual loss, ophthalmoplegia and other neurological complications. Tumour recurrence is also a possibility. CNS metastases and, rarely, distant metastases occur with pituitary tumours. Endocrine abnormalities are amenable to correction. However, damage in many organ systems as a result of long-standing uncorrected deficiencies may be irreversible.

Neurological morbidity may be related to the mass effect of the pituitary lesion on the neighbouring structures, the underlying medical pathology affecting CNS structures other than the pituitary, and the associated features of

congenital/developmental syndromes in which the pituitary is involved along with other systems.

No racial predilection is known. Symptomatic prolactinomas are found more frequently in women. Cushing's disease also is more frequent in women (female-to-male ratio 3:1). Most pituitary tumours occur in young adults, but they may be seen in adolescents and elderly persons. Acromegaly is usually seen in the fourth and fifth decades of life.

Examination

Neuro-ophthalmological examination

Visual acuity can be decreased in one or both eyes. The pupillary light reaction can be abnormal. Colour vision can be affected. Bitemporal hemiachromatopsia to red may be localized to the optic chiasm. This can be tested easily at the bedside. The hallmark abnormality associated with chiasmal compression is a bitemporal superior quadrant anopsia. Larger lesions may be associated with a bitemporal hemianopsia. Since the optic chiasm is usually adjacent to the tuberculum sellae, chiasmal compression is commonly seen. Less frequently, the chiasm may be anterior or posterior to the tuberculum sellae (i.e. prefixed or post-fixed chiasm). Thus, the pattern of the visual field defect can be varied. Any form of temporal field defect, even if monocular, can result from chiasmal compression. The anterior chiasmal syndrome is not usually caused by pituitary adenomas. However, bitemporal scotomata and, infrequently, homonymous defects due to optic tract compression may be seen.

Ophthalmoscopic examination

Optic atrophy is seen frequently. It is generally a horizontal-oriented atrophy (i.e. bow-tie) that corresponds to the topographic localization of the nasal retina within the optic nerve. Drop-out of the nerve fibre layer in the nasal retina also may be noted. Papilloedema is exceptional, seen only in patients with pituitary apoplexy. Less frequently, optic atrophy can occur, with increased cup-to-disk ratio resembling glaucomatous optic atrophy.

Work-up

Laboratory studies

- *Pituitary mass:* Categorize into micro- and macroadenoma
- Anatomical and functional evaluation
  —Anatomical
  —Visual fields and ophthalmological evaluation are critical in confirming the presence of a chiasmal syndrome
  —Neuroimaging would be appropriate (*see* imaging studies)
- Functional evaluation
- Prolactinomas

Serum prolactin levels should be measured in any patient with a suspected sellar or suprasellar mass. Prolactin is collected in the fasting state and pooled. If elevated, the possibility of pharmacological and other factors should be investigated before ordering extensive neuroimaging studies. Generally, a single pooled fasting elevated prolactin level may confirm the diagnosis. Minor elevations may be somewhat difficult to interpret, since breast manipulation can elevate the serum level. The first level obtained serves as a baseline and guides the course of dopamine–agonist therapy. In idiopathic hyperprolactinaemia the level is <100 ng/ml. A reading of >100 ng/ml should be evaluated. However, resperidol is known to cause an elevation of prolactin to the tune of 200 ng/dl.

- Growth hormone abnormalities

Growth hormone (GH) levels are raised in acromegaly but can fluctuate significantly. Intravenous GH levels done every 5 minutes for 24 hours may show consistent elevation of GH. This is not a practical diagnostic method, but does indicate that a single GH value is not sufficient to make a diagnosis. Serum IGF-1 level is the best endocrinological test for acromegaly. IGF-1 reflects the GH concentration in the past 24 hours. Technical factors may limit its usefulness in some laboratories. An oral glucose tolerance test is the definitive test for the diagnosis of acromegaly; a positive result is the failure of GH to decrease to <1 mcg/L 1 hour after ingestion of 75 g of glucose.

- Cushing's disease and Cushing's syndrome

Twenty-four-hour urine is collected for estimation of free cortisol. Usually, 2 baseline values are obtained. *Dexamethasone suppression test:* the physiological basis of this test is a decrease in ACTH secretion by the pituitary because of exogenous glucocorticoid administration. Dexamethasone is administered at a dose of 1 mg. The serum cortisol level is measured the next morning; it should be <138 nmol/L (i.e. <5 mcg/dl). *Standard low-dose dexamethasone:* Two-day baseline serum and urine cortisol levels are determined. The patient is then given 4 doses of 0.5 mg of dexamethasone at 6-hour intervals. Normal suppression is a serum cortisol level of <138 nmol/L or a urine level of <55 nmol/L. High-dose dexamethasone suppression confirms the diagnosis of a pituitary adenoma. It suppresses the pituitary gland even in the presence of an adenoma. If cortisol levels remain unchanged, the cause of the increased cortisol is not a pituitary adenoma. Instead, it could be a pituitary macroadenoma. *Serum levels of ACTH:* the basal serum concentration of ACTH, if >10 pg/ml, indicates ACTH-dependent Cushing's syndrome whereas a value <5 pg/ml indicates an adrenal cause. Venous sampling of ACTH from the petrosal sinuses by means of cerebral venography may be valuable when the diagnosis is difficult. Baseline petrosal sinus levels of CRF distinguish patients with Cushing's disease from those with ectopic ACTH secretion.

- Glycoprotein hormones—Thyroid-stimulating hormone (TSH), follicle-stimulating hormone (FSH), luteinizing hormone (LH)

Pituitary adenomas that are associated with TSH hypersecretion are uncommon. These patients have increased T3 and T4 levels, hyperthyroidism, and goitre with inappropriately high levels of TSH. The best way to diagnose the condition would be to carry out a thyroid scan, which shows an increased uptake in spite of a high or a high-normal TSH. Increased FSH levels may be apparent from the histological examination of a pituitary adenoma in patients without apparent preoperative endocrine abnormalities and in some patients with hypogonadism. Increased LH levels also may be seen in patients with hypogonadism. The secreted hormone is not intact LH, and serum testosterone levels are not increased. Free alpha and beta subunits of FSH are secreted by pituitary tumours that are thought to be inactive. A high percentage of these tumours have a paradoxical release of FSH subunits in response to TRH stimulation (200 mcg). Rarely, these tumours are associated with precocious puberty or resumption of bleeding in a postmenopausal woman. The initial screening endocrine tests should include levels of prolactin, IGF-1, LH, FSH, TRH and alpha subunit, cortisol, and T4; men should have the testosterone level determined.

- *Pituitary apoplexy:* CSF may be xanthochromic, with crenated RBCs and a high protein level.

Imaging studies

MRI of the brain and sellar region with multiplanar thin sections is of critical importance. This provides axial, coronal and sagittal sections of the sellar contents. Generally, the relationship between the lesion and the optic chiasm and visual pathways is recognized easily. Pregadolinium and post-gadolinium images are recommended to ensure that primarily isointense lesions do not escape detection. CT scan of the brain with sellar images may be sufficiently specific and can detect tumour calcifications. However, the detail is generally inferior to that of MRI. Cerebral angiography is not performed routinely in the work-up of sellar mass lesions. It is generally performed when vascular lesions are suspected.

Other tests

A final diagnosis generally is not made until the lesion is resected. If a granulomatous or infectious process is the primary concern, other systemic and neurological testing may be required.

Procedures

Inferior petrosal sinus sampling

This is a specialized test done at a few centres in India. The test is to be ordered only when the diagnosis is in doubt or localization of the lesion in the pituitary is required. According to the results, hemihypophysectomy is performed. Patients who are suspected of having a pituitary tumour resulting in Cushing's syndrome may be referred for inferior petrosal sinus sampling if findings on MRI examination of the pituitary do not reveal a tumour or are inconclusive.

The inferior petrosal sinus sampling procedure is performed in the radiology department. With the patient on the angiography table, both groin regions are partially shaved, sterilized, and a local anaesthetic is injected into the skin to provide pain relief. A tiny incision is made within the skin and a needle is inserted to puncture the femoral vein. A small catheter is then inserted into the vein and flushed with an intravenous solution. Longer catheters are passed into the shorter catheters and advanced through the large veins traversing the torso into the neck and then into the base of the skull. Thereafter, a microcatheter is advanced through each of these larger guiding catheters and threaded into the inferior petrosal sinuses which lie along the internal aspect of the skull base and drain blood from the pituitary gland. Once these microcatheters have been positioned, contrast dye is injected and X-rays are taken to verify their position in the inferior petrosal sinuses. Next, blood samples are collected from both the catheters in the inferior petrosal sinuses and from a peripheral (usually arm) vein. Thereafter, CRH (not available in India so antidiuretic hormone [ADH] is used instead) is administered through the peripheral vein. Repeat blood samples are drawn at 2, 5 and 10 minutes after the injection. Additional X-rays are taken to confirm that the catheters have not been dislodged from the site during the sampling procedure. Thereafter, the catheters are removed and direct pressure is applied to the groin region to decrease the likelihood of bruising. Patients are observed for 4 hours following the procedure to ensure that there is no bleeding from the femoral vein puncture site. Normal non-strenuous activity may be resumed after 48 hours of the procedure. ACTH levels are measured in each of the blood samples obtained during the procedure. The ratios of ACTH levels between blood obtained from the petrosal sinus sampling and the peripheral vein samples are compared. The results are used to determine whether ACTH production is due to a pituitary or non-pituitary source.

Histological findings

The role of pathological examination of pituitary tumours is critical. Routinely, standard histological examination, electromicroscopy and immuno-histochemistry are performed on these lesions. The findings then are correlated with clinical and imaging results. At times, the differentiation of hyperplasia from adenoma may be difficult. Other non-pituitary mass lesions may be identified easily on pathological examination.

Treatment

Treatment of the majority of pituitary tumours is surgical (except prolactin-secreting ones). However, with advances in pharmacotherapeutics, GH-secreting tumours are increasingly being managed with drugs.

Medical care

The majority of prolactinomas respond to dopamine receptor agonists. Improvement in visual field abnormalities, resolution of symptoms associated with hyperprolactinaemia, and visible diminution of the actual mass can result with treatment. Drugs such as bromocriptine and cabergoline can be used. Cabergoline can be used in bromcriptine resistance as well. The surgical option is used only when there is visual impairment or domaminergic resistance. Somatostatin analogues (octreotide) can be helpful in the treatment of increased post-operative levels of GH in acromegaly. In some cases, the tumour may shrink modestly. Gallstones are a frequent complication of somatostatin-analogue therapy. Dopamine agonists have also been used. Replacement therapy for decreased or absent hormones should be instituted as needed. All hormone-based treatment should be directed by a consulting endocrinologist.

Somatostatin analogues

These agents are used to treat disorders associated with acromegaly.

Octreotide (Sandostatin)

Hypothalamic polypeptide that inhibits production of GH. Acts primarily on somatostatin receptor subtypes II and V. Has multitude of other endocrine and nonendocrine effects, including inhibition of glucagon, VIP, and GI peptides. More effective than dopamine agonists in acromegaly.

Dosing
- *Adult:* 100–500 mcg subcutaneous tid
- *Pediatric:* Administer lower limit of adult dosing range

May reduce effects of cyclosporine; patients on insulin, oral hypoglycemics, beta-blockers, or calcium channel blockers may need dosage adjustment

Documented hypersensitivity

Pregnancy

C–Fetal risk revealed in studies in animals but not established or not studied in humans; may use if benefits outweigh risk to fetus.

Precautions

Adverse effects related primarily to altered GI motility and include nausea, abdominal pain, diarrhea, increased incidence of gallstones, and biliary sludge; because of alteration in counter-regulatory hormones (ie, insulin, glucagon, GH), hypoglycemia or hyperglycemia may be seen; bradycardia, cardiac conduction abnormalities, and arrhythmias have been reported; because of inhibition of TSH secretion, hypothyroidism may occur; use caution in patients with renal impairment; cholelithiasis may occur.

Long-acting derivatives of octreotide are available which can be used once a month.

Dopamine agonists

Dopamine receptors in the hypothalamus exert an inhibitory action on some pituitary cells, particularly those producing prolactin and, to a lesser extent, GH.

Bromocriptine (Parlodel)

Ergot alkaloid derivative with dopaminergic properties. Inhibits prolactin secretion.

Dosing
- *Adult:* 2.5 mg PO tid
- *Pediatric:* Not established

- *Interactions:* Ergot alkaloids may increase toxicity; amitriptyline, butyrophenones, imipramine, methyldopa, phenothiazines, and reserpine may decrease effects.
- *Contraindications:* Documented hypersensitivity; ischemic heart disease; peripheral vascular disorders

Precautions

Pregnancy
C–Fetal risk revealed in studies in animals but not established or not studied in humans; may use if benefits outweigh risk to fetus.

Precautions
Caution in renal or hepatic disease; many females with prolactinomas become pregnant while using dopamine–agonist therapy (once conception takes place, dopamine agonist may be discontinued 4 weeks after confirmation of pregnancy); occasionally, enlargement of prolactinoma may occur with symptomatic visual loss, transient diabetes insipidus, and, rarely, pituitary apoplexy.

Transsphenoidal surgery can be performed, if necessary, with continuation of pregnancy and successful full-term delivery; dopamine–agonist therapy may be reinitiated

Cabergoline can be used in pregnancy and has been used with good results by us in micro and macroprolactinomas.

Pegvisomant

- Growth hormone receptor antogonistist
- Given subcutaneously
- May cause tumour enlargement.

Cabergoline (Quinazoline, Dostinex)

Formerly CV205–502. Long-acting dopamine receptor agonist with high affinity for D2 receptors. Prolactin secretion by anterior pituitary predominates under hypothalamic inhibitory control exerted through dopamine.

Dosing
- *Adult:* 125 mcg to 1 mg PO twice weekly
- *Pediatric:* Not established
- *Interactions:* May increase effects of antihypertensive medications (adjust dose accordingly); other dopamine agonists may reduce effects
- *Contraindications:* Documented hypersensitivity; uncontrolled hypertension

Precautions

Pregnancy
B–Fetal risk not confirmed in studies in humans but has been shown in some studies in animals

Precautions
Caution when patient is taking hypertensives; do not use to inhibit physiologic lactation because of relatively high incidence of stroke, seizures, hypertension; monitor prolactin levels monthly; caution in hepatic impairment

Pergolide (Permax)

Pergolide was withdrawn from the US market in March 2007, because of heart valve damage resulting in cardiac valve regurgitation. It is important not to abruptly stop pergolide. Healthcare professionals should assess patients' need for dopamine agonist (DA) therapy and consider alternative treatment. If continued treatment with a DA is needed, another DA should be substituted for pergolide. (For more information, see FDA MedWatch Product Safety Alert and Medscape Alerts: Pergolide Withdrawn From US Market.)

Potent dopamine receptor agonist at both D1 and D2 receptor sites. Approximately 10–1000 times more potent than bromocriptine on mg per mg basis. Inhibits secretion of prolactin; causes transient rise in serum concentrations of GH and decrease in serum concentrations of LH.

Dosing
- *Adult:* 50 mcg to 1 mg PO tid
- *Pediatric:* Not established

Corticosteroids

These agents are used in the management of adrenocortical insufficiency.

Hydrocortisone (Efcorlin, Hydrocort)

DOC because of mineralocorticoid activity and glucocorticoid effects.

- *Interactions:* Corticosteroid clearance may decrease with estrogens; may increase digitalis toxicity secondary to hypokalemia
- *Contraindications:* Documented hypersensitivity; viral, fungal, or tubercular skin infections

Precautions

Pregnancy
C–Foetal risk revealed in studies in animals but not established or not studied in humans; may use if benefits outweigh risk to foetus.

Precautions
Caution in hyperthyroidism, osteoporosis, peptic ulcer, cirrhosis, nonspecific ulcerative colitis, diabetes, and myasthenia gravis

Dosing
- *Adult:* 100 mg i.v. bolus, followed by continuous infusion of 100 mg q8h for 24–48 h; once patient is stable, initiate PO hydrocortisone (50 mg q8h for another 48 h; may taper dose to 30–50 mg/d in divided doses)
- *Pediatric:*
  <12 years: 1–2 mg/kg IV bolus, followed by 25–150 mg/d divided q6–8h
  >12 years: 1–2 mg/kg IV bolus, followed by 150–250 mg/d divided q6–8h

Thyroid products

These agents are used as supplemental therapy in hypothyroidism.

Levothyroxine (Eltroxin, Thyronorm, etc.)

DOC. Rapidly inhibits the release of thyroid hormones via a direct effect on the thyroid gland and inhibits the synthesis of thyroid hormones. Iodide also appears to attenuate cAMP-mediated effects of thyrotropin. In active form, influences growth and maturation of tissues. Involved in normal growth, metabolism, and development.

Dosing
- *Adult:* 12.5–50 mcg/d PO and increase by 25–50 mcg/d q2–4 week to a maximum of 100–200 mcg/day
- *Pediatric:*
  Neonate to 6 months: 25–50 mcg/d PO
  6–12 months: 50–75 mcg/d PO
  1–5 years: 75–100 mcg/d PO
  6–12 years: 100–150 mcg/d PO
  >12 years: 150 mcg/d PO
- *Interactions:* Cholestyramine may decrease liothyronine absorption; estrogens may decrease response to thyroid hormone therapy in patients with nonfunctioning thyroid glands; effect of anticoagulants increased when administered with liothyronine; activity of some beta-blockers may decrease when hypothyroid patient is converted to a euthyroid state
- *Contraindications:* Documented hypersensitivity; uncorrected adrenal insufficiency

Precautions

Pregnancy
A–Foetal risk not revealed in controlled studies in humans.

Precautions
Caution in angina pectoris or cardiovascular disease; monitor thyroid status periodically.

Estrogen derivatives

These agents are used in the treatment of hypoestrogenism.

Estrogens (Premarin)

Contains a mixture of estrogens obtained exclusively from natural sources, occurring as the sodium salts of water-soluble estrogen sulfates blended to represent the average composition of material derived from pregnant mares' urine. Mixture of sodium estrone sulfate and sodium equilin sulfate. Contains as concomitant components, sodium sulfate conjugates, 17-alpha-dihydroequilenin, 17-alpha-oestradiol, and 17-beta-dihydroequilenin.

Restores estrogen levels to concentrations that induce negative feedback at gonadotrophic regulatory centers, which, in turn, reduces release of gonadotropins from pituitary. Increases synthesis of DNA, RNA, and many proteins in target tissues.

Important in developing and maintaining female reproductive system and secondary sex characteristics; promotes growth and development of vagina, uterus, fallopian tubes, and breasts. Affects release of pituitary gonadotropins; causes capillary dilatation, fluid retention, and protein anabolism; increases water content of cervical mucus; and inhibits ovulation. Predominantly produced by the ovaries.

Dosing
- *Adult:* 0.3–1.25 mg PO qd; may use higher doses depending on tissue response of patient
- *Pediatric:*
  <12 years: Not established
  >12 years: 0.3 mg PO qod for up to 6 months, slowly (at 6-month intervals) increasing to adult dose
- *Interactions:* May reduce hypoprothrom-

binemic effect of anticoagulants; coadministration of barbiturates, rifampin, and other agents that induce hepatic microsomal enzymes may reduce estrogen levels; pharmacologic and toxicologic effects of corticosteroids may occur as a result of estrogen-induced inactivation of hepatic *P450* enzyme; loss of seizure control has been noted when administered concurrently with hydantoins

- *Contraindications:* Documented hypersensitivity; known or suspected pregnancy; breast cancer, undiagnosed abnormal genital bleeding, active thrombophlebitis, or thromboembolic disorders; history of thrombophlebitis, thrombosis, or thromboembolic disorders associated with previous oestrogen use (except when used in treatment of breast or prostatic malignancy)

Precautions

Pregnancy
X–Contraindicated; benefit does not outweigh risk

Precautions
Certain patients may develop undesirable manifestations of excessive oestrogenic stimulation, such as abnormal or excessive uterine bleeding or mastodynia; estrogens may cause some degree of fluid retention (exercise caution); prolonged unopposed estrogen therapy may increase risk of endometrial hyperplasia.

Androgens

These agents are used in the treatment of male hypogonadism.

Testosterone (Depo-Testosterone)

Promotes and maintains secondary sex characteristics in androgen–deficient males.

Dosing
- *Adult:*
  75–150 mg IM q7–10d or 100–200 mg IM q2week
  Buccal adhesive (Striant): Apply 1 buccal adhesive system (30 mg) to gum q12h
- *Pediatric: >13 years:* 50–100 mg IM every mo initially followed by 50–100 mg IM q2week after 1 year of treatment, with gradual increase to adult dose
- *Interactions:* May increase effects of anticoagulants
- *Contraindications:* Documented hypersensitivity; severe cardiac or renal disease; benign prostatic hypertrophy with obstruction; males with carcinoma of the breast, undiagnosed genital bleeding

Precautions

Pregnancy
X–Contraindicated; benefit does not outweigh risk

Precautions
Anabolic effects may enhance hypoglycemia; monitor hand and wrist every 6 mo to determine rate of bone maturation. Rotate buccal adhesive system application site; do not chew or swallow buccal adhesive system

Growth Hormone (GH)

These agents are used in the replacement of endogenous growth hormone in patients with adult growth hormone deficiency.

Human GH (Genotropin, Humatrope, Nutropin)

Stimulates growth of linear bone, skeletal muscle, and organs. Stimulates erythropoietin, which increases red blood cell mass.

Currently widely available in SC injection form. Adjust dose gradually based on clinical and biochemical responses assessed at monthly intervals, including body weight, waist circumference, serum IGF-1, IGFBP-3, serum glucose, lipids, thyroid function, and whole body dual-energy X-ray absorptiometry. In children, assess response based on height and growth velocity. Continue treatment until final height or epiphysial closure or both have been recorded.

Dosing

- *Adult:* Usual starting dose is 2–5 mcg/kg/d or about 0.1–0.3 mg/d subcutaneous
- *Pediatric:* 0.15–0.3 mg/kg/week subcutaneous initially; divide into equal doses to be given daily or 6 times/week
- *Interactions:* Glucocorticoids may decrease growth promoting effects
- *Contraindications:* Documented hypersensitivity; closed epiphyses; actively growing intracranial tumor; any underlying intracranial lesion

Precautions

Pregnancy

C-Fetal risk revealed in studies in animals but not established or not studied in humans; may use if benefits outweigh risk to the foetus.

Precautions

Caution in diabetes; reconstitute with sterile water for injection if administering to newborns

Vasopressin analogues

These agents are used in the treatment of diabetes insipidus.

Desmopressin (DDAVP, Stimate)

Synthetic analogue of hypothalamic/posterior pituitary hormone 8-arginine vasopressin (antidiuretic hormone [ADH]). Has no effect on V1 receptors, which are responsible for vasopressin-induced vasoconstriction. Instead, acts on V2 receptors at renal tubuli, increasing cellular permeability of collecting ducts, which are responsible for antidiuretic effect. Effect is prevention of nocturnal diuresis and elevated BP in the mornings, resulting in reabsorption of water by kidneys. Formulated as a tab and a nasal spray. Tab is more convenient to administer.

Dosing

- *Adult:* 2–4 mcg i.v./subcutaneous divided bid
- *Pediatric:*
  <3 months: Not established
  3 months to 12 years: 5–30 mcg/d intranasally qd or divided bid
  >12 years: Administer as in adults
- *Interactions:* Coadministration with demeclocycline and lithium decrease effects; fludrocortisone and chlorpropamide increase effects of desmopressin; loperamide increases bioavailability and absorption of desmopressin, thus potentially increasing effect
- *Contraindications:* Documented hypersensitivity; platelet-type von Willebrand's disease

Precautions

Pregnancy

B-Foetal risk not confirmed in studies in humans but has been shown in some studies in animals.

Precautions

Avoid overhydration in patients using desmopressin to benefit from its hemostatic effects.

Surgical care

A detailed description of surgical management is beyond the scope of this chapter.

The goal of surgery is total resection limited to the lesion, without compromising post-operative endogenous pituitary function. Thus, a skilled neurosurgeon carefully balances maximally effective tumour removal with the requirement to preserve non-tumorous pituitary trophic function. Trans-sphenoidal microscopic surgery is the most frequent surgical approach for the resection of pituitary tumours. With larger lesions, a transfrontal approach may become necessary to decompress the visual pathways. Minimally invasive endoscopic surgery using a 4 mm endoscope through a nostril is a possibility in selected cases. Open low-field intra-operative MRI monitoring during trans-sphenoidal surgical resection to monitor the precise extent of tumour resection is gaining acceptance.

Radiation therapy

A detailed description of radiotherapy is beyond the scope of this chapter. Delivery of supervoltage photons from cobalt 60 or linear acclearator devices is useful in tumour recurrence or prophylactically after resection if there is evidence of residual tumour on postoperative neuroimaging. Traditionally, radiotherapy had been given in a fractionated manner at standard doses of 1.8–2 Gy per fraction daily. Radiation therapy (RT) is complementary to surgery in preventing progression or recurrence. Standard radiation techniques involve the use of three fields (parallel opposed fields with a coronal field) or rotational techniques to avoid unnecessary radiation to the temporal lobes. Dosages of 4500–5000 cGy delivered in 180 cGy fractions are recommended. In general, patients with subtotally resected tumours are given RT. Although radiation reduces the risk of recurrence or delays recurrence after gross total resection, we follow these patients with serial MRI scans and visual field examination, and withhold radiation unless there is documented tumour regrowth. Side-effects include hypopituitarism; within 10 years of radiation, 80% of patients have gonadotrophic, somatotrophic, thyrotrophic or corticotrophic defects. Radiosurgery by Gamma-knife using focused Co–60 emissions and a linear

accelerator delivers high-dose radiation that spares the surrounding tissue.

Inpatient care

Care of patients is primarily on an outpatient basis. Only those undergoing surgery are kept as inpatients. Additionally, a small percentage of patients with pituitary apoplexy present with a clinical picture similar to that of subarachnoid haemorrhage.

Careful hormonal control of patients undergoing surgery is essential, under the direction of an endocrinologist. A syndrome of inappropriate antidiuretic hormone secretion (SIADH) may be seen transiently, followed by diabetes insipidus (DI). DI is defined as a urine output >50 ml/kg/day. If DI is established, the patient is started on ADH intranasally or orally. The drug is given 6 days a week with one drug holiday. Before labelling somebody as having DI, it is important to always see the amount of fluid given pre- and intraoperatively. Postoperative hypoadrenalism is a possibility that requires careful monitoring. Hormonal levels should be assessed and replacement provided when appropriate. In most cases, CSF rhinorrhoea should be diagnosed and addressed promptly. In most cases, trans-sphenoidal hypophysectomy has a low risk and good prognosis.

Further outpatient care

Adjustment of hormonal therapy is necessary following trans-sphenoidal resection of the adenoma. This may be done in the weeks following surgery by the consulting endocrinologist. *Steroid replacement:* If a macroadenoma has been operated upon it is assumed that the patient will require steroid replacement. In microadenoma, steroid replacement can wait and is given only when absolutely essential. The usual steroid given is prednisolone. The dose is 7.5 mg/day in two divided doses at 8 am and 4 pm. A smaller dose is given in the evening so as to not suppress endogenous secretion of ACTH. The need for further steroid is evaluate by the short syncathene test. For the replacement of thyroid hormones free T4 and TSH are evaluated. If free T4 is low, replacement is started. In young women, if the menses do not resume, oestrogen and progesterone are started. For men, similarly, if there is a reduction in libido or a low serum testosterone level, replacement is started. In recent years, GH replacement is also being given to adults. Those who can afford it can be given the hormone.

Periodic follow up by a neuro-ophthalmologist is essential, particularly when there is residual tumour. Visual fields and fundus photographs should be obtained before and immediately after tumour resection. These parameters provide a baseline for follow-up examinations. RT is often necessary for managing the local mass effects of large macroadenomas. The indications for RT at this time are controversial. In a recent study, Alameda *et al.* followed 51 patients with pituitary tumour who underwent surgery; 22 with complete macroscopic resections judged by imaging were tumour-free 3–6 years postoperatively. Twenty-seven patients with residual tumours after surgical resection were treated with RT. Fourteen residual tumours decreased in size, 11 remained stable, 1 increased in size, and 1 patient was lost to follow up.[4] RT is thus a useful treatment alternative for patients with residual tumours after surgery. Fractionated stereotactic radiotherapy (FSR) was found to be safe and effective by Colin *et al.* in 110 consecutive patients.[5] Moreover, it may reduce the possibility of post-radiation optic neuropathy.

Initial hormonal deficiencies may improve over time. Therefore, frequent endocrine re-evaluation is necessary. Pre-radiation and post-radiation endocrinological and neuro-ophthalmological evaluations must be performed. A postoperative cerebral imaging study is important to determine the possibility of residual tumour. If residual tumour is present, serial imaging is required. Adverse effects of radiation on the hypothalamus, pituitary and visual pathways require close monitoring.

Complications

Pituitary apoplexy

As its name indicates, the apoplectic onset of haemorrhage within a pituitary adenoma may lead to hypothalamic, chiasmal, cavernous sinus and brainstem compression. Meningeal irritation results from blood in the subarachnoid space. On occasion, the degree of subarachnoid haemorrhage is significant, and a spinal tap may show evidence of acute or subacute bleeding. The acute panhypopituitarism is associated with shock and hypothalamic–brainstem compression, which could lead to coma and even death. Headache, vomiting, visual loss, blindness, ophthalmoplegia and altered consciousness may be present. In a series involving 62 patients, Semple *et al.* found that headache was the most common symptom in 87% of their cases, visual loss occurred in 56% of the patients, ophthalmoplegia in 45%, and altered level of consciousness in 13%. Hypopituitarism was present in 73% of patients and DI in 8%.[2]

In most cases, surgical intervention is required, which gives excellent results. Candidates for emergency surgery include patients with rapidly deteriorating vision, altered mental status and hypothalamic compression. Pituitary apoplexy may be fatal in a few instances. Conservative treatment is an option in stable cases, particularly if they have prolactinomas. Factors leading to haemorrhage within a pituitary adenoma identified by Biousse *et al.* include the following: reduced blood flow to the gland, sudden increment of blood flow, stimulation of the gland by endocrine mechanisms, anticoagulation and trauma.[3] An upper respiratory tract infection with frequent coughing and sneezing also may trigger an apoplectic event. The best method to make the diagnosis of pituitary apoplexy is cerebral imaging. MRI is preferred but CT scan is an acceptable option if MRI is not available.

Other complications

Some patients may present to a neurologist with complications following surgery and RT. Surgery for pituitary tumours, particularly those resected via a trans-sphenoidal approach, has an excellent outcome with successful decompression of the visual pathways, cavernous sinus and hypothalamus. Transfrontal resections are associated with more complications. In cases handled by a skilled surgeon, surgical complications are minimal but can include any of the following:

- Incomplete resection of large adenomas
- Transient or permanent DI
- CSF rhinorrhoea
- Monohormonal or polyhormonal deficiencies
- Residual permanent visual field defects

Empty sella syndrome: An empty sella may occur after trans-sphenoidal surgery and is generally benign. Generally, herniation of the chiasm inside the sella does not typically cause visual field defects. Radiation toxicity may occur as a rare complication of the treatment of pituitary adenomas, resulting in hypothalamic and chiasmal necrosis.

Prognosis

In prolactin-secreting microadenomas, surgical resection is curative. Dopamine agonists provide symptom control for micro- and prolactin-secreting macroadenomas, Surgical resection is curative in 60% of patients with acromegaly; octreotide therapy controls symptoms. Surgical resection is curative in Cushing's disease. Rarely, invasive tumours produce metastatic deposits within the neuraxis via the CSF pathways. Rarely, distant metastases may occur.

Patient education

The successful management of pituitary adenomas requires a highly motivated and compliant patient. The most important hormone replaced is steroid. Stress doses are advised to patients in a language which they understand. There have been deaths when stress doses have not been explained properly or the patient has not complied with the instructions. Hormone-replacement therapy is demanding, and a non-compliant patient is at risk for complications due to misuse of these agents. Interaction of a team of specialists is required to manage these lesions. One of the specialists should serve as a team leader and coordinate the patient's care. Prompt reporting of new symptoms is important in addition to routine follow-up visits. If the patient has no new symptoms or problems after 5 years of beginning treatment, follow-up visits can be less frequent. The frequency of follow-up visits depends on the presence of residual tumour, visual deficit, hormonal needs, history of RT, or other complicating circumstances.

Other lesions of the pituitary

Inflammatory and granulomatous expansive lesions of the pituitary

Inflammatory and granulomatous diseases of the pituitary are rare causes of sellar masses. Lymphocytic hypophysitis is the most relevant of these disorders, and it is characterized by an autoimmune pathogenesis with focal or diffuse inflammatory infiltration and varying degrees of pituitary gland destruction. It is most common within 2 months of parturition, or even in the last month of pregnancy. Most patients present with field defects, headache and hyperprolactinaemia. Endocrine symptoms may include partial or total hypopituitarism, with ACTH deficiency being the earliest and most frequent alteration. Treatment is with steroids and replacement of deficient hormones. Trans-sphenoidal biopsy for a histopathological diagnosis may be done. Pituitary abscess is a rare but potentially life-threatening disease and, in 30%–50% of patients, anterior pituitary hormone deficiencies or central DI at onset may be observed: the earliest manifestation being GH deficiency, followed by FSH/LH, TSH and ACTH deficiencies.

Fungal infections of the pituitary are rare and include aspergillosis and coccidioidomycosis. The pituitary may be involved in systemic diseases; in sarcoidosis, endocrine complications are rare, but the hypothalamus and pituitary are the glands most commonly affected. DI is reported in approximately 25%–33% of all cases of neurosarcoidosis and is the most frequently observed endocrine disorder. Hyperprolactin-aemia and anterior pituitary deficiencies may also occur. Rarely, partial or global anterior pituitary dysfunction may be present in Wegener's granulomatosis, either at onset or during the course of the disease, resulting in the deficiency of one or more of the pituitary hormones.

Other forms of granulomatous pituitary lesions include idiopathic giant cell granulo-matous hypophysitis, Takayasu's disease, Cogan's syndrome and Crohn's disease. The hypothalamic–pituitary system is involved mainly in children with Langerhans' cells histiocytosis who develop DI, which is the most common endocrine manifestation. Anterior pituitary dysfunction is found more rarely and is almost invariably associated with DI. Pituitary involvement may also be observed in another form of systemic histiocytosis, Erdheim–Chester disease. Tuberculosis is a rare cause of hypo-physitis, which may present with features of anterior pituitary dysfunction, such as hypo-pituitarism with hyperprolactinaemia.

Sheehan's syndrome

This is also known as postpartum hypo-pituitarism or postpartum pituitary necrosis, is hypopituitarism caused by necrosis due to blood loss and hypovolaemic shock during and after childbirth. It is a rare complication of pregnancy, usually occurring after excessive blood loss. The presence of disseminated intravascular coagulation (i.e. in amniotic fluid embolism or the HELLP syndrome [haemolytic anaemia, elevated liver enzymes, low platelet count]) also appears to be a factor in its development.

The most common initial symptoms of Sheehan's syndrome are the absence of lactation and/or difficulties with lactation. Many women also report amenorrhoea or oligomenorrhoea after delivery. In some cases, a woman with Sheehan's syndrome might be relatively asympto-matic, and the diagnosis is not made until years later, when features of hypopituitarism appear. Such features include secondary hypothyroidism with tiredness, intolerance to cold, constipation, weight gain, hair loss and slowed thinking, as well as a slowed heart rate and low blood pressure. Another such feature is secondary adrenal insufficiency which, in the rather chronic case, is similar to Addison's disease with symptoms including fatigue, weight loss, hypoglycaemia (low blood sugar levels), anaemia and hypo-natraemia (low sodium levels). In such a woman, however, the condition may become acutely exacerbated when her body is stressed by, for example, a severe infection or surgery years after her delivery, a condition equivalent to an Addisonian crisis.[6] Gonadotrophin deficiency will often cause amenorrhoea, oligomenorrhoea, hot flashes or decreased libido. GH deficiency causes may vague symptoms including fatigue and decreased muscle mass. Uncommonly, Sheehan's syndrome may also appear acutely after delivery, mainly by hyponatremia. There are several possible mechanisms by which hypo-pituitarism can result in hyponatremia, including decreased free-water clearance by hypothyro-idism, direct syndrome of inappropriate antidiuretic hormone (ADH) hypersecretion, decreased free-water clearance by glucocorticoid deficiency (independent of ADH). The potassium level inthese situations is normal, because adrenal production of aldosterone is not dependent on the pituitary. There have also been cases with acute hypoglycemia.[7]

Pathophysiology: Hypertrophy and hyperplasia of the lactotrophs during pregnancy results in the enlargement of the anterior pituitary, without a corresponding increase in blood supply. Secondly, the anterior pituitary is supplied by a low-pressure portal venous system.[8] These vulnerabilities, when affected by major haemorrhage or hypotension during the peripartum period, can result in ischaemia of the affected pituitary regions leading to necrosis. The posterior pituitary is usually not affected due to its direct arterial supply.

History: The specific association with postpartum shock or haemorrhage was described in 1937 by the British pathologist Harold Leeming Sheehan (1900–1988),[9] whereas Simmond's syndrome occurs in either sex due to causes unrelated to pregnancy.[10]

Treatment: Replacement of hormones secreted by the target glands is the most effective treatment for hypopituitarism. Hormone replacement therapy includes cortisol, T4, and androgen or cyclic oestrogen. Prolactin need not be replaced. A patient of reproductive age may benefit from administration of FSH and human chorionic gonadotrophin to boost fertility. GH replacement is recommended for adults as well as children.

The future: Gene therapy

The current treatment for pituitary tumours includes surgery, radiation and pharmacotherapy. In spite of the advances in this field, success rates have not been satsifactory. Gene therapy, which uses nucleic acids as drugs, has emerged as an attractive therapeutic option for tumours which do not respond to the classical treatment strategies. One would use gene therapy along with the best currently available treatment option. The development of animal models of pituitary tumours and hormonal hypersecretion has proven critical in the implementation of gene therapy. Preclinical trials using several gene therapy approaches have been successfully implemented.[11]

References

1. Talkad AV, Kattah JC, Xu MY, *et al.* Prolactinoma presenting as painful postganglionic Horner syndrome. *Neurology* 2004;**62**:1440–1 [Medline].
2. Semple PL, Webb MK, de Villiers JC, *et al.* Pituitary apoplexy. *Neurosurgery* 2005;**56**:65–72; discussion 72–3 [Medline].
3. Biousse V, Newman NJ, Oyesiku NM. Precipitating factors in pituitary apoplexy. *J Neurol Neurosurg Psychiatry* 2001;**71**:542–5 [Medline].
4. Alameda C, Lucas T, Pineda E, *et al.* Experience in management of 51 non-functioning pituitary adenomas: Indications for postoperative radiotherapy. *J Endocrinol Invest* 2005;**28**:18–22 [Medline].
5. Colin P, Jovenin N, Delemer B, *et al.* Treatment of pituitary adenomas by fractionated stereotactic radiotherapy: A prospective study of 110 patients. *Int J Radiat Oncol Biol Phys* 2005;**62**:333–41 [Medline].
6. Schrager S, Sabo L. Sheehan syndrome: A rare complication of postpartum hemorrhage. *J Am Board Fam Pract* 2001;**14**:389–91. PMID 11572546.
7. Bunch TJ, Dunn WF, Basu A, *et al.* Hyponatremia and hypoglycemia in acute Sheehan's syndrome. *Gynecol Endocrinol* 2002;**16**:419–23. PMID 12587538.
8. http://www.ncbi.nlm.nih.gov/bookshelf/br.fcgi?book=endocrin&part=A1257 under heading Sheehan's syndrome.
9. Sheehan HL. Post-partum necrosis of anterior pituitary. *The Journal of Pathology and Bacteriology, Chichester* 1937;**45**:189–214.
10. Sheehan's syndrome at Who Named It?
11. Seilicovich A, Pisera D, Sciascia SA, *et al.* Gene therapy for pituitary tumors. *Curr Gene Ther* 2005;**5**:559–72.

26

Evidence-based management of neurotuberculosis

R. LAKSHMI NARASIMHAN, GNANA SHANMUGAM

Tuberculosis (TB) is the most important and common infectious disease in the world, with an estimated one-third of the population infected with the TB bacillus. Each year, an estimated 8 million individuals around the world develop active TB and 70,000 of these patients acquire TB meningitis. In immune-competent individuals, CNS TB accounts for about 1% of all cases of TB and 6% of extrapulmonary TB.[1] The incidence of CNS TB is directly proportional to the incidence of TB infection in the general population; 10% of all patients with TB are estimated to have CNS involvement.[2] CNS manifestations of TB primarily include three clinical categories: meningitis, tuberculoma brain and spinal tuberculous arachnoiditis. In spite of effective treatment regimens, the case–fatality rate remains high at 15%–40%.[3] The emergence of multidrug-resistant (MDR) TB and co-infection with HIV have complicated the management of TB.

Classification

Classifying the entire spectrum of neuro-tuberculosis is difficult, but it can be broadly divided into intracranial and spinal TB. Further classification into several subtypes can be done according to the anatomical structures involved and the mode of clinical presentation. This classification[4] has included all the well-accepted forms of CNS TB.

Intracranial

- TB meningitis—acute, subacute, chronic
- Tuberculous meningitis (TBM) with miliary TB
- Tuberculous vasculitis
- Tuberculous encephalopathy
- Hypertrophic pachymeningitis
- Tuberculoma brain (single or multiple)
- Tuberculous abscess
- Calvarial TB (less common)

Spinal

- Pott's spine with paraplegia
- Tuberculous arachnoiditis with myelo-radiculopathy
- Spinal meningitis
- Non-osseous spinal tuberculoma

Pathophysiology of neurotuberculosis

CNS TB may occur during the stage of primary infection or more commonly as a consequence of reactivation of latent tuberculous foci. Usually, this happens by a two-stage process.[5] First, during primary infection, tubercle bacilli reach the brain or spinal cord through haematogenous spread from the lung or other organs and form tubercles (rich focus). At a later stage the tubercle ruptures into the subarachnoid space[6] or ventricle, or grows[7] further. CNS TB can also occur during the course of miliary TB or from parameningeal infection such as calvarial TB or tuberculous otitis. The neurological damage resulting from discharge from the tubercles is dependent not only on the number and virulence of the bacilli, but also on the response of the host immune system.

TB meningitis

Pathology

Rupture of the tubercle into the subarachnoid space produces an intense inflammatory reaction, which is more prominent in the base of the brain. This results in the formation of thick exudates in the basal cisterns, cerebellum and brainstem (Fig. 1). These basal exudates are more severe around the circle of Willis[8] and produce vessel wall inflammation, and narrowing and occlusion of the vessels by thrombus. Tuberculous vasculitis predominantly affects the deep penetrating branches (lenticulostriate, medial striate, thalamo-perforating branches) and produce infarcts in the basal ganglia and thalamus (Fig. 2). Large vessels such as the ICA and proximal MCA are also affected. Hydrocephalus may occur due to CSF flow obstruction at the level of the basal cisterns, fourth ventricle or aqueduct of Sylvius.

Clinical features

The clinical features of TBM are protean. Most often, the diagnosis is missed in the early stages and clinical suspicion is necessary in any patient presenting with headache and fever of acute, subacute or chronic onset. Most patients present with non-specific clinical features in the form of

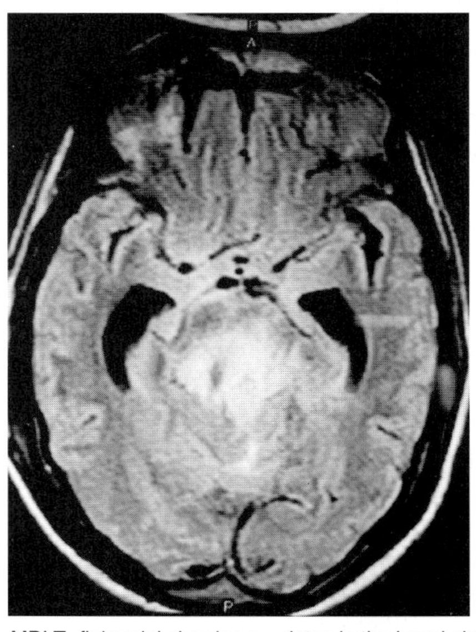

Fig. 1. MRI T$_2$ flair axial showing exudates in the basal cisterns

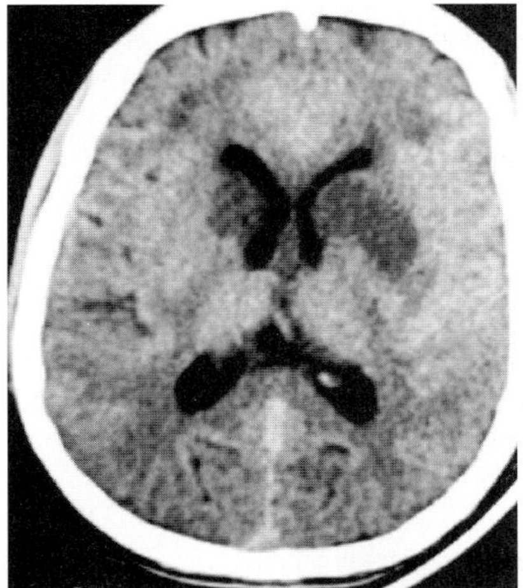

Fig. 2. CT Brain axial of a patient with tuberculous meningitis showing bilateral basal ganglionic infarcts, predominantly in the bilateral head of caudate nucleus and left lentiform nucleus

fever (60%–95%), headache (50%–80%), vomiting (30%–60%), photophobia (5%–10%) and anorexia (60%–80%).[9] TBM typically follows a sub-acute course with neck stiffness, altered sensorium and cranial neuropathies. The six different clinical syndromes of TBM are acute meningitis syndrome, chronic meningitis syndrome, serous meningitis, specific meningeal TB, tuberculoma en plaque and tuberculous encephalopathy. Other presentations include behaviour disorder without meningeal signs, seizures, isolated cranial neuropathies, stroke and recurrent aseptic meningitis. Classically, TBM is characterized by 3 stages;[10] these are (i) the prodromal stage, (ii) the stage of meningeal irritation and (iii) the stage of diffuse or focal cerebral involvement. The prodromal stage lasts for a few weeks and is characterized by apathy, anorexia, nausea, vomiting, restlessness and behavioural changes. The meningitic phase is characterized by headache, vomiting and fever. Neck stiffness is generally not as severe as in pyogenic meningitis. In infants, a tense fontanelle is a more important sign than neck stiffness. In the third stage, raised intracranial tension (ICT) dominates the clinical picture and is characterized by an altered sensorium, deterioration in vision, pupillary dilatation and pyramidal signs.

Diagnosis

Early diagnosis of TBM is crucial, because early initiation of treatment will prevent disabling and irreversible complications. Empirical anti-tuberculous therapy (ATT) should be initiated in any patient with meningitis with lymphocytic pleocytosis and elevated CSF protein.

Diagnostic features of tuberculous meningitis[11]

Clinical
- fever and headache (for more than 14 days)
- vomiting
- altered sensorium or focal neurological deficit

CSF

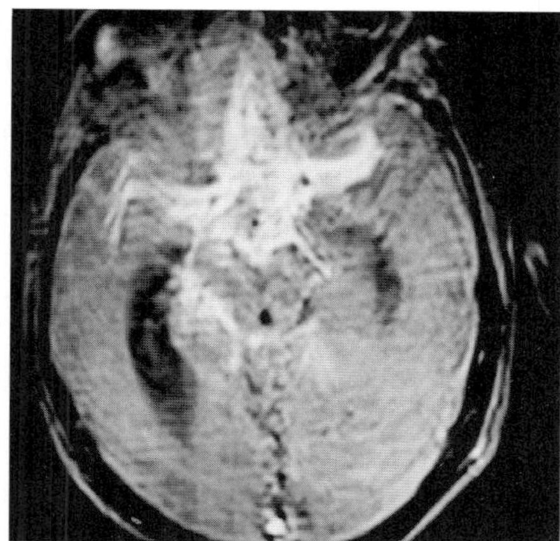

Fig. 3. MRI brain T$_1$ axial contrast of a patient with tuberculous meningitis showing the exudates in the cisterns with hydrocephalus

- pleocytosis (more than 20 cells, of which more than 60% are lymphocytes)
- increased proteins (more than 100 mg/dl)
- low sugar (less than 60% of the corresponding blood sugar level)
- low chloride levels especially in HIV coinfection. Normal CSF chloride levels are 116–130 mmol/L as against serum levels of 95–105 mmol/L. A chloride level of less than 100 mmol/L is virtually diagnostic of TBM.
- India-ink studies and microscopy for malignant cells should be negative.

Imaging
- exudates in the basal cisterns (Fig. 3) or Sylvian fissure, hydrocephalus
- infarcts (basal ganglionic) (Fig. 2)
- gyral enhancement
- tuberculoma formation.

What is the evidence for CSF cytology

Usually, there is a predominant lymphocytic reaction (60–400 WBC/ml) with raised protein levels.[12] CSF proteins range between 100 mg% and 500 mg% in 65% of cases; less than 100 mg% in 10% of cases; more than 500 mg% in 10% of cases. Cases with subarachnoid block develop an extremely high protein content (2–8 g%).[13] In the early stages of infection, a significant number of polymorphonuclear[14] cells may be observed, but over the course of several days to weeks, they are typically replaced by lymphocytes. The CSF is typically clear or slightly turbid. If the CSF is left to stand, a fine clot resembling a pellicle or cobweb may form. This faintly visible 'spider's web clot' is due to the very high level of protein in the CSF (i.e. 1–8 g/L, or 1000–8000 mg/dL) typical of this condition.

The CSF may be acellular in HIV-positive patients. For patients with HIV and/or immuno-suppression, while the mean WBC count in the CSF is 230 cells/μl, as many as 16% of HIV-infected patients may have an acellular CSF, compared with 3%–6% of HIV-negative patients.[15] While HIV-infected patients generally have a mean protein level of 125 mg/dl (range 50–200 mg/dl), as many as 43% of these patients may have a normal CSF protein content.[15]

There is a gradual decrease in the sugar concentration of the CSF, which is usually less than 50% of the serum glucose concentration; the values may vary between 18 and 45 mg/dl. In a study of 232 cases of TBM, a characteristic tubercular pattern of CSF was found in only 143 cases.[16]

A comparative study[17] was done in 110 children with TBM and 94 children with pyogenic meningitis. The clinical features predictive of TBM from this study include (i) symptoms for more than 6 days, (ii) optic atrophy, (iii) focal neurological deficits, (iv) abnormal movements, and (v) neutrophils constituting less than half of the total CSF leukocytes. The diagnostic sensitivity and specificity of these criteria were 55% and 98%, respectively, if three or more features were present, 98% and 44%, respectively, when only one feature was present.

What is the evidence for bacteriological diagnosis of the CSF

A definitive diagnosis of TBM depends upon the detection of the tubercle bacilli in the CSF, either by smear examination or by bacterial culture. It has been claimed that if large volumes of CSF are carefully examined, the organism can be found in over 90% of centrifuged CSF specimens,[18] the highest detection rates being achieved in ventricular fluid. With repeated sequential examinations of the CSF, Kennedy and Fallon[19] reported tubercle bacilli in 87% of patients. In their study, AFB were visible in stained CSF sediments (Zeihl–Neelson technique) in 37% of patients during initial examinations, but the yield was 87% when the CSF from four serial spinal taps was examined. In another study,[18] bacteriological diagnosis was made in 107 of 132 adults with clinically suspected TBM. To increase the positive yield, a centrifuged sediment of more than 10 ml of CSF should be used for acid-fast staining and 200–500 high power fields should be examined of each specimen for at least 30 minutes, preferably by more than one observer. Serial CSF examinations and examination of the ventricular CSF will increase the yield further.

Traditional culture methods are time-consuming and the sensitivity is low. The statistics from the National Institute of Mental Health and Allied Neuro Sciences (NIMHANS) showed that the number of CSF samples positive with AFB culture ranged from 41 to 148 per year with a mean of 115±37. Because of the poor sensitivity and delay in getting results from conventional culture methods, several other techniques were devised for early bacteriological confirmation.[20]

What is the evidence for other techniques and PCR

The tuberculin test: Negative results from the purified protein derivative (PPD) test do not rule out TB. The Centers for Disease Control and Prevention (CDC) and American Thoracic Society (ATS) guidelines stress that, in general, a tuberculin skin test should not be obtained unless treatment would be offered in the event of a positive test result.[21] Cut-off points for induration (5 mm, 10 mm or 15 mm) to determine a positive test result vary, based on the pretest category into which the patient falls. While this approach might decrease the specificity of the test, it increases the sensitivity for capturing those at highest risk for developing the disease in the short-term.

Biochemical assays such the CSF adenosine deaminase level are raised in the CSF in patients with TBM, with a reported sensitivity and specificity of 99%.[22] The clinical utility of other biochemical tests such as CSF tuberculostearic acid estimation and bromide partition test is low. In a study of 2325 specimens processed by the BACTEC system, the isolation rates were 93% and 39% for BACTEC and conventional Lowenstein–Jensen (LJ) medium, respectively.[23]

A revolutionary method for the rapid detection of *M. tuberculosis* is nucleic acid amplification test (NAT) using polymerase chain reaction (PCR). In this method, DNA probes are used to identify mycobacterial RNA or DNA sequences in the CSF. The sensitivity of PCR is not superior to that of conventional microscopy and culture methods. In a study comparing PCR with microscopy and cultures of the CSF, the sensitivity of PCR testing was only 60% in patients classified as having definite or probable TBM.[24] In another meta-analysis of PCR assay[25] in TBM, the sensitivity was 56% and specificity was 98%. After initiating ATT, the sensitivity of culture methods falls further, but mycobacterial DNA is detectable by CSF PCR[26] assays until one month after the start of treatment. A prospective blinded study conducted in NIMHANS.[27] On 677 CSF samples from patients with suspected TBM using PCR revealed that all culture-positive samples were also positive by the PCR assay. The sensitivity was 76.5% and specificity was 89.2%.[27]

Another new immunological technique for rapid diagnosis involves demonstrating the presence of IgG antibodies to a 30 kD protein[28] antigen (30 kDpa) and culture filtrate protein (CFP). In a study conducted on 20 suspected cases of TBM, the sensitivity and specificity of

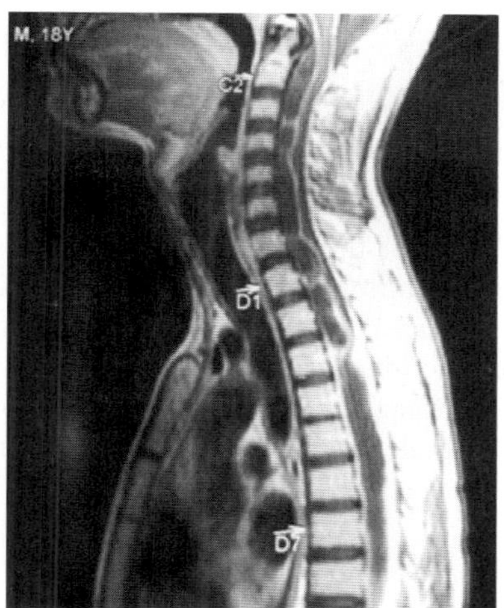

Fig. 4. MRI T₂ sag spine showing loculated fluid collection in the anterior thecal space compressing the cord

IgG antibodies to 30 kDpa was 80% and 91%, respectively and the corresponding figures for CFP were 85% and 94%, respectively.

A dot-immunobinding assay (Dot-Iba)[29] has been standardized to measure circulating antimycobacterial antibodies in CSF specimens for rapid laboratory diagnosis of TBM. Specific CSF IgG antibody to *M. tuberculosis* from a patient with culture-proven TBM was isolated and coupled with activated cyanogen bromide-Sepharose 4B. A 14-kD antigen present in the culture filtrates of *M. tuberculosis* was isolated by immunosorbent affinity chromatography and used in the Dot-Iba to quantitate specific antimycobacterial antibodies. The Dot-Iba gave positive results in all 5 patients with culture-proven TBM; no false-positive results were obtained from CSF specimens from patients with partially treated pyogenic meningitis. Sumi *et al.* have developed a Dot-Iba in their laboratory, which is a simple, rapid and specific method and, more importantly, is suited for routine application in laboratories with limited resources.[29]

Demonstration of mycobacterial antigen 14-kD by rapid Dot-Iba proved to be sensitive for rapid diagnosis. In a study[30] conducted on 30 suspected cases of TBM, the sensitivity and specificity were 83.5% and 95%, respectively.

What is the evidence for neuro-imaging in diagnosis

Certain findings in neuro-imaging give a clue that the possible cause for meningitis is TB. The findings[31] include the presence of basal meningeal exudates (commonly seen in the perimesencephalic cisterns), hydrocephalus, tuberculomas and vasculitic infarct. Gadolinium-enhanced T_1-weighted images demonstrate prominent leptomeningeal and basal cistern enhancement (Fig. 5). With ependymitis, linear periventricular enhancement is present. Deep grey-matter nuclei, deep white matter and pontine infarctions resulting from vasculitis are hyperintense on T_2-weighted images. The majority of infarcts are located in the basal ganglia, internal capsule, thalamus, and are rare in the large vessel territories. Contrast CT and MRI are better at demonstrating the abnormalities than plain CT.[32] Diffusion-weighted MRI is especially sensitive in depicting early ischaemic lesions when findings on T_2-weighted MRI are normal. In two large community-based series, hydrocephalus was seen in approximately 75% of patients, basilar meningeal enhancement in 38%, cerebral infarcts in 15%–30%, and tuberculomas in 5%–10%.[33,34] Diffusion tensor imaging (DTI)-derived fractional anisotropy (FA) has the potential for delineating meningeal infection.[35]

Tuberculoma brain

Tuberculomas[36] are circumscribed, avascular, granulomatous masses of tubercular origin, located in the brain parenchyma. They are well delineated from the surrounding brain tissue and surrounded by oedema and gliosis. The necrotic ore of the mass is composed of caseous material in which acid-fast bacilli (AFB) can be demonstrated. They may present either as meningitis or intracranial space-occupying lesions. They occur in 4.5%–28% of patients with TBM.[37] The symptoms are low-grade fever, headache, vomiting, seizures, focal neurological deficit and

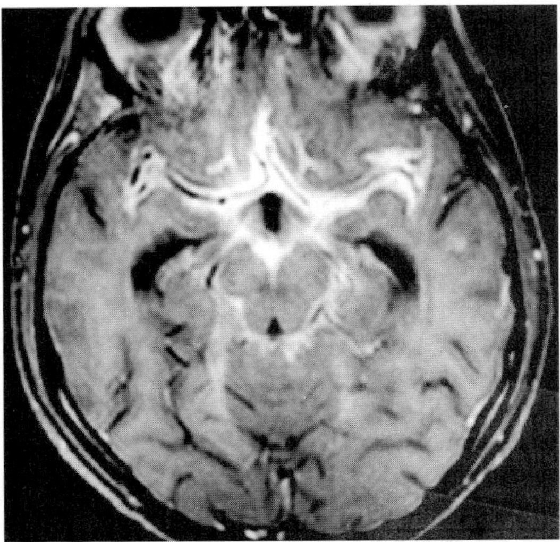

Fig. 5. MRI gadolinium T1 axial of same patient in Fig. 4 - basal exudates enhancing with contrast

papilloedema. Children may present with brainstem syndromes, cerebellar manifestations and multiple cranial nerve palsies.[38]

On CT, tuberculomas are visible as low- or high-density rounded or lobulated masses. They show intense homogeneous or ring enhancement after contrast administration. They have an irregular wall of varying thickness. Moderate-to-marked perilesional oedema is frequently present. Non-caseating granulomas are homogeneously enhancing lesions. Caseating granulomas are rim enhancing; if these have a central calcific focus, they may form a target-like lesion.[39] Granulomas may also form a miliary pattern with multiple tiny nodules scattered throughout the brain. All lesions are surrounded by hypoattenuating oedema.

Tuberculomas may be single or multiple, and are more common in the frontal and parietal lobes, usually in the parasagittal areas. On CT scanning,[40] a tuberculoma measures more than 20 mm in diameter. They are frequently irregular in outline, and are always associated with marked cerebral oedema (leading to midline shift) and progressive focal neurological deficit. The MRI features of tuberculoma depend on whether the lesion is non-caseating, caseating with a solid centre, or caseating with a liquid centre.

The non-caseating granulomas[41] are hypo-intense on T_1-weighted images and hyperintense on T_2-weighted images; after contrast administration, the lesion usually shows homogeneous enhancement. The second type of tuberculoma is hypointense or isointense on T_1-weighted images and T_2-weighted images. After contrast administration, there is ring enhancement (Fig. 6). These types of granulomas have a variable degree of perilesional oedema. A tuberculoma with central liquefaction of the caseous material appears centrally hypointense on T_1- and hyperintense on T_2-weighted images with a peripheral hypointense ring, which represents the capsule of the tuberculoma. Images after contrast administration show ring enhancement.

MR spectroscopy with a single-voxel proton technique can be used to characterize tuberculomas and differentiate them from neoplasms. Tuberculomas show an elevated lipid peak that is best seen by using the stimulated-echo acquisition mode technique and a short echo time.[42] Necrosis of the waxy walls of mycobacteria within the granuloma is believed to cause the elevation in lipid peaks.[43] The lactate peak is caused by anaerobic glycolysis and is found in inflammatory, ischaemic and neoplastic lesions of the brain; this finding is non-specific (Fig. 7).[43]

Tuberculous encephalopathy

This condition is mentioned by Dastur and Udani,[44] and is common in infants and children. Tuberculous encephalopathy is characterized by diffuse swelling of the brain in the absence of infarction, meningitis, tuberculoma or hydrocephalus. The pathological changes are probably due to a delayed type of hypersensitivity to tubercular protein. The disease starts acutely in the form of seizures, altered sensorium, neurological deficits such as hemiplegia and coma. Meningeal signs are usually absent. The diagnosis can be suspected in a child with miliary

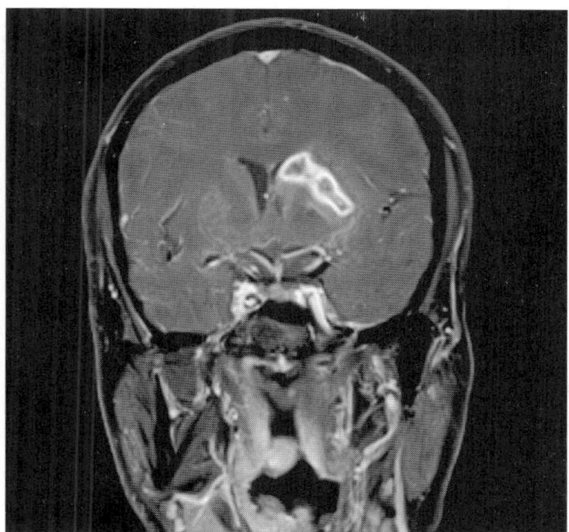

Fig. 6. Post-contrast T_1 coronal view—tuberculoma in the left basal ganglionic region with thick peripheral rim of enhancement

TB, a positive tuberculin test, or contact with a case of pulmonary TB. The CSF may be normal or may show elevated protein and lymphocytes. Sometimes, brain biopsy is needed to confirm the diagnosis.

Tuberculous abscess

Tuberculous brain abscess is a distinct and uncommon condition. It has been reported in 4%–7.5% of patients with neurotuberculosis. To diagnose tuberculous abscess, the following histopathological criteria should be fulfilled:[45] Microscopic evidence of pus in the abscess cavity, microscopic changes in the abscess wall, isolation of *M. tuberculosis*, and absence of the typical giant cells and epithelioid granulomatous reaction of tuberculomas.

Abscesses are usually solitary and large; rarely, they may be multiple and progress much more rapidly than tuberculomas. CT and MRI pictures of a tuberculous abscess show a lesion with a liquid centre; however, they are much larger than tuberculoma, frequently multiloculated and surrounded by marked oedema. Clinical features include partial seizures, rapidly progressive focal

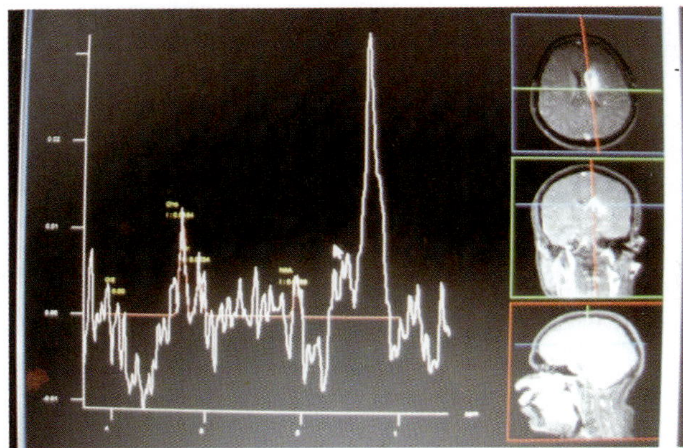

Fig. 7. MR spectroscopy of the same patient showing elevated lipid and lactate peak and decreased NAA peak at the site of lesion conforming the diagnosis of tuberculoma

neurological deficit and raised ICT. Surgical exploration and drainage of the pus may produce excellent long-term results.

Calvarial tuberculosis

Among the various forms of CNS TB, calvarial TB is rare. This rarity may be related to the paucity of lymphatics in the calvarium.[46] It usually occurs secondary to haematogenous spread from primary foci such as the lungs, or from cervical or hilar lymphadenitis. The most common sites of involvement are the frontal and parietal bones, and the most common presentation is a painless, fluctuant, soft scalp swelling. Skin attachment, sinus formation and discoloration are late features. Headache, if present, is localized to the site of infection. Seizures and motor deficit are rare features. An extensive area of destruction occurs before clinical presentation. Batuk *et al.*[46] reported 11 cases of calvarial TB. The treatment is surgery and ATT.[46]

Pott's spine

Involvement of the spine occurs in less than 1% of patients with TB. It is a leading cause of paraplegia in developing countries such as India. The thoracic spine is involved in about 65% of cases, and the lumbar, cervical and thoracolumbar spine in about 20%, 10% and 5%, respectively. The atlanto-axial region may also be involved in less than 1% of cases.[47] Young males are generally affected. Infection in the vertebral bodies usually starts in the cancellous bone adjacent to an intervertebral disc or anteriorly under the periosteum of the vertebral body; the neural arch is rarely affected. Vertebral destruction leads to collapse of the body of the vertebra along with anterior wedging. Spinal cord compression in Pott's spine is mainly caused by pressure from a paraspinal abscess.

The typical clinical features are local pain, paraspinal muscle spasm, tenderness over the affected spine or kyphotic deformity in the form of a gibbus. A paravertebral abscess may be palpated on the back of a number of patients. These patients usually have acute or subacute progressive, spastic type of sensorimotor paraparesis. The incidence of paraparesis in patients with Pott's spine varies from 27% to 47%.[48] MRI is the imaging modality of choice. A plain film shows decreased bone density and joint space destruction in long-standing disease. CT-guided biopsy may be useful for making an aetiological diagnosis.[49] Surgical decompression is needed for most patients.

Spinal arachnoiditis

This is characterized by painful root and spinal cord symptoms that can mimic an intraspinal tumour. It is a common cause of myeloradiculopathy in endemic countries such as India. Inflammatory exudates encase the spinal cord and nerve roots, and there is associated inflammation of the small vessels.[50] Thus, the spinal cord is damaged both by compression and ischaemia (Fig. 4). The changes of arachnoiditis may be focal, multifocal or diffuse. The hallmark of diagnosis is the characteristic myelographic picture showing poor flow of contrast material with multiple irregular filling defects, cyst formation and sometimes spinal block (Fig. 4). The CSF changes are those of chronic meningitis. Frequently, the CSF sugar concentration is normal.[51]

Treatment of neurotuberculosis

Antituberculous therapy

The primary goal of ATT is to kill the tuberculous bacilli rapidly, prevent the emergence of drug resistance and eliminate persistent bacilli from the host's tissues to prevent relapse. TBM should be considered a medical emergency and ATT should be initiated as soon as possible when there is a strong clinical suspicion of TBM. The decision to start ATT should be based solely on clinical judgement and it should not be delayed by waiting for bacteriological confirmation. Delay in initiating treatment, even by a few days, can be potentially harmful to the patient and result in serious irreversible morbidities or mortality.

There are no randomized, controlled trials to establish the optimal drug combination, dosage or duration of ATT for CNS TB. The recommendations[52] of the American and British Thoracic Societies (BTS), Infectious Disease Society of America (IDSA) and CDC are an initial two-month period of intensive therapy with four drugs, followed by a prolonged continuation phase lasting 7–10 months, depending on the clinical response and established drug sensitivity of the isolate.

First-line drugs are isoniazid (INH), rifampicin (RIF), pyrazinamide (PZA) and ethambutol (EMB). They are bactericidal, can be administered orally, penetrate the inflamed meninges, and achieve CSF levels that exceed the inhibitory concentration needed for sensitive strains. INH has excellent CNS penetration irrespective of meningeal inflammation, and is more active against rapidly dividing than dormant organisms.[53] The initial dose is 10 mg/kg per day (up to 300 mg/day) for adults and children. RIF is active against both rapidly dividing organisms and semidormant sub-populations of organisms. The dose is 10 mg/kg per day (up to 600 mg/day in adults). PZA readily penetrates the CSF and is highly active against intracellular mycobacteria. Within the dose range of 15–30 mg/kg per day (maximum 2 g dose), PZA augments the regimen without added risk for hepatotoxicity when the drug's use is limited to 2 months.

Streptomycin (15 mg/kg per day IM in adults to a maximum dose of 1 g; 20–40 mg/kg per day in children) was added to INH in order to enhance sterilization and reduce the risk of clinical relapse from resistant organisms. With the availability of newer, less toxic agents (e.g. RIF and PZA), reliance on streptomycin is generally limited to regions of the world with a high prevalence of INH resistance. EMB (15–25 mg/kg per day) achieves moderate CSF concentrations but carries the risk of optic neuritis at higher doses. Ocular toxicity is rare at the recommended dose of 15 mg/kg per day. Patients receiving EMB should undergo baseline Snellen visual acuity and red–green colour perception testing, and should be referred to an ophthalmologist if visual complaints develop while on therapy.[54]

The choice of a fourth drug in the intensive phase is controversial. According to the BTS guidelines, either streptomycin or EMB may be used. The IDSA/ATS recommends the use of EMB considering the increasing reports of resistance to streptomycin.[55] The recommended duration of therapy is 9–12 months in drug-sensitive infections. If PZA is omitted or cannot be tolerated, treatment should be extended to 18 months. A number of other studies report varying experiences with short-course (6 months) treatment.[56] As the emergence of neurological deficit has been seen in some of these studies, a minimum of 12 months of treatment would be worthwhile. A similar drug regimen has been recommended for all forms of CNS TB.[57]

Directly observed therapy, short-course (DOTS)

Poor compliance with the ATT regimen is the most common cause of treatment failure, relapse and emergence of drug-resistant bacilli. Administering ATT on an intermittent basis improves adherence to the drugs and, consequently, treatment outcome. Several clinical trials have been conducted to compare daily and intermittent ATT therapy and have demonstrated that the intermittent regimen is as effective as a daily regimen.[58] Directly observed therapy, short-course (DOTS) has now become the World Health Organization (WHO) strategy for effective control of TB. WHO advocates directly observed high-dose intermittent therapy given thrice weekly. The Category I DOTS regimen is followed for the treatment of CNS TB.[59] Venugopal *et al.* conducted an observational study in 32 patients with neurotuberculosis and concluded that intermittent short-course chemotherapy is efficacious in curing the disease.[60] Large comparative clinical trials are necessary to compare intermittent therapy with daily therapy.

Drug-resistant tuberculosis

How common is MDR TB?

The prevalence of CNS infection caused by drug-resistant strains is increasing. WHO estimates that worldwide, approximately 10% of clinical isolates of *M. tuberculosis* are resistant to one or more first-line anti-TB drugs.[61] Risk factors for the development of drug resistance include a previous history of ATT, exposure to drug-resistant organisms, poor drug compliance and prescribing an improper drug regimen by healthcare professionals. Strains of *M. tuberculosis* resistant to both INH and RIF are termed as multidrug-resistant (MDR) strains. A prospective study[62] from Viet Nam of 180 adults with TBM examined the effect of drug resistance on response to treatment and outcome. Resistance to at least one anti-TB drug was identified in 72 of 180 (40%) isolates and 10 isolates (5.6%) were resistant to both INH and RIF (multidrug resistance [MDR]).

How to manage MDR TB

INH and streptomycin resistance was significantly associated with slower CSF bacterial clearance, but not with any difference in clinical response or outcome.[63] Combined INH and RIF resistance, however, was strongly predictive of death (relative risk of death 11.6 [95% CI: 5.2–26.3]) and independently associated with HIV infection.[63]

LJ culture medium or the more recent radiometric assays can be used to assess drug sensitivity. Cases with isolated INH resistance should be treated for an extended period of time (18–24 months). Second-line drugs such as ethionamide, cycloserine, aminoglycosides and quinolones can be used to treat drug-resistant cases.[64] When treating MDR CNS TB, a single drug should never be added to a failing regimen. The initial regimen should contain at least 4–5 drugs to which the bacilli are sensitive and which have not been used previously.

Role of corticosteroids

Corrticosteroids reduce the inflammation and

neurological complications, and shorten the time to recovery.[65] There is considerable experimental evidence and a growing base of clinical data that adjunctive glucocorticoid therapy is beneficial in both adults and children with TBM.[66] A randomized, double-blind trial in Viet Nam compared dexamethasone (for the first 6–8 weeks of treatment in a tapering dosage regimen) with placebo in 545 patients more than 14 years of age.[67] Mortality was significantly reduced in the dexamethasone-treated group (32% versus 41%). The mortality benefit was most evident for patients with early disease. There was no demonstrable reduction in residual neurological deficits and disability among surviving patients. No mortality benefit from dexamethasone was evident in 98 HIV-infected patients included in the study.

A Cochrane review by Prasad *et al.* analysed seven trials involving 1140 participants (with 411 deaths).[68] All used dexamethasone or prednisolone. Overall, corticosteroids reduced the risk of death (RR 0.78, 95% CI: 0.67–0.91; 1140 participants, 7 trials). Data on disabling residual neurological deficit from three trials showed that cortico-steroids reduce the risk of death or disabling residual neurological deficit (RR 0.82, 95% CI: 0.70–0.97; 720 participants, 3 trials). Adverse events included gastrointestinal bleeding, bacterial and fungal infections, and hyper-glycaemia, but these were mild and treatable.

The glucocorticoid drug[69] used is either dexamethasone or prednisone. Dexamethasone is used at a total dose of 8 mg/day for children weighing <25 kg; 12 mg/day for adults and children >25 kg, for 3 weeks, then tapered gradually over the following 3–4 weeks. Prednisone is used at a dose of 2–4 mg/kg per day for children; 60 mg/day for adults for 3 weeks, then tapered gradually over the following 3 weeks.

A study[70] conducted in 141 children with TBM randomly assigned them to either a steroid (oral prednisolone 2 or 4 mg/kg/day) or a non-steroid group. The administration of corticosteroid significantly improved the survival and intellectual outcome of children with TBM. No significant difference was noticed between the two treatment groups with regard to motor deficit, blindness or deafness, and the clinical outcome of children receiving high- and low-dose prednisolone did not differ significantly. No significant difference in intracranial pressure or degree of hydrocephalus was noted between the two groups after the first month of treatment. Both the response of the tuberculoma to treatment and the incidence of delayed occurrence of tuberculomas were significantly improved after steroid therapy.

Other indications for steroid therapy include (i) patients presenting with an acute 'encephalitis', especially if the CSF opening pressure is ≥400 mm H_2O or if there is clinical or CT evidence of cerebral oedema, (ii) patients who demonstrate a 'therapeutic paradox', an exacerbation of clinical signs (e.g. fever, change in mentation) after beginning ATT, (iii) patients with intracerebral tuberculoma, where the oedema is out of proportion to the mass effect and there are clinical neurological signs (altered mentation or focal deficits), (iv) those with focal neurological deficit, (v) those with spinal block (CSF protein >400 mg/dl), and (vi) basilar exudates.

Role of surgery

Hydrocephalus

Hydrocephalus is a frequent complication of TBM, which occurs in the first 4–6 weeks of illness. If left untreated, it may result in permanent neurological damage or even death.[71] Hydrocephalus occurs due to obstruction of the ventricular pathway and subarachnoid space by inflammatory exudates. A communicating hydro-cephalus is more common than an obstructive hydrocephalus. Shoeman *et al.* found that the hydrocephalus was of communicating type in 82% of patients with TBM.[72] Surgical intervention is required for the management of obstructive hydrocephalus, although in the absence of obstruction, hydrocephalus may be managed medically. When reducing elevated intracranial pressure in the latter instance, the use of mannitol, furosemide and acetazolamide was significantly more effective than antituberculous drugs alone. Mannitol is effective for acute decompensation. Early placement of a ventriculo-peritoneal (VP) shunt was the treatment of choice in a large number of series.[73] The outcome is better in patients with a normal sensorium than in those with an altered sensorium.[74] In patients with poor-grade hydrocephalus (comatose patients), the altered sensorium may be due to multiple factors, such as vasculitic infarct and coexisting encephalitis; hence, the outcome may not be good in these patients. These patients can be subjected to a trial of external ventricular drainage for 48 hours. If the sensorium improves, the patient can be taken for VP shunting.

Endoscopic third ventriculostomy (ETV) is a recently introduced and alternative approach to VP shunting. As even minor bleeding can obscure the endoscopic field, ETV is better avoided in acute hydrocephalus. The procedure is also difficult when the floor of the third ventricle is obliterated by thick exudates. This procedure is thus reserved for those who have been treated with ATT at least for 4 weeks or in whom the disease has burned out and hydrocephalus developed as a late complication. Chugh *et al.* found that the outcome was better in those who received ATT for 4 weeks prior to ETV than those who were operated upon earlier.[75]

Tuberculoma

Unlike other CNS mass lesions, medical management is preferred for clinical tuberculomas, unless the lesion produces obstructive hydrocephalus or compression of the brainstem. In the past, surgical resection was often complicated by severe, fatal meningitis. Intracranial tuberculomas that act as single space-occupying lesions with midline shifts and increased intracranial pressure, and that fail to respond to chemotherapy, should be surgically removed.[76] If the tuberculoma is totally removed, about 80% of patients will enjoy long-term recovery, particularly if they were treated in the early stages of the disease.

It has frequently been observed that intracranial tuberculomas appear to paradoxically increase in size while patients are being treated for TBM.[77] These lesions are usually discovered accidentally when follow-up CT scan is performed routinely or when new neurological signs develop during the course of ATT. A recent study noted that about 8% of patients developed asymptomatic tuberculoma during the first month of treatment.[77] Concomitant steroid therapy probably has a preventive action against the development of these focal lesions. Paradoxical enlargement has also been observed in isolated intracranial tuberculoma while the patient was on ATT.[78] However, with continued treatment, there is eventual resolution of these tuberculomas.[78]

Thalidomide is recommended by British Infectious Disease Society for treating patients with tuberculoma who do not respond to treatment with ATT and steroids.

Management of spinal arachnoiditis

Treatment of spinal arachnoiditis is difficult, as there may not be any satisfactory response to either to ATT or steroids, and the disease often progresses despite therapy. A study conducted by Gourie Devi and Satishchandra showed that patients treated with intrathecal hyaluronidase had significantly lesser functional disability.[79]

Management in HIV infection

CNS involvement occurs in 10%–20% of AIDS-related TB and carries a high mortality rate.[80] Once infected with *M. tuberculosis*, HIV coinfection is the strongest risk factor for progression to active TB; the risk has been estimated to be as high as 10% per year, compared with a 5%–10% lifetime risk among persons with TB but not HIV infection.[80] Although patients who are HIV-infected and also have TB are at increased risk for TBM, the clinical features, response to therapy and outcomes of TB do not seem to be altered by HIV.[81] Tuberculous granulomas are less common than meningitis, and intravenous drug users are at higher risk.[81] Patients infected with HIV, especially those with AIDS, are at very high risk for developing active TB when exposed to a person with infectious drug-susceptible or drug-resistant TB. They have a higher incidence of drug-resistant TB, in part due to Mycobacterium avium intracellulare, and have worse outcomes.[82]

Because of the severely reduced immune response in HIV-positive patients with TBM, formation of basal exudates is scanty. Tuberculous arteritis, phlebitis and cerebral infarcts are common in HIV-positive patients.[83] Due to the scant exudates, hydrocephalus and meningeal enhancement are uncommon in HIV-positive patients. In a study of HIV-positive patients with neurotuberculosis, meningeal enhancement was present in 36%, hydrocephalus in 32%, tuberculoma in 24%, tuberculous abscess in 20% and infarcts in 36%.[83]

Cytological diagnosis from the CSF is difficult in TBM, because the CSF is often acellular and sometimes a neutrophilic response is observed. The yield of tubercle bacilli from the CSF of HIV-infected patients is high due to the high bacterial load in these patients.[84] ATT and duration of treatment is essentially the same in these patients as in HIV-uninfected patients.[85] A study conducted by Karande *et al.* to assess the outcome of children with TBM with or without HIV infection concluded that there were no significant differences between HIV-infected and HIV-negative children admitted with TBM in terms of outcome and treatment response.[86] The role of corticosteroid therapy is controversial in HIV-infected patients with TBM. A controlled trial showed that outcome is better in patients treated with corticosteroids.[87]

TB IRIS

Immune reconstitution inflammatory syndrome (IRIS) is an inflammatory reaction to infection with *M. tuberculosis* occurring during anti-retroviral therapy (ART)-mediated immune reconstitution. TB IRIS can present in two ways: (i) Paradoxical deterioration in a patient established on TB treatment (paradoxical TB IRIS); (ii) unmasking of untreated TB. In paradoxical TB IRIS, which occurs in a patient with HIV infection and TB, initially there is a stable response to ATT. However, paradoxical worsening of tuberculous manifestations occurs within 3 months of starting or changing ART. New or worsening meningitis or focal neurological deficits may be seen after starting ART. The treatment of TB IRIS is controversial. The usual recommendation is to interrupt ART temporarily, continue ATT and to reintroduce ART after the patient has been stabilized and there is no neurological worsening. This approach carries the risk of progression of HIV infection. The role of steroids during neurological worsening is controversial. Sharma *et al.* studied 237 patients who had TB at the start of ART.[88] In total, 18 (7.5%) of 237 patients with TB at baseline had paradoxical TB-associated IRIS and most IRIS occurred within 30 days of initiating highly active antiretroviral therapy (HAART).

Conclusion

The clinical, pathological and radiological features of neurotuberculosis vary widely. Early diagnosis and management of TBM is critical. Empirical ATT is often initiated on the basis of clinical suspicion and a typical CSF picture, but bacteriological confirmation is challenging. The increasing problem of drug resistance and HIV co-infection has added a new challenge. Large, randomized controlled trials are necessary to establish the evidence for the diagnosis and management of neurotuberculosis.

References

1. CDC. Reported tuberculosis in the United States, 2004. Atlanta, GA: US Department of Health and Human Services, CDC; September 2005.
2. Wood M, Anderson M. Chronic meningitis. In: *Neurological infections; major problems in neurology*, vol 16. Philadelphia: WB Saunders; 1998:169–248.
3. Farer LS, Lowell AM, Meador MP. Extrapulmonary tuberculosis in the United States. *Am J Epidemiol* 1979;**109**:205.
4. Karg RK. Tuberculosis of the central nervous system. *Postgrad Med J* 1999;**75**:133–40.
5. Rich AR, McCordock HA. Pathogenesis of tubercular meningitis. *Bull John Hopkins Hosp* 1933;**52**:5–13.
6. Berger JR. Tuberculous meningitis. *Curr Opin Neurol* 1994;**7**:191–200.
7. Sheller JR, Des Prez RM. CNS tuberculosis. *Neurol Clin* 1986;**4**:143–58.
8. Bhargava S, Gupta AK, Tandon PN. Tuberculous meningitis: A CT scan study. *Br J Radiol* 1982;**55**:189–96.
9. Thwaites GE, Hien TT. Tuberculous meningitis: Many questions, too few answers. *Lancet Neurol* 2005B;**4**:160–70.
10. Tandon PN. Tuberculous meningitis (cranial and spinal). In: Vinken PJ, Bruyen GW (eds). *Handbook of clinical neurology*. Infections of the nervous system, Vol 33. Amsterdam: North Holland; 1978:185–262.
11. Ahuja GK, Mohan KK, Prasad K, *et al.* Diagnostic criteria for tuberculous meningitis and their validation. *Tubercle Lung Dis* 1994;**75**:149–52.
12. Thwaites GE, Chau TT, Farrar JJ. Improving the bacteriological diagnosis of tuberculous meningitis. *J Clin Microbiol* 2004;**42**:378.
13. Leonard JM, Des Prez RM. Tuberculous meningitis. *Infect Dis Clin North Am* 1990;**4**:769–87.
14. Newton RW. Tuberculous meningitis. *Arch Dis Child* 1994;**70**:364–6.
15. Katrak SM, Shembalkar PK, Bijwe SR, *et al.* The clinical, radiological, and pathological profile of tuberculous meningitis in patients with and without HIV infection. *J Neurol Sci* 2000;**181**:118–26.
16. Merritt HH, Fremont-Smith F. *The cerebrospinal fluid*. Philadelphia: WB Saunders; 1938.
17. Kumar R, Singh SN, Kohli N. A diagnostic rule for tuberculous meningitis. *Arch Dis Child* 1999;**81**:221–4.
18. Molavi A, LeFrock JL. Tuberculous meningitis. *Med Clin North Am* 1985;**69**:315–31.
19. Kennedy DH, Fallon RJ. Tuberculous meningitis. *JAMA* 1979;**241**:264–8.
20. Daniel TD. New approaches to the rapid diagnosis of tuberculous meningitis. *J Infect Dis* 1987;**155**:599–607.
21. American Thoracic Society. Targeted tuberculin testing and treatment of latent tuberculosis infection. *Am J Respir Crit Care Med* 2000;**161**:S221–S247.
22. Blake J, Berman P. The use of adenosine deaminase assays in diagnosis of tuberculosis. *S Afr Med Journ* 1982;**62**:19.
23. Tortoli E, Cichero P, Chirillo MG, *et al.* Multicenter comparison of ESP culture medium II with BACTEC 460 TB and with LJ medium for the recovery of mycobacteria from different clinical specimens. *J clinical microbial* 1998;**36**:1378–81.
24. Kox LF, Kuijper S, Kolk AH. Early diagnosis of tuberculous meningitis by polymerase chain reaction. *Neurology* 1995;**45**:2228–32.
25. Pai M, Flores LL, Pai N, *et al.* Diagnostic accuracy of nucleic acid amplification tests for tuberculous meningitis; a systematic review and meta-analysis. *Lancet Infect Dis* 2003;**3**:633–43.
26. Nguyen LN, Fox LFF, Pham LD, *et al.* The potential contribution of polymerase chain reaction to the diagnosis of tuberculous meningitis. *Arch Neurol* 1996;**53**:771–6.
27. Rafi W, Venkataswamy MM, Nagarathna S, *et al.* Role of IS6110 uniplex PCR in the diagnosis of tuberculous meningitis: experience at a tertiary neurocentre. *Int J Tuberc Lung Dis* 2007;**11**:209–14.
28. Kashyap RS, Kainthla RP, Satpute RM. Demonstration of IgG Antibodies to 30 Kd protein antigen in CSF for diagnosis of tuberculous meningitis by antibody capturing ELISA. *Neurol India* 2004;**52**:359–62.
29. Sumi MG, Annamma M, Sarada C, *et al.* Rapid diagnosis of tuberculous meningitis by a dot-immunobinding assay. *Acta Neurol Scand* 2000;**101**:61–4.
30. Mathai A, Radhakrishnan VV, Saradha C. Detection of heat stable mycobacterial antigen in cerebrospinal fluid by dot-immunobinding assay. *Neurol India* 2003;**51**:52–4.
31. Eide FF, Gean AD, So IT. Clinical and radiographic findings in disseminated tuberculosis of the brain. *Neurology* 1993;**43**:1427–9.
32. Gee GT, Bazan C III, Jinkins JR. Miliary tuberculosis involving the brain: MR findings. *AJR* 1992;**159**:1075–6.

33. Bhargava, S, Gupta, AK, Tandon, PN. Tuberculous meningitis—a CT study. *Br J Radiol* 1982;**55**:189.

34. Ozates M, Kemaloglu S, Gurkan F, *et al*. CT of the brain in tuberculous meningitis. A review of 289 patients. *Acta Radiol* 2000;**41**:13.

35. Le Bihan D, Mangin JF, Poupon C, *et al*. Diffusion tensor imaging: Concepts and applications. *J Magn Reson Imaging* 2001;**13**:534–46.

36. Talamas O, Del Brutto OH, Garcia-Ramos G. Brainstem tuberculoma. *Arch Neurol* 1989;**46**:529–35.

37. Rajshekhar V, Chandy MJ. Tuberculomas presenting as isolated intrinsic brain stem masses. *Br J Neurosurg* 1997;**11**:127–33.

38. Vengsarkar US, Pisipati RP, Parekh B, *et al*. Intracranial tuberculoma and CT scan. *J Neurosurg* 1986;**64**:568–74.

39. Van Dyk A. CT of intracranial tuberculomas with special reference to the 'target sign'. *Neuroradiology* 1988;**30**:329.

40. Rajshekhar V, Haran RP, Prakash SG, *et al*. Differentiating solitary small cystiorcus granulomas and tuberculomas in patients with epilepsy: Clinical and computed tomographic criteria. *J Neurosurg* 1993;**78**:402–7.

41. Jinkins JR, Gupta R, Chang KH, *et al*. MR imaging of central nervous system tuberculosis. *Radiol Clin North Am* 1995;**33**:771–86.

42. Offenbacher, H, Fazekas, F, Schmidt, R, *et al*. MRI in tuberculous meningoencephalitis: Report of four cases and review of the neuroimaging literature. *J Neurol* 1991;**238**:340.

43. Trivedi R, Suksena S, Gupta RK. MRI in central nervous system tuberculosis. *Indian J Radiol Imaging* 2009:**19**:256–65.

44. Udani PM, Dastur DK. Tuberculous encephalopathy with and without meningitis: Clinical features and pathological correlations. *J Neurol Sci* 1970;**10**:541–61.

45. Farrar DJ, Flanigan TP, Gordon NM, *et al*. Tuberculous brain abscess in patient with HIV infection: Case report and review. *Am J Med* 1997;**102**:297–301.

46. Diyora B, Kumar R, Sharma A. Calvarial tuberculosis a report of 11 cases. *Neurol India* 2009;**57**:607–12.

47. Razai AR, Lee M, Cooper PR, *et al*. Modern management of spinal tuberculosis. *Neurosurgery* 1995;**36**:87–98.

48. Miller JD. Pott's paraplegia to day. *Lancet* 1995;**340**:264.

49. Nussbaum ES, Rockswold GL, Bergman TA, *et al*. Spinal tuberculosis: A diagnostic and management challenge. *J Neurosurg* 1995;**83**:243–7.

50. Wadia NH. Radiculomyelopathy associated with spinal meningitis (arachnoiditis) with special reference to spinal tuberculous variety. In: Spillane JD (ed). *Tropical neurology*. London: Oxford University Press; 1973:63–72.

51. Shaw MDM, Russel JA, Grossart KW. The changing pattern of spinal arachnoiditis. *JNNP* 1978;**41**:97–107.

52. Blumberg HM, Burman WJ, Chaisson RE, *et al*. American Thoracic Society/Centers for Disease Control and Prevention/Infectious Diseases Society of America: Treatment of tuberculosis. *Am J Respir Crit Care Med* 2003;**167**:603.

53. Donald PR, Gent WL, Seifart HI, *et al*. Cerebrospinal fluid isoniazid concentrations in children with tuberculous meningitis: The influence of dosage and acetylation status. *Pediatrics* 1992;**89**:247–50.

54. Chatterjee B, Friedman G. Ocular toxicity following ethambutol in standard dosage. *Br J Dis Chest* 1986;**80**:288.

55. Centers for Disease Control. Treatment of tuberculosis. *MMWR Recomm Rep* 2003;**52**:1–77.

56. Van Loenhout-Rooyackers JH, Keyser A, Laheij RJ, *et al*. Tuberculous meningitis: Is a 6 months treatment regimen sufficient? *Int J Tuberc Lung Dis* 2001;**5**:1028–35.

57. Chemotherapy and management of tuberculosis in the United Kingdom: Recommendations 1998. Joint Tuberculosis Committee of the British Thoracic Society. *Thorax* 1998;**53**:536.

58. Ramachandran P, Duraipandian M, Nagarajan M, *et al*. Three chemotherapy studies of tuberculous meningitis in children. *Tubercule* 1986;**67**:17–29.

59. Harries A, Maher D. TB: A clinical manual for South-East Asia. Geneva: WHO; 1997.

60. Venugopal K, Sreelatha PR, Philip S, *et al*. Treatment outcome of neurotuberculosis patients put on DOTS —An observation study from the field. *Indian J Tuberc* 2008;**55**:199–202.

61. World Health Organization (WHO). Global tuberculosis control: Surveillance, planning, financing. Geneva: WHO; 2004.

62. Thwaites GE, Lan NT, Dung NH, *et al*. Effect of antituberculous drug resistance on response to treatment and outcome in adults with tuberculous meningitis. *J Infect Dis* 2005;**192**:79.

63. Patel VB, Padayatchi N, Bhigjee AI, *et al*. Multidrug-resistant tuberculous meningitis in KwaZulu-Natal, South Africa. *Clin Infect Dis* 2004;**38**:851–6.

64. Sharma SK, Mohan A. Multidrug-resistant tuberculosis. *Indian J Med Res* 2004;**120**:354–76.

65. Schoeman JF, Vanzyl LF, Laubscher JA, *et al.* Effect of cortico-steroids on intracranial pressure, computed tomographic findings, and clinical outcome in young children with tuberculous meningitis. *Pediatrics* 1997;**99**:226–31.

66. Kumarvelu S, Prasad K, Khosla A, *et al.* Randomized controlled trial of dexamethasone in tuberculous meningitis. *Tubercle Lung Dis* 1994;**75**:203–7.

67. Thwaites GE, Nguyen DB, Nguyen HD, *et al.* Dexamethasone for the treatment of tuberculous meningitis in adolescents and adults. *N Engl J Med* 2004;**351**:1741–51.

68. Prasad K, Singh MB. Corticosteroids for managing tuberculous meningitis. *Cochrane Database of Systematic Reviews* 2008, Issue 1, CD002244, pub 3.

69. Kaojarern S, Supmonchai K, Phuapradit P, *et al.* Effects of steroids on cerebrospinal fluid penetration of antituberculous drugs in tuberculous meningitis. *Clin Pharmacol Ther* 1991;**49**:6–12.

70. Karak B, Garg RK. Corticosteroids in tuberculous meningitis. *Indian Pediatrics* 1998;**35**:193–4.

71. Holdiness MR. Management of tuberculous meninglitis. *Drugs* 1990;**39**:224–33.

72. Schoeman J, Donald P, Keet M, *et al.* Tuberculous hydrocephalus, comparison of different treatments with regard to ICP, ventricular size and clinical outcome. *Dev Med Child Neurol* 1991;**33**;396–405.

73. Palur R, Rajasekar V. Shunt surjery for tuberculous meningitis, A long-term follow up study. *J Neurosurg* 1991;**74**:64–69.

74. Lamprecht D, Schoeman J, Donald P. Ventriculo peritoneal shunt in childhood tuberculous meningitis. *Br J Neurosurg* 2001;**15**:119–25.

75. Chugh A, Hussain M, Gupta RK. Surgical outcome of tuberculous meningitis hydrocephalus treated by endoscopic third ventriculostomy. *J Neurosurg Pediatr* 2009;**3**:371–7.

76. Razai AR, Lee M, Cooper PR, *et al.* Modern management of spinal tuberculosis. *Neurosurgery* 1995;**36**:87–98.

77. Teoh R, Humhrie MJ, O'Mahoney G. Symptomatic intracranial tuberculomas developing during treatment of tuberculosis. A report of 10 patients and review of literature. *Q J Med* 1987;**63**:449–53.

78. Pauranik A, Behari M, Maheshwari MC. Appearance of tuberculoma during treatment of tuberculous meningitis. *Jpn J Med* 1987;**26**:332.

79. Gourie-Devi M, Satishchandra P. Hyaluronidase as an adjuvant in the treatment of cranial arachnoiditis (hydrocephalus and optochiasmatic arachnoiditis) complicating tuberculous meningitis. *Acta Neurol Scand* 1980;**62**:368–81.

80. Yechoor VK, Shandera WX, Rodriguez P, *et al.* Tuberculous meningitis among adults with or without HIV infection. *Arch Intern Med* 1996;**156**:1710–16.

81. Silber E, Sonnenberg P, Ho KC, *et al.* Meningitis in a community with a high prevalence of tuberculosis and HIV infection. *J Neurol Sci* 1999;**162**:20–6.

82. Bishburg E, Sunderam G, Reichman LB, *et al.* Central nervous system tuberculosis with the acquired immunodeficiency syndrome and its related complex. *Ann Intern Med* 1986;**105**:210–13.

83. Whiteman M, Espinoza LM, Post JD, *et al.* Central nervous system tuberculosis in HIV-infected patients: Clinical and radiographic findings. *Am J Neuroradiol* 1995;**16**:1319–27.

84. Berenguer J, Moreno S, Laguna F, *et al.* Tuberculous meningitis in patients infected with human immunodeficiency virus. *N Engl J Med* 1992;**326**:668–72.

85. Dube MP, Holtom PD, Larsen RA. Tuberculous meningitis in patients with and without human immunodeficiency virus infection. *Am J Med* 1992;**93**:520–4.

86. Karande S, Gupta V, Kulkarni M, *et al.* Tuberculous meningitis and HIV. *Indian J Pediatr* 2005;**72**:755–60.

87. Smith AW, Smith EW. Tuberculous meningitis and corticosteroids: A review. *Neurol J Southeast Asia* 1998;**3**:57–60.

88. Sharma SK, Dhooria S, Barwad P, *et al.* A study of TB-associated immune reconstitution inflammatory syndrome using the consensus case-definition. *Indian J Med Res* 2010;**131**:804–8.